Understanding OCT Angiography

From Pathophysiology to Clinical Imaging

Understanding OCT Angiography

From Pathophysiology to Clinical Imaging

Bruno Lumbroso MD
President of the Italian Society of OCT Angiography, Centro Italiano Macula
Rome, Italy

David Huang MD, PhD
Peterson Professor of Ophthalmology and Professor of Biomedical Engineering
Casey Eye Institute, Oregon Health & Science University (OHSU), USA

Eric H Souied MD, PhD
Head of Department of Ophthalmology
Centre Hospitalier Intercommunal de Créteil, Université Paris Est Créteil, France

Maria Cristina Savastano MD PhD
Centro Italiano Macula,
Rome Italy

Yali Jia PhD
Jennie P. Weeks Professor of Ophthalmology and Associate Professor of Biomedical Engineering
Casey Eye Institute, Oregon Health & Science University (OHSU), USA

Marco Rispoli MD
Ospedale Oftalmico di Roma and Centro Italiano Macula
Rome, Italy

JP medical publishers

London • New Delhi

Published by Jaypee Brothers Medical Publishers,
4838/24 Ansari Road, New Delhi, India
Tel: +91 (011) 43574357 Fax: +91 (011)43574390
Email: info@jpmedpub.com, jaypee@jaypeebrothers.com
Web: www.jpmedpub.com, www.jaypeebrothers.com

JPM is the imprint of Jaypee Brothers Medical Publishers.

ISBN: 978-1-909836-93-8

British Library Cataloguing in Publication Data
A catalogue record for this book is available from the British Library

Library of Congress Cataloging in Publication Data
A catalog record for this book is available from the Library of Congress

Development Editor:	Harsha Madan
Editorial Assistant:	Keshav Kumar
Artwork:	Donata Piccioli
Cover Design:	Seema Dogra

Preface

Optical coherence tomography (OCT) angiography and structural OCT are, at the present, time necessary for understanding pathogenesis, clarifying morphology and structure of retina and choroid, and refining diagnosis and management of ocular conditions. OCT imaging evolution presents us with an exponential increase of the quantity of data we have to classify, sift, assess, count, and preserve. OCT assessment and interpretation activity encompass both a technical and an intellectual aspect.

This handbook is the result of close collaboration of an international group of specialists: David Huang and Yali Jia (Portland, Oregon), Eric H Souied (Creteil France), Francesco Bandello and Giuseppe Querques, Milan, Italy, Marco Rispoli, Maria Cristina Savastano and myself in Rome Italy. I thank Donata Piccioli, the artist who illustrated all our scientific works and textbooks, for her beautiful drawings.

We wrote this handbook to help and guide the clinician in assessing, classifying, sifting and selecting information. After exposing the pathophysiology of the diseases, we describe the basic lesions, and then explain how these elementary lesions combine together to form clinical situations. Finally, we rapidly outline the disorders management.

All our OCT and OCT angiography figures were obtained with Optovue OCT. This practical handbook is extensively illustrated with cross sectional and "*en face*" OCT images, drawings, and several tables.

Bruno Lumbroso
David Huang, Eric H Souied
Maria Cristina Savastano
Yali Jia, Marco Rispoli
November 2019

Contents

Contributors

Luca Agnifili MD, PhD
Ophthalmology Department University
"G. d'Annunzio" of Chieti-Pescara,
Center of Excellence, National High-Tech Center
(CNAT), Italian School of Robotic Surgery in
Ophthalmology, Italy

Federico Anselmucci MD
Ophthalmology, University "Sapienza" of Rome,
"Polo Pontino" Terracina, Italy

Steven T Bailey MD
Associate Professor of Ophthalmology
Casey Eye Institute, Oregon Health & Science
University (OHSU), USA

Francesco Bandello MD, FEBO
Professor & Chairman
Department of Ophthalmology University
Vita Salute, IRCCS Ospedale San Raffaele
Milan, Italy

Enrico Borrelli MD, FEBO
Department of Ophthalmology,
University Vita-Salute, IRCCS Ospedale San
Raffaele, Milan, Italy

Lorenza Brescia MD
Ophthalmology Department University
"G. d'Annunzio" of Chieti-Pescara,
Center of Excellence, National High-Tech Center
(CNAT), Italian School of Robotic Surgery in
Ophthalmology, Italy

Maria A Burnasheva MD
Department of Ophthalmology
Military Medical Academy
St. Petersburg, Russia

Vittorio Capuano MD
Department of Ophthalmology
Centre Hospitalier Intercommunal de Créteil
Université Paris Est Créteil, France

Lorenzo Casillo MD
Ophthalmology, University "Sapienza" of Rome,
"Polo Pontino" Terracina, Italy

Gilda Cennamo MD, PhD
Assistant Professor
Eye Clinic Federico II University, Naples, Italy

Adele Chiaravalloti MD
Medical Retinal Unit IRCCS-Fondazione Bietti
Rome, Italy

Luca Di Antonio MD, PhD
Ophthalmology Department University
"G. d'Annunzio" of Chieti-Pescara
Center of Excellence, National High-Tech Center
(CNAT), Italian School of Robotic Surgery in
Ophthalmology, Italy

Tristan T Hormel PhD
Postdoctoral fellow
Casey Eye Institute, Oregon Health & Science
University (OHSU), USA

David Huang MD, PhD
Peterson Professor of Ophthalmology and
Professor of Biomedical Engineering
Casey Eye Institute, Oregon Health & Science
University (OHSU), USA

Yali Jia PhD
Jennie P. Weeks Professor of Ophthalmology and
Associate Professor of Biomedical Engineering
Casey Eye Institute, Oregon Health & Science
University (OHSU), USA

Alexei N Kulikov MD
DSc Department of Ophthalmology
Military Medical Academy
St. Petersburg, Russia

Bruno Lumbroso MD
President of the Italian Society of OCT Angiography,
Centro Italiano Macula, Rome, Italy

Dmitrii S Maltsev MD, PhD
Department of Ophthalmology
Military Medical Academy
St. Petersburg, Russia

Leonardo Mastropasqua MD
Professor in Ophthalmology
University "G. d'Annunzio" of Chieti-Pescara
Head of the Ophthalmology Department
Head of the Center of Excellence, National High-Tech Center (CNAT) Head of Italian School of Robotic Surgery in Ophthalmology
President of the Italian Society of University Ophthalmologists (SOU), Italy

Daniela Montorio MD, PhD
Fellow Eye Clinic Federico II
University, Naples, Italy

Mariacristina Parravano MD
Head – Medical Retinal Unit IRCCS-Fondazione Bietti Rome, Italy

Giuseppe Querques MD, PhD
Head – Medical Retina & Imaging Unit Department of Ophthalmology University Vita Salute IRCCS Ospedale San Raffaele Milan, Italy

Lea Querques MD
Department of Ophthalmology University Vita Salute, IRCCS Ospedale San Raffaele
Milan, Italy

Marco Rispoli MD
Ospedale Oftalmico di Roma and Centro Italiano Macula, Rome, Italy

Riccardo Sacconi MD, FEBO
Department of Ophthalmology
University Vita-Salute, IRCCS Ospedale San Raffaele, Milan, Italy

Maria Cristina Savastano MD PhD
Centro Italiano Macula,
Rome, Italy

Barbara Scatena MD
Ophthalmology Department University "G. d'Annunzio" of Chieti-Pescara
Center of Excellence, National High-Tech Center (CNAT), Italian School of Robotic Surgery in Ophthalmology, Italy

Eric H Souied MD, PhD
Head of Department of Ophthalmology
Centre Hospitalier Intercommunal de Créteil,
Université Paris Est Créteil, France

Massimiliano Tedeschi MD
Medical Retinal Unit IRCCS-Fondazione Bietti
Rome, Italy

Enzo Maria Vingolo MD, PhD
Ophthalmology, University "Sapienza" of Rome, "Polo Pontino" Terracina, Italy

Ilaria Zucchiatti MD
Department of Ophthalmology University Vita Salute, IRCCS Ospedale San Raffaele
Milan, Italy

Acknowledgements

Thanks to

Jay Wei of Optovue Inc., who is always close to us and gave us intellectual and practical help since the first day of "*en face*" OCT and OCT Angiography.

Nicolas Bruel of Optovue Inc., for his collaboration

Donata Piccioli for making artwork out of rudimentary schematic outlines.

Aldo Armeni for his precious collaboration in producing impeccable OCT and OCTA scans.

All Jaypee Publishers team in New Delhi, (specifically Harsha Madan) for their inestimable patience and relentless help in preparing this handbook.

Bruno Lumbroso
David Huang, Eric H Souied
Maria Cristina Savastano
Yali Jia, Marco Rispoli

Introduction

Bruno Lumbroso, David Huang, Eric H Souied, Maria Cristina Savastano, Yali Jia, Marco Rispoli

Understanding OCT angiography, from pathophysiology to clinical imaging

Ophthalmology stride of progress largely outperforms other medical domains. Our understanding of the diseases strictly trails the new possibilities of analysis and deduction that the new instruments bring us. Imaging and treatment of retinal diseases have been profoundly renewed these last 15 years. The pace of innovation in our subspecialty is astonishing. Advances in imaging technologies such as "*en face*" optical coherence tomography (OCT); structural OCT, optical coherence tomography angiography (OCTA), and wide-field retinography and their extensive application in everyday practice have improved diagnosis, treatment, and monitoring of most retinal disorders. OCTA brings a new understanding in the pathological process of ophthalmological disorders. These treatments and technologies that are currently standard did not even exist 15 years ago.

There is a continuous feedback between industries and clinicians leading to renewed assessment of well-known diseases. Successful use of intravitreal injections for neovascularization, diabetic macular edema, and other syndromes has not only improved prognosis but also transformed acute diseases in chronic disorders and thus intensely increased the global patient quantity. Our knowledge of diseases has greatly improved and the patient's number exponentially increased. This progression has generated the necessity of more qualified retina specialists.

Most clinicians have begun translating the new OCTA technology into clinical practice. These 3D imaging tools are safer, faster, cheaper, and better than fluorescein angiography. They offer a wealth of facts that combine the data provided by dye angiography to structural OCT imaging. OCTA provides, in everyday clinical use, clearer and more detailed imaging of the vascular networks than other imaging techniques. Since it is entirely noninvasive, it can be used on a routine basis to screen for diseases and monitor the efficacy of treatment. Quantitative OCTA vascular evaluation is nowadays part of the basic assessment of most retinal disorders and integral part of the follow-up.

In addition to the benefits offered by the noninvasive OCTA over invasive dye angiography in macular diseases, it has been progressively used in glaucoma diagnosis. OCTA of the disc and peripapillary area is also available with all systems.

This volume will bring the incredibly fast changes in this field to residents in ophthalmology, postgraduate students and to all ophthalmologists who want to keep abreast with the relevant advances in their field. It will interest also orthoptists and optometrists who are attracted in using the latest devices.

This handbook intends to teach OCTA interpretation for routine everyday use, documenting and diagnosing retinal pathologies. In each chapter are included sections on: pathophysiology, clinical features, imaging (structural OCT, "*en face*" OCT, OCTA) and updated management. In each section all essential clinical and imaging elements are analyzed, integrated, synthetized, summarized, simplified when needed, and always updated. This book is illustrated with numerous drawings, outlines, structural, and functional OCT figures.

Simplified outlines, numerous flowcharts, and many tables offer guidance through difficult diagnoses and facilitate interpretation of morphological alterations.

We believe that ophthalmologists and technicians will find this book valuable and useful. We wish this manual also to be suitable for a general audience of eye specialists seeking a clear, state-of-the-art, and comprehensive description of OCTA.

1 Technology principles and terminology

David Huang, Yali Jia

Structural optical coherence tomography

Conventional structural optical coherence tomography (OCT) is based on reflectance signal backscattered from tissue structures. The reflectance signal provides information on variations in intrinsic tissue reflectivity on a microstructural level, but is also affected by shadowing, pupil vignetting, media opacity, defocus, incidence angle, and other factors that affect the signal strength.

Optical coherence tomographic angiography

Optical coherence tomographic angiography (OCTA) methodology has evolved over the past decade. It is a functional extension of OCT, which allows for the visualization of both transverse and axial flow in blood vessels down to the capillary level. OCTA images display flow signal instead of reflectance signal. The flow signal is computed based on the variation of the speckle pattern between a series of consecutive OCT B-scans. The speckle pattern could be analyzed in terms of amplitude, phase, or complex signals.

Split-spectrum amplitude-decorrelation angiography

Recognising that speckle patterns in different spectral (wavelength) bands contain independent flow information, the split-spectrum amplitude-decorrelation angiography (SSADA) algorithm[1] spectrally splits each B-scan into multiple image frames for the purpose of flow signal calculation. SSADA has been show to improve the signal-to-noise ratio of flow detection by up to a factor of 4, using only 2 consecutive B-scans at each location to obtain high-quality angiograms.[2]

Relationship between decorrelation and velocity

Optical coherence tomographic angiography is sensitive to both axial and transverse flow, with a slightly higher sensitivity for the axial component. The decorrelation value increases monotonically with higher flow velocity. The relationship is nonlinear, with the decorrelation value reaching an upper limit beyond a saturation velocity. For the typical OCTA scan pattern, the inter-B-scan time ranges between 2 and 10 milliseconds, and saturation occurs in larger retinal and choroidal vessels.[3] Even in capillaries, it is difficult to measure flow velocity using OCTA because the OCT beam's focal spot diameters are typically larger than the capillary width, causing the decorrelation value to vary with capillary width as well as flow velocity.

Cross-sectional and *en face* OCTA

Optical coherence tomographic angiography data takes the form of 3-dimensional (3D) volumes containing both reflectance and flow signals. This could be display in cross sections or *en face* slabs. Cross-sectional OCTA typically displays vascular flow in colour and nonvascular reflectance in grey scale. *En face* OCTA is usually generated by maximum flow projection, where the highest flow signal value over the axial range of the slab is used for display. The slabs are based on tissue boundaries identified by image segmentation software. They should ideally enclose a single plexus or several adjacent plexuses. Slabs could also be designed to optimize the detection of abnormal blood vessels in normally avascular layers.

Retinal plexuses

Projection-resolved OCTA[1] shows there are up to four retinal plexuses (depending on location), which could be organized into two complexes (**Figure 1**). The boundary between the superficial and deep vascular plexuses lies in the middle of the inner plexiform layer (IPL). The earliest OCTA software incorrectly divided the retinal circulation into the superficial and deep plexuses at the junction between the IPL and the inner nuclear layer (INL), which would split the IPL and cause vessel density measurements to be highly sensitive to segmentation errors. The correct segmentation boundaries should be used going forward.

OCTA artifacts

Bulk motion causes artifactual flow signal that appears as bright line artifacts on *en face* OCTA. Bulk motion artifacts could be reduced using real-time tracking during acquisition,[4,5] post-processing registration,[6] and post-processing subtraction algorithms (**Figures 2a** to **c**).[7] Flow projection artifacts (**Figures 3a** to **c**) are the result of flickering shadows cast by flowing blood in superficial vasculature that causes reflectance variations in deeper layers, which are then detected as a flow signal by the OCTA algorithm. The artifact manifests as tails below blood vessel on cross-sectional OCTA and the replication of superficial vascular pattern on *en face* OCTA of deeper slabs. Projection-resolved OCTA (PR-OCTA) uses a post-processing algorithm to resolve the ambiguity between flow signal due to in-situ flow (real vessels) and projected flow, thereby removing tails and providing clean visualization of vessels in deeper slabs.[8] The OCTA flow signal is also dependent on reflectance signal strength on a log-linear fashion[7] and thus vessel density measured from OCTA images with low signal strength could be artifactually decreased, unless compensation were made.[9] Shadows from iris vignetting, cataract, and vitreous floaters could cause artifactual retinal and choroidal perfusion defects on OCTA. And

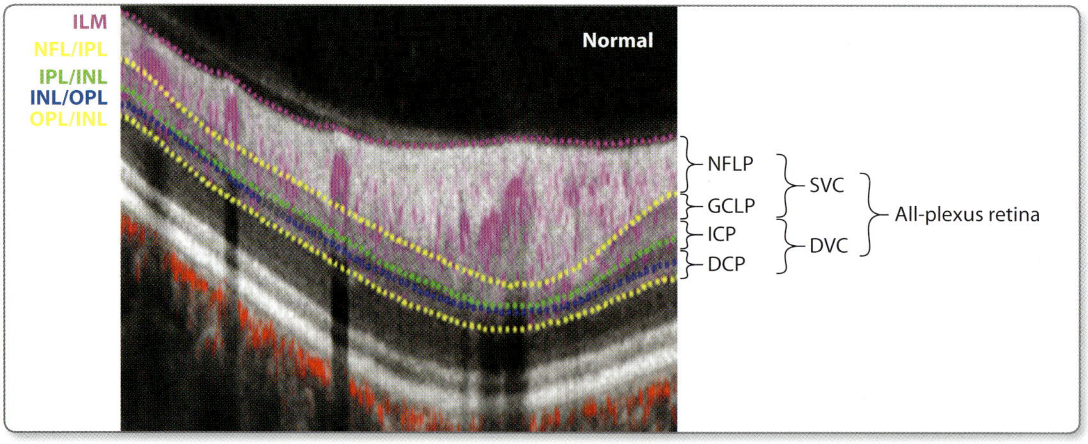

Figure 1 Anatomic localization of vascular plexuses in the human retina in the macula, and current and proposed optical coherence tomography angiography segmentation boundaries. Cross-sectional projection-resolved optical coherence tomography angiograms (PR-OCTA) of a normal eye. Flow signals (purple for retinal and red for choroidal blood flow) were overlaid on reflectance signal (grey scale).
The ICP exists between the IPL and INL. The DCP exists between the INL and OPL. The GCLP/ICP boundary lies in the middle of the IPL and the ICP/DCP boundary lies in the middle of the INL.
(ILM, inner limiting membrane; NFL, nerve fibre layer; GCL, ganglion cell layer; IPL, inner plexiform layer; INL, inner nuclear layer; OPL, outer plexiform layer; ONL, outer nuclear layer; NFLP, NFL plexus; GCLP, GCL plexus; ICP, intermediate capillary plexus; DCP, deep capillary plexus; SVC, superficial vascular complex; DVC, deep vascular complex)

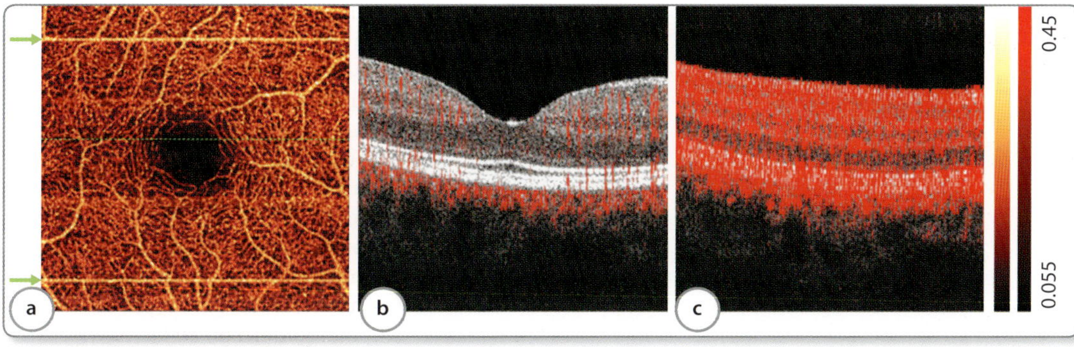

Figure 2 Examples of bulk motion artifacts. (a) *En face* inner retinal angiogram. Two bright lines in the image are the result of microsaccades (green arrows), disrupting vessel continuity. (b) Typical cross-sectional angiogram [from the green, dotted line in panel (a) without motion artifact]. (c) Cross-sectional angiogram at the position of the larger microsaccade shows high flow signal at all reflective structures.

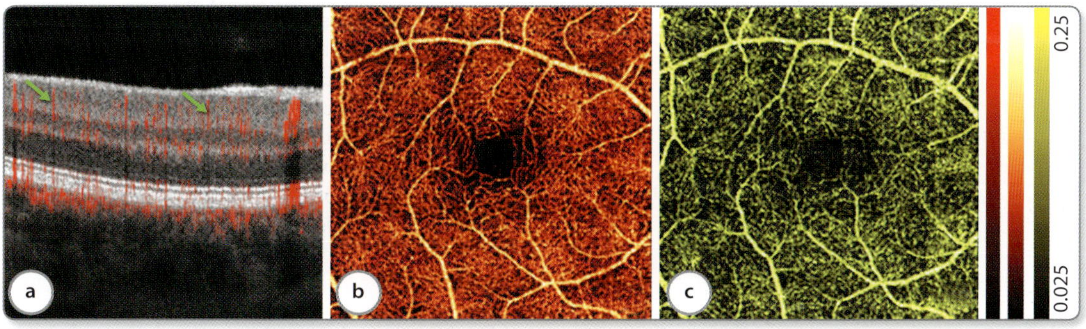

Figure 3 Examples of projection artifacts. (a) Cross-sectional angiogram showing tails trailing beneath vessels (green arrows). (b) Inner retinal angiogram. (c) Outer retinal angiogram shows projection of the inner retinal vasculature.

shadows from drusens could cause artifactual choroidal defects on OCTA (**Figures 4a** to **c**). Care should be taken to distinguish capillary dropout from shadow artifacts.

OCTA parameters quantifying perfusion and ischemia

The flow index is calculated as the average flow signal value in the region of interest on an *en face* OCTA.[10] The vessel area density is calculated as the percentage area occupied by vessels in the selected region.[11] The vessel length density is the length of the vascular network divided by the area of interest in units of mm^{-1}.[12] It is calculated from skeletonized *en face* OCTA. The avascular area or nonflow area sums abnormally large gaps between flow pixels on an *en face* angiogram.[13] Nonperfusion or capillary dropout area refers to an avascular area that should normally be vascular.[14,15] For example, on an OCT angiogram of the macula, any retinal avascular area outside of the FAZ is considered retinal nonperfusion area.

Quantification of neovascularization

In proliferative diabetic retinopathy, neovascular membrane is measured in the preretinal vitreous slab. In age-related macular degeneration, neovascularization is measured in the outer retinal slab after the removal of projection

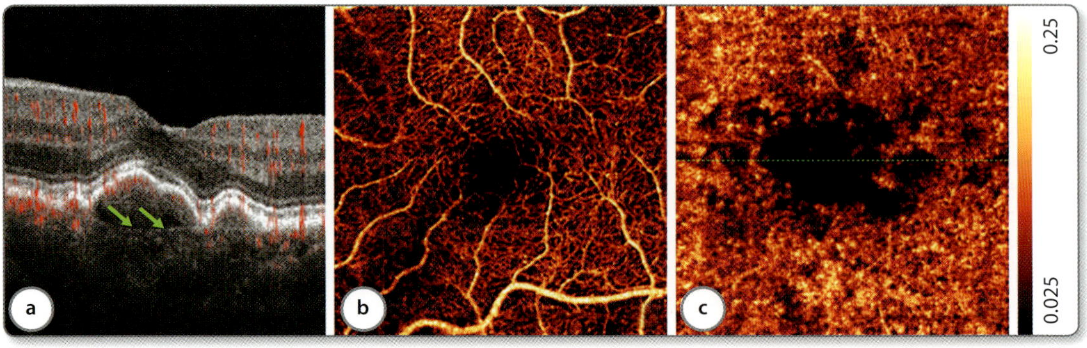

Figure 4 Examples of shadow artifacts. (a) Cross-sectional angiogram showing shadow artifacts caused by drusens (green arrows). (b) Inner retinal angiogram. (c) Choriocapillaris angiogram shows artifactual flow defects (black area in the middle).

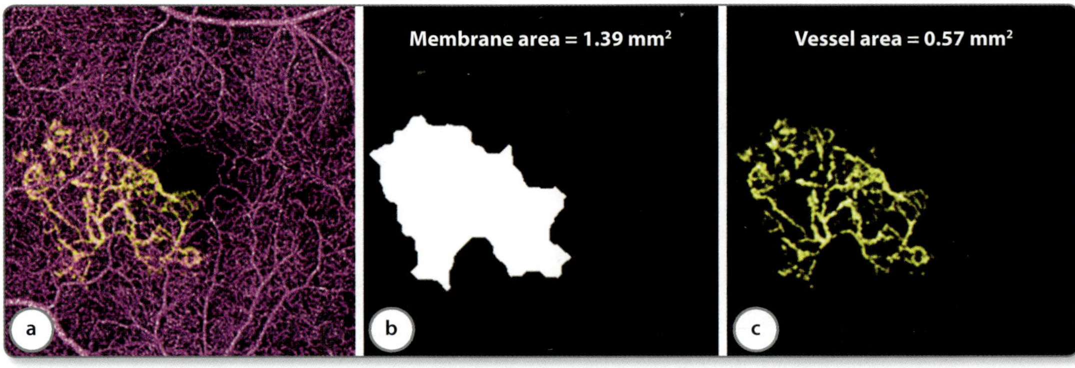

Figures 5 An example to show the quantification on neovascularization in age-related macular degeneration. (a) Choroidal neovascularization (CNV, yellow) overlaid by inner retinal vasculature (purple). (b) CNV membrane area (white) delineated automatically. (c) CNV vessel area showing flow pixels only.

artifacts. On the *en face* angiogram, lesion or membrane area measures the area occupied by both the flow pixels (vessels) and the intervening nonflow pixels (fibrous tissue).[16] The vessel area only counts the flow pixels (**Figures 5a** to **c**).[17]

Optovue angiovue technology

The AngioVue OCTA system Avanti (Optovue, Inc., Freemont, CA) is a high-speed (70 kHz) spectral-domain OCT system. Using the efficient SSADA algorithm, each standard OCTA volume is acquired in 3 seconds. Two image volumes are registered and merged using the patented motion correction technology (MCT) to minimise motion artifacts and improve image quality.[6,18] The AngioAnalytics software maps and measures vessel density and nonflow area to measure ischemia, and vessel area to quantify neovascularization. Video tracking and high-definition (400 × 400) OCTA have been recently added to further improve image quality.

Clinical applications of OCTA technology

Optical coherence tomographic angiography uses intrinsic motion contrast to detect flow, and therefore does not require injection of a contrast agent like conventional fluorescein angiography (FA). The noninvasive nature of OCTA allows for routine use to detect disease and monitor treatment efficacy. Therefore, OCTA is likely to be used more than FA ever was. OCTA does not detect dye leakage or staining, therefore the recognition of abnormal vessels such as retinal or choroidal neovascularization is based on their distinct patterns and occurrence in normally nonvascular layers. Because OCTA is 3D, it is possible to separately visualise retinal vascular plexuses and choroidal layers by *en face* projection of segmented slabs. In diabetic retinopathy, retinal venous occlusion, and other retinal vascular diseases, OCTA is used to detect and quantify retinal neovascularization and ischemia (increased avascular area and decrease vessel density).[19] In age-related macular degeneration, inherited retinal degenerations, and other outer retina/choroidal diseases, OCTA is used to detect and quantify choroidal neovascularization and choriocapillary defects.[11,20,21] In glaucoma and other optic neuropathies, OCTA is used to detect decreased perfusion in the optic disc, peripapillary retina and choroid, and macular ganglion cell complex.[22-24]

References

1 Jia Y, Tan O, Tokayer J, et al. Split-spectrum amplitude-decorrelation angiography with optical coherence tomography. Opt Express 2012; 20:4710–4725.

2 Gao SS, Liu G, Huang D, et al. Optimization of the split-spectrum amplitude-decorrelation angiography algorithm on a spectral optical coherence tomography system. Opt Lett 2015; 40:2305–2308.

3 Su JP, Chandwani R, Gao SS, et al. Calibration of optical coherence tomography angiography with a microfluidic chip. J Biomed Opt 2016; 21:86015.

4 Braaf B, Vienola KV, Sheehy CK, et al. Real-time eye motion correction in phase-resolved OCT angiography with tracking SLO. Biomedical optics express 2013; 4:51–65.

5 Zhang Q, Huang Y, Zhang T, et al. Wide-field imaging of retinal vasculature using optical coherence tomography-based microangiography provided by motion tracking. J Biomed Opt 2015; 20:066008.

6 Kraus MF, Potsaid B, Mayer MA, et al. Motion correction in optical coherence tomography volumes on a per A-scan basis using orthogonal scan patterns. Biomed Opt Express 2012; 3:1182–1199.

7 Camino A, Jia Y, Liu G, et al. Regression-based algorithm for bulk motion subtraction in optical coherence tomography angiography. Biomedical optics express 2017; 8:3053–3066.

8 Zhang M, Hwang TS, Campbell JP, et al. Projection-resolved optical coherence tomographic angiography. Biomed Opt Express 2016;7:816–828.

9 Gao SS, Jia Y, Liu L, et al. Compensation for Reflectance Variation in Vessel Density Quantification by Optical Coherence Tomography Angiography. Invest Ophthalmol Vis Sci 2016; 57:4485–4492.

10 Jia Y, Morrison JC, Tokayer J, et al. Quantitative OCT angiography of optic nerve head blood flow. Biomed Opt Express 2012; 3:3127–137.

11 Jia Y, Bailey ST, Hwang TS, et al. Quantitative optical coherence tomography angiography of vascular abnormalities in the living human eye. Proc Natl Acad Sci USA 2015; 112:E2395–2402.

12 Gao SS, Liu L, Bailey ST, et al. Quantification of choroidal neovascularization vessel length using optical coherence tomography angiography. J Biomed Opt 2016; 21:076010.

13 Hwang TS, Gao SS, Liu L, et al. Automated Quantification of Capillary Nonperfusion Using Optical Coherence Tomography Angiography in Diabetic Retinopathy. JAMA Ophthalmol 2016; 134:367–73.

14 Zhang M, Hwang TS, Dongye C, et al. Automated Quantification of Nonperfusion in Three Retinal Plexuses Using Projection-Resolved Optical Coherence Tomography Angiography in Diabetic RetinopathyQuantification of Retinal Ischemia in Three Plexuses. Invest Ophthalmol Vis Sci 2016; 57:5101–5106.

15 Hwang TS, Zhang M, Bhavsar K, et al. Visualization of 3 Distinct retinal plexuses by projection-resolved optical coherence tomography angiography in diabetic retinopathy. JAMA Ophthalmol 2016; 134:1411–1419.

16 Liu L, Gao SS, Bailey ST, et al. Automated choroidal neovascularization detection algorithm for optical coherence tomography angiography. Biomed Opt Express 2015; 6:3564–3576.

17 Jia Y, Bailey ST, Wilson DJ, et al. Quantitative optical coherence tomography angiography of choroidal neovascularization in age-related macular degeneration. Ophthalmology 2014; 121:1435–1444.

18 Camino A, Zhang M, Gao SS, et al. Evaluation of artifact reduction in optical coherence tomography angiography with real-time tracking and motion correction technology. Biomed Opt Express 2016; 7:3905–3915.

19 Hwang TS, Hagag AM, Wang J, et al. Automated quantification of nonperfusion areas in 3 vascular plexuses with optical coherence tomography angiography in eyes of patients with diabetes. JAMA Ophthalmol 2018; 136:929–936.

20 McClintic SM, Jia Y, Huang D, et al. Optical coherence tomographic angiography of choroidal

neovascularization associated with central serous chorioretinopathy. JAMA Ophthalmol 2015; 133:1212–1214.

21 Patel RC, Wang J, Hwang TS, et al. Plexus-Specific Detection of Retinal Vascular Pathologic Conditions with Projection-Resolved OCT Angiography. Ophthalmol Retina 2018; 2:816–826.

22 Liu L, Jia Y, Takusagawa HL, et al. Optical coherence tomography angiography of the peripapillary retina in glaucoma. JAMA Ophthalmol 2015; 133:1045–1052.

23 Jia Y, Wei E, Wang X, et al. Optical Coherence Tomography Angiography of Optic Disc Perfusion in Glaucoma. Ophthalmology 2014; 121:1322–1332.

24 Takusagawa HL, Liu L, Ma KN, et al. Projection-Resolved Optical Coherence Tomography Angiography of Macular Retinal Circulation in Glaucoma. Ophthalmol 2017; 124:1589–1599.

2 Performing a correct OCTA examination

Marco Rispoli, Bruno Lumbroso

Performing a valuable optical coherence tomographic angiography (OCTA) involves a multifactorial method that relies on numerous interrelated evaluations, scheduling, and implementation processes. Carrying out a correct OCTA examination requires concrete and theoretical skills: good device handling and appropriate knowledge. The operator must study to acquire the knowledge necessary for a correct handling of the device. It is mandatory to know how the machine and the algorithm work in order to avoid false-positive and false-negative flow signals.

The operator needs to perform examination and choose protocol: macula and/or nerve head, define the angiography scan size basing on the diagnostic suspicious or diagnosis. Handling an OCTA instrument may change depending from device (joystick, servo drive, full/semiautomatic, etc.). Warming up device and beam tuning should be very fast processes in order not to stress the patient.

Thresholding

Optical coherence tomographic angiography image is made by selecting time variations between two consecutive acquisitions. There are diverse time variations in optical coherence tomography (OCT), moving erythrocytes peristaltic action, and the noise. The noise is a fast time variation and may be decorrelated by OCTA algorithm becoming a false flow signal. Fortunately, the OCT signal of the retina is far greater than the noise signal.

In certain areas of the eye [vitreous and subretinal pigment epithelium (RPE) space], the OCT signal may decrease significantly so the noise may have a more important influence in OCTA algorithm generating false flow signals. For this reason, a thresholding algorithm works on every OCT device. Below a defined threshold, angiography algorithm will not operate and there will not be any decorrelation processes.

It is very difficult to choose the noise level in order to cut it because it depends from a lot of parameters. In absence of additional information, low OCTA signal in a thresholded OCTA image does not mean that in a certain area there is a low or no flow and conversely.

Examining vitreous, we will have a low OCT signal and low noise, so we will not have a flow signal. Examining choroid, we will have a low OCT signal and high noise that will be thresholded. In this case, choroidal flows will appear dark (low blood flow) because of thresholding process.

In case of geographic atrophy, we will see choroidal vessels bright through atrophy (high OCT signal above threshold) and dark below the RPE (low OCT signal below threshold). However, do not forget that OCTA signal depends both upon the threshold and the examination level.

Threshold or not threshold?

Thresholded OCTA: It is useful for retinal vasculature (high OCT signal and low noise).

Unthresholded OCTA: It is useful for inferring the absence of blood flow on the basis of the absence of an OCTA signal: absence of an unthresholded OCTA signal definitively implies the absence of blood flow.

In general, there are two risks that need to be balanced when choosing a threshold: eliminating true flow in vasculature (false negative) and including noise (false positive).

If the threshold is set higher, then OCTA devices may threshold out vasculature in low-signal areas. If the threshold is set lower, then there may be excess noise in the OCTA image. In the choriocapillaris, noise is especially problematic because the vascular features of the choriocapillaris are smaller than the transverse resolution of standard OCT systems, they cannot be resolved.

Commercial devices are all thresholded.

Practical problems of OCTA: Technical tips

Patient should feel comfortable and relaxed. Room atmosphere should be quiet with no noise.

Positioning correctly the patient's head is very important. Chin and front should be in, pressed to the device's rests. Sometimes, it will be needed to rotate the head on the left or on the right to avoid nose contact with the instrument optics.

Mydriasis is not always necessary if the compliance is good. Sometimes, a moderate mydriasis allows to get around lens opacities.

Optical coherence tomographic angiography is born from the structural OCT, thus it will be necessary to acquire first the structural examination imaging, then the functional cube. OCTA is the end result of a three-dimensional (3D) functional cube. This cube is obtained by acquiring structural scans and, the better is signal/noise ratio, the better will be the resulting OCTA data.

There is a specified number of pixels in the OCTA examination field, thus with a wider field, resolution will decrease. The best fields in relation to pixel density are the 3 × 3 mm and the 6 × 6 mm with more (HD) lines. It is possible to acquire OCTA scans that include the middle periphery, if the patient cooperates. In this case, the physiologically tilted retinal profile could change some layers reflectivity and consequently the boundaries assignment.

The eye tracker is very useful even in the highly compliant patient in order to obtain remarkable images. In low compliance cases or in patients affected by nystagmus, the eye tracker allows to get a useful examination.

Fixation problems

If a patient cannot fix properly the fixation dot, the eye tracker could not be able to track all the movements and may induce artifacts.

There are two possible solutions:

1. The first is to deactivate the motion correction technology algorithm (if present on the device) working individually on the fast X or fast Y image. This trick works only on research-dedicated devices because this procedure does not allow image standardization procedures. The OCTA image will have a lower resolution, but image interpretation will be possible but without quantitative data (analytics tool)
2. The second solution is to deactivate the eye tracker. In this way the acquisition time decreases consistently and will generate less artifacts than with the tracking is on

Mistakes to be avoided

Projection artifact

Flow projections artifacts are the result of fluctuating shadows cast by flowing blood in a superficial vascular network that causes variation of the OCT signal in deeper, highly reflective layers, mainly in RPE. Flow from the retinal circulation is projected, as a shadow, on the RPE or the outer plexiform layer (OPL).

This projection artifact can be removed by software in the OCT device, but it may work differently from device to device. This algorithm is able to decrease the density of each voxel that lies below the same Z axis. In this way all projected flow signals will be decreased in intensity.

Fixing some practical problems

No structural OCT signal, no OCTA image: OCTA algorithm works on variations on beam amplitude, phase or other parameters. If we have no OCT signal on certain area, we will not have any decorrelation process. Be sure to have the best OCT signal by setting up the beam manually (centring, focusing, and referencing).

Decreased OCT signal: Low structural OCT contrast leads to low quality OCTA. Dry eye, corneal scars, lens opacities, and vitreous opacities may lower the OCT signal on the retina, projecting some shadows on it. In these cases, *en face* OCTA shows some dark areas with smooth borders due to low structural signal on structural B-scan. Systems that work on amplitude decorrelation have a good tolerance on low signals. However, in some cases, the signal may be too low to be decorrelated.

Dry eye may decrease the OCT signal, but also media opacities.

To improve low contrast: Artificial tears will increase tear quality. Better pupil dilatation gives more space to bypass opacities. Focus/polarize manually if the automated setting is not satisfactory.

Motion artifacts in OCTA image

All movements are processed as motion. OCTA algorithms work on motion contrast, so every movement will be decorrelated. Heartbeat, saccades, and unstable fixation, may give motion signals on OCTA and should be avoided. Those artifacts may appear during acquisition or in the postprocessing phase.

Systems with severe eye tracking usually take a very long time to acquire an angio scan if the patient has low compliance; but on the other side, a too fast and tolerant tracker will produce lot of artifacts.

Some devices combine two or more acquisitions in order to reduce motion artifacts, despite the time.

Segmentation problems: Not always the default segmentation is the best segmentation

Default settings are excellent to study normal retina. If retinal layers are distorted (edema or atrophy), automated segmentation gives inappropriate results. It will be necessary to use manual segmentations.

If one or more boundaries seem to be positioned incorrectly, we will have to correct boundaries properly, and then reprocess the data.

Boundaries control is mandatory before evaluating an OCTA examination.

The most important boundaries are the inner limiting membrane (ILM) and the Bruch's membrane.

Inner limiting membrane allows to separate retinal from preretinal flows [e.g. proliferative diabetic retinopathy (PDR) and central retinal vein occlusion (CRVO)] while Bruch's membrane allows to define choroidal neovascularization (CNV) type (1, 2, 3, and mixed).

Usually the Bruch's membrane boundary fails to be properly traced by the software.

3 OCT angiography: Prospects and challenges

Tristan T Hormel, Yali Jia

While providing similar diagnostic capabilities as other ophthalmic angiographic imaging modalities such as fluorescein angiography,[1,2] optical coherence tomographic angiographic (OCTA) offers the additional advantages of three-dimensional, high-resolution, rapid, and noninvasive imaging. While these facets of the technology already represent clinically useful capabilities, as a developing technology, OCTA still retains areas that could be improved. The depth-resolved and high-resolution nature of the technology imbues it with the potential to acquire clear and plexus-specific images for perusal by clinicians. In the same way, plexus-specific quantification of OCTA metrics should also be possible. Research already indicates that embedding plexus-specific analytic capabilities within the technology would yield advantages for disease diagnosis and monitoring.[3-7]

Artifacts

That it has only limited ability to cleanly resolve different retinal plexuses, despite being an inherently volumetric approach to imaging, is due to the many types of artifacts that afflict OCTA images. Three types of artifacts are especially prominent in OCTA: projection, signal reduction, and bulk motion.[8] Improvements in OCTA technology must confront the effect of these artifacts on OCTA data analysis. Two complementary approaches are possible: (1) artifacts can be compensated for to provide clearer two-dimensional (2D) *en face* or three-dimensional (3D) cross-sectional or volumetric OCTA visualization.[9-12] However, even in artifact-free images, quantification of different parameters may be difficult to achieve manually or with simple algorithms. Therefore, to achieve better OCTA quantification, in addition to artifact compensation, (2) image analysis methods can be improved. Many powerful approaches in structural optical coherence tomography (OCT)[13-15] and OCTA[16,17] are based on artificial intelligence (AI). AI-enhanced algorithms have proven capable in the context of automating measurements that would either be infeasible to perform manually or are difficult to automate with traditional image processing techniques.

To illustrate these ideas, we will consider two examples, starting with the effect of projection artifacts on imaging choroidal neovascularization (CNV). Because projection artifacts mimic the appearance of superficial vessels in deeper anatomic layers, they can give a false impression of CNV development. Of course, projection artifacts are problematic for many more reasons that just complicating CNV quantification. Because signal from superficial layers overlays true signal in deep plexuses, projection artifacts also prevent clear plexus-specific imaging and quantification. This is in many ways a larger concern than the disruption of CNV visualization, since by smearing information across several plexuses, projection artifacts prevent pathophysiological investigation in an isolated plexus.

Projection artifacts

As projection artifacts are a frequent complication in OCTA imaging, multiple methods focused on their removal exist. In slab subtraction, superficial vascular signal is subtracted from deeper layers in order to remove the projection artifacts.[18-21] However, this technique also removes true flow signal when projection artifacts overly real vasculature. Furthermore, as it does not provide volumetric compensation, slab subtraction is only useful for cleaning *en face* images. In the projection-resolved OCTA (PR-OCTA) approach, detail from the reflectance OCT volume as well as the OCTA volume is incorporated in order to remove projection artifacts without also removing real signal from deeper layers (**Figure 1**).[22,23] The resulting angiograms are largely free of projection artifacts and enable plexus-specific imaging. Using their relative position to RPE, we are able to classify CNV into type I, type II, type III or mixed (**Figure 2**).[24] Several studies using PR-OCTA have confirmed heterogeneous disease progression in different layers.[3,5,6,25-27] Furthermore, PR-OCTA enables clear visualization of four separate plexuses in the human retina,[28] an organization corroborated by histology.[29]

Even with state-of-the-art artifact removal, some residual projection artifacts can remain in OCTA images. Saliency-based approaches to CNV lesion detection will often confuse these artifacts for true CNV.[18] Our recent work (unpublished) is instead based on a convolutional neural network (CNN), an important AI technique in image analysis. A CNN learns from many examples of manually graded data, which affords it the ability to interpret high-level image features such as a CNV lesion or a residual projection artifact. The result is an algorithm that can correctly differentiate between residual artifacts and the true lesion, which can help not only diagnose the scans with CNV but also segment CNV membrane area and CNV vascular area (**Figure 3**).

Signal reduction artifacts

The second class of important artifacts in OCTA imaging are signal reduction artifacts. Due to vignetting or vitreous floaters that attenuate OCTA illumination, shadow artifacts appear as regions with low signal in OCTA images. Artifacts of this sort are especially confounding for measurements of avascular area, as they can render even vascular regions apparently vessel-free. This is an important limitation, since capillary dropout is implicated in such prevalent diseases as diabetic retinopathy (DR)[30-34] and glaucoma.[6,35-38] One way to circumvent this issue is to include information from the OCT reflectance dataset in the input to a CNN. Since the reflectance image will also lose signal from shadowing, but not from avascular areas, it can be used to distinguish true vessel loss. In this way, our group developed a CNN capable of accurately quantifying avascular area even in the presence of shadow artifacts (**Figure 4**).[17]

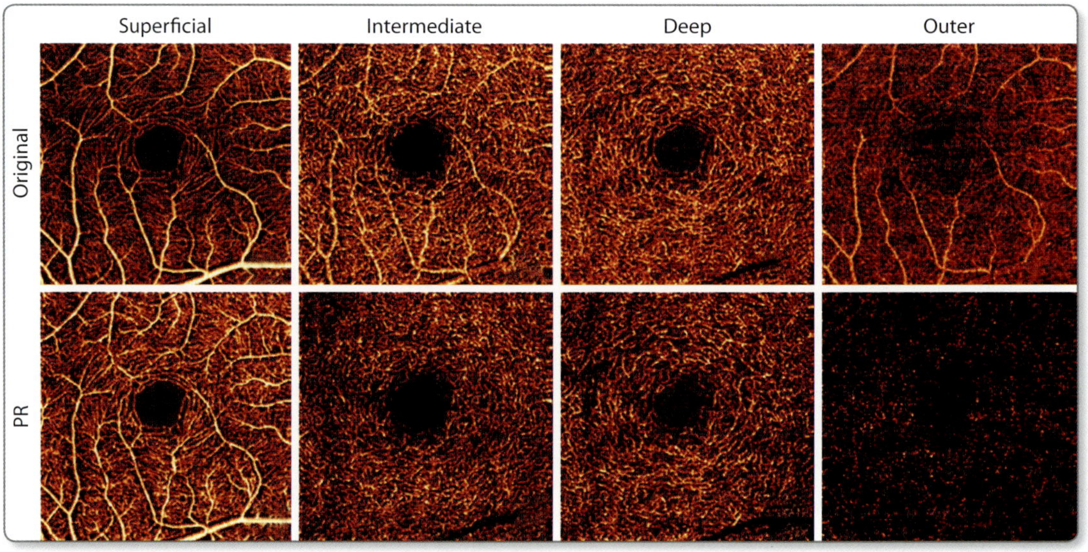

Figure 1 Projection-resolved optical coherence tomographic angiography (PR-OCTA) of a healthy eye. Shown are the superficial vascular complex (SVC), intermediate capillary plexus (ICP), the deep capillary plexus (DCP), and the outer retina. The original OCTA data (top row) shows large vessels from the SVC projected into other plexuses and the outer retina; these artifacts are largely absent after PR-OCTA processing (bottom row).
Adapted from Wang et al.[23]

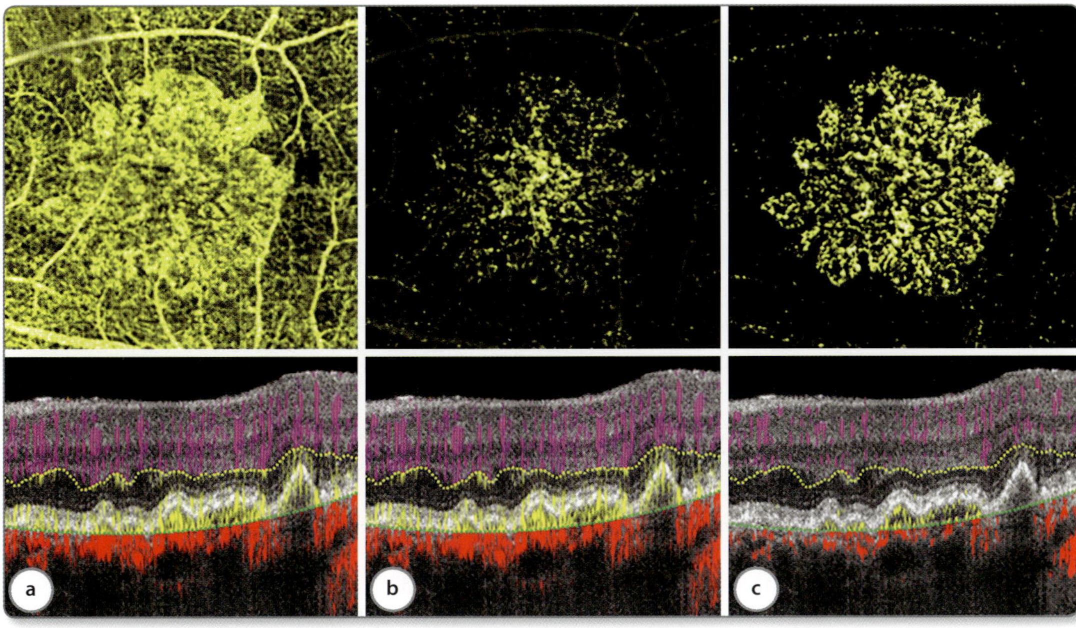

Figure 2 Choroidal neovascularization (CNV) imaged using (a) uncorrected optical coherence tomographic angiography (OCTA), (b) slab subtraction, and (c) projection resolved optical coherence tomographic angiography (PR-OCTA). Row 1: *en face* images, row 2: cross-sectional images with inner retinal (violet), choroidal (red), and pathological outer retinal (yellow) flow overlaid. The uncorrected OCTA images (a) show a large amount of spurious signal, while the slab-subtraction method, in which superficial flow is simply subtracted from deeper anatomic slabs, leaves the CNV lesion fragmented. PR-OCTA, on the other hand, removes projection artifacts while leaving the CNV intact. PR-OCTA also enables classification of CNV by type, due to its ability to accurately resolve the depth of the lesion.
Reprinted from Patel et al.[3]

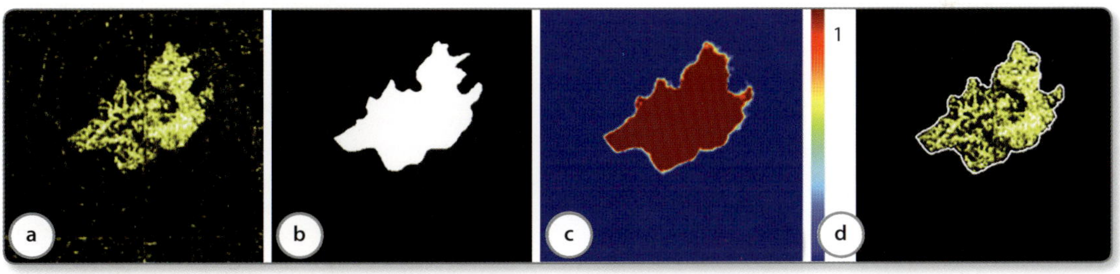

Figure 3 Automated choroidal neovascularization (CNV) detection using artificial intelligence (AI). (a) Projection-resolved optical coherence tomographic angiography (PR-OCTA) outer retinal angiogram; (b) Manually graded CNV lesion area; (c) Algorithm output probability map; (d) AI-generated lesion area, with signal outside of the lesion area suppressed.

In summary, the combination of artifact compensation and advanced AI-driven image analysis allows for the visualization and quantification of retinal vasculature in health and disease. This chapter has showcased just two prominent artifacts (projection and signal reduction artifacts) and their effect on imaging of two pathologies (CNV and capillary dropout). But merging clean, plexus-specific imaging and advanced image processing techniques is a clear way forward to improve the biomedical utility of OCTA technology in general. We suspect that soon more OCTA measurements will be capable of accurate, automated quantification at levels of anatomic specificity.

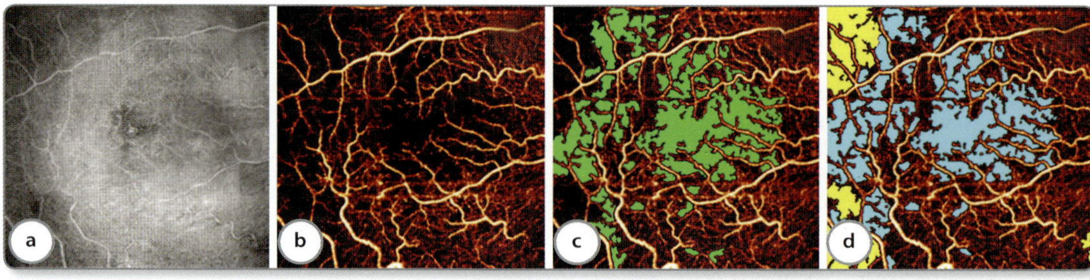

Figure 4 Automated avascular area detection. (a) Reflectance optical coherence tomography (OCT) image, with shadow artifacts visible to the left; (b) Optical coherence tomographic angiography (OCTA) image of the superficial vascular complex, with some apparently avascular area actually caused by shadow artifacts; (c) Manually graded ground avascular area (green) overlaid on the angiogram; (d) Artificial intelligence produced avascular area (blue) and area identified as shadow artifact (yellow) by the algorithm.
Reprinted from Guo et al.[17]

References

1. Hwang TS, Jia Y, Gao SS, et al. Optical coherence tomography angiography features in diabetic retinopathy. Retina 2015; 35:2371–2376.
2. Salz DA, de Carlo TE, Adhi M, et al. Select Features of Diabetic Retinopathy on Swept-Source Optical Coherence Tomographic Angiography Compared With Fluorescein Angiography and Normal Eyes. JAMA Ophthalmol 2016; 134:644–650.
3. Patel RC, Wang J, Hwang TS, et al. Plexus-Specific Detection of Retinal Vascular Pathologic Conditions with Projection-Resolved OCT Angiography. Ophthalmol Retina 2018; 2:816–826.
4. Onishi AC, Nesper PL, Roberts PK, et al. Importance of considering the middle capillary plexus on OCT angiography in diabetic retinopathy. Invest Ophthalmol Vis Sci 2018; 59:2167–2176.
5. Takusagawa HL, Liu L, Ma KN, et al. Projection-resolved optical coherence tomography angiography of macular retinal circulation in glaucoma. Ophthalmol 2017; 124:1589–1599.
6. Liu L, Edmunds B, Takusagawa H, et al. Projection-resolved optical coherence tomography angiography of the peripapillary retina in glaucoma. Am J Ophthalmol 2019; 207:99–109.
7. Bhavsar KV, Jia Y, Wang J, et al. Projection-resolved optical coherence tomography angiography exhibiting early flow prior to clinically observed retinal angiomatous proliferation. Am J Ophthalmol Case Rep 2017; 8:53–57.
8. Spaide RF, Fujimoto JG, Waheed NK. Image artifacts in optical coherence angiography. Retina 2015; 35:2163–180.
9. Camino A, Jia Y, Liu G, et al. Regression-based algorithm for bulk motion subtraction in optical coherence tomography angiography. Biomed Opt Express 2017; 8:3053–3066.
10. Gao SS, Jia Y, Liu L, et al. Compensation for reflectance variation in vessel density quantification by optical coherence tomography angiography. Invest Ophthalmol Vis Sci 2016; 57:4485–4492.
11. Yu JJ, Camino A, Liu L, et al. Signal strength reduction effects in OCT angiography. Ophthalmol Retina 2019; 3:835–42.
12. Zang P, Liu G, Zhang M, et al. Automated motion correction using parallel-strip registration for wide-field en face OCT angiogram. Biomed Opt Express 2016; 7:2823–2836.
13. Lee CS, Baughman DM, Lee AY. Deep learning is effective for classifying normal versus age-related macular degeneration OCT images. Ophthalmol Retina 2017; 2:322–327.
14. Lee CS, Tyring AJ, Deruyter NP, et al. Deep-learning based, automated segmentation of macular edema in optical coherence tomography. Biomed Opt Express 2017; 8:530–533.
15. Halupka KJ, Antony BJ, Lee MH, et al. Retinal optical coherence tomography image enhancement via deep learning. Biomed Opt Express 2018; 9:6205–6221.
16. Guo Y, Camino A, Wang J, et al. MEDnet, a neural network for automated detection of avascular area in OCT angiography. Biomed Opt Express 2018; 9:5147.
17. Guo Y, Hormel TT, Xiong H, et al. Development and validation of a deep learning algorithm for distinguishing the nonperfusion area from signal reduction artifacts on OCT angiography. Biomed Opt Express 2019; 10:3257–3268.
18. Liu L, Gao SS, Bailey ST, et al. Automated choroidal neovascularization detection algorithm for optical coherence tomography angiography. Biomed Opt Express 2015; 6:3564.
19. Jia Y, Bailey ST, Wilson DJ, et al. Quantitative optical coherence tomography angiography of

choroidal neovascularization in age-related macular degeneration. Ophthalmol 2014; 121:1435–1444.
20. Jia Y, Bailey ST, Hwang TS, et al. Quantitative optical coherence tomography angiography of vascular abnormalities in the living human eye. Proc Nati Acad Sci 2015; 112:e2395–2402.
21. Zhang A, Zhang Q, Wang RK, Minimizing projection artifacts for accurate presentation of choroidal neovascularization in OCT micro-angiography. Biomed Opt Express 2015; 6:4130.
22. Zhang M, Hwang TS, Campbell JP, et al. Projection-resolved optical coherence tomographic angiography. Biomed Opt Express 2016; 7:816–828.
23. Wang J, Zhang M, Hwang TS, et al. Reflectance-based projection-resolved optical coherence tomography angiography. Biomed Opt Express 2017; 8:1536–48.
24. Patel R, Wang J, Campbell JP, et al. Classification of choroidal neovascularization using projection-resolved optical coherence tomographic angiography. Invest Ophthalmol Vis Sci 2018; 59:4285–91.
25. Chen X, Rahimy E, Sergott RC, et al. Spectrum of retinal vascular diseases associated with paracentral acute middle maculopathy. Am J Ophthalmol 2015; 160:26–34.e21.
26. Hagag AM, Wang JI, Lu K, et al. Projection-resolved optical coherence tomographic angiography of retinal plexuses in retinitis pigmentosa. Am J Ophthalmol 2019; 204:70–9.
27. Nelis P, Kleffner I, Burg MC, et al. OCT-angiography reveals reduced vessel density in the deep retinal plexus of CADASIL patients. Sci Rep 2018; 8:1–7.
28. Campbell JP, Zhang M, Hwang TS, et al. Detailed vascular anatomy of the human retina by projection-resolved optical coherence tomography angiography. Sci Rep 2017; 7:1–11.
29. Stone J, van Driel D, Valter K, et al. The locations of mitochondria in mammalian photoreceptors: Relation to retinal vasculature. Brain Res 2008; 1189:58–69.
30. Couturier A, Mané V, Bonnin S, et al. Capillary plexus anomalies in diabetic retinopathy on optical coherence tomography angiography. Retina 2015; 35:2384–91.
31. Hwang TS, Gao SS, Liu L, et al. Automated quantification of capillary nonperfusion using optical coherence tomography angiography in diabetic retinopathy. JAMA Ophthalmol 2016; 134:367–373.
32. Hwang TS, Hagag AM, Wang J, et al. Automated quantification of nonperfusion areas in 3 vascular plexuses with optical coherence tomography angiography in eyes of patients with diabetes. JAMA Ophthalmol 2018; 97239:929–936.
33. Kim AY, Chu Z, Shahidzadeh A, et al. Quantifying microvascular density and morphology in diabetic retinopathy using spectral-domain optical coherence tomography angiography. Invest Ophthalmol Vis Sci 2016; 57:362–370.
34. Nesper PL, Roberts PK, Onishi AC, et al. Quantifying microvascular abnormalities with increasing severity of diabetic retinopathy using optical coherence tomography angiography. Invest Ophthalmol Vis Sci 2017; 58:BIO307–BIO315.
35. Yarmohammadi A, Zangwill LM, Diniz-filho A, et al. Optical coherence tomography angiography vessel density in healthy, glaucoma suspect, and glaucoma eyes. Invest Ophthalmol Vis Sci 2016; 57:OCT451–459.
36. Yarmohammadi A, Zangwill LM, Diniz-filho A, et al. Relationship between Optical Coherence Tomography Angiography Vessel Density and Severity of Visual Field Loss in Glaucoma. Ophthalmology 2016; 123:2498–2508.
37. Yarmohammadi A, Zangwill LM, Manalastas PI, et al. Peripapillary and Macular Vessel Density in Patients with Primary Open-Angle Glaucoma and Unilateral Visual Field Loss. Ophthalmology 2017; 125:578–87.
38. Jia Y, Wei E, Wang X, et al. Optical coherence tomography angiography of optic disc perfusion in glaucoma. Ophthalmology 2014; 121:1322–32.

4 OCT angiography quantitative assessment

Bruno Lumbroso, Marco Rispoli

Introduction

Optical coherence tomography (OCT) angiography quantitative assessment is currently an obligatory phase in any optical coherence tomographic angiography (OCTA) examination whereas dye angiography cannot provide quantitative data. Dye staining and leakage conceal the neovascular network morphology.

Flow qualitative imaging should be associated in the same examination to quantitative analysis for immediate assessment and follow-up. AngioAnalytics software allows to measure quantitatively OCT angiography data. Quantitative parameters may be measured dependably and recurrently. Comprehensive analysis of OCTA parameters is not limited to flow area, nonflow area and vessel density map, but it includes other important factors: vessel diameter, vessel perimeter index, blood vessel tortuosity, area of foveal avascular zone, and parafoveal avascular density.

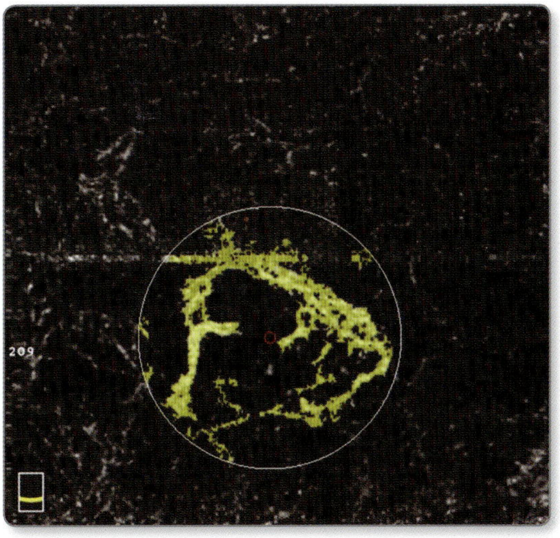

Figure 1 The choroidal neovascularization area is delimited by a ring line, inside which the new vessels flow appears in yellow. The software prints the value of the area outlined by the operator alongside with the value of the neovascular yellow area. (Optovue)

Flow area

The OCT angiography quantifies flow in the vascular structures of the segmented volume. The operator outlines the neovascular membrane after selecting the right volume and segmentation slab (**Figure 1**). The software automatically identifies and measures the outlined area and the flow it contains. Measurements should be made to help monitoring (**Figure 2**). This is useful in the follow-up of neovascular membranes, before and after treatment and in the study of the evolution of preretinal and prepapillary new vessels (treated or not treated).

Nonflow area, vascular dropout area

After selecting the right volume, the operator should click any point in the nonflow area and the software automatically delimits the area where pixels have the same value (**Figures 3** and **4**). The nonperfused areas may be highlighted in yellow. This technique allows measuring vascular "dropout" in areas where blood flow is lower than normal due to relative or total ischemia. It is possible and useful clinically to study separately dropout areas in the superficial and in the deep vascular networks. Dropout measurement is advantageous in all vascular disorders.

Flow density map

The flow density map measures the flow in vascular areas on *en face* angiograms. Density map shows areas of flow and no flow. The ratio is expressed numerically and shown on a scale of false colors (**Figure 5**). The warm colors are given

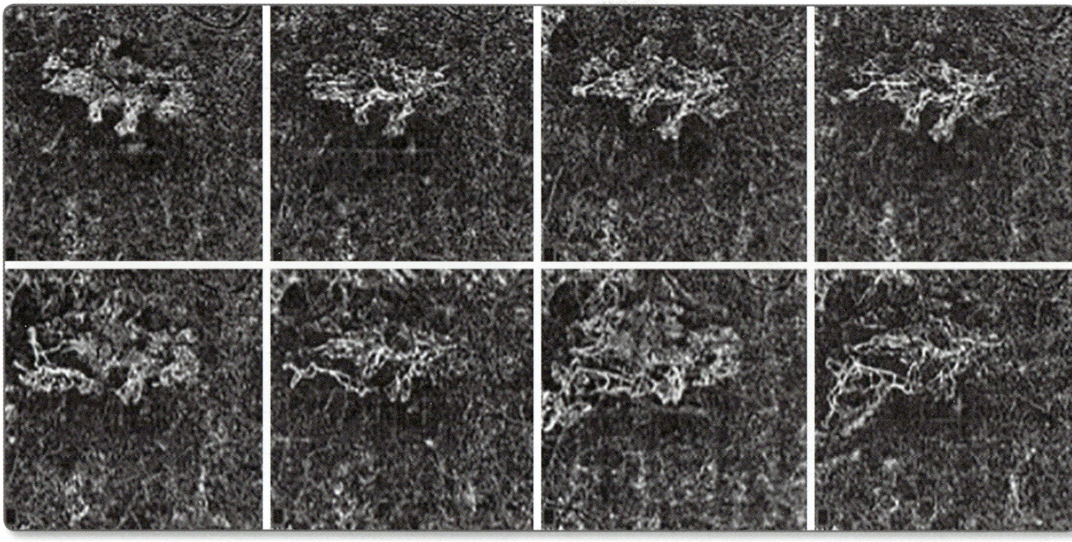

Figure 2 Monitoring CNV evolution during treatment. In this choroidal neovascularization (CNV) case, the successive images allow to follow vascular growth areas and areas of regression. Measurement of the neovascular area made at every examination allows immediate qualitative and quantitative comparison. (Optovue)

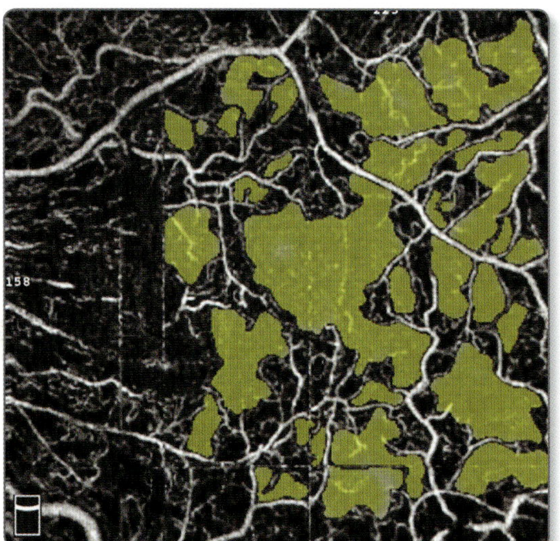

Figure 3 Branch venous occlusion of a branch with vascular dropout in the superficial vascular plexus. The nonflow areas are highlighted in yellow, measured in square millimeters and may be compared with successive examinations. (Optovue)

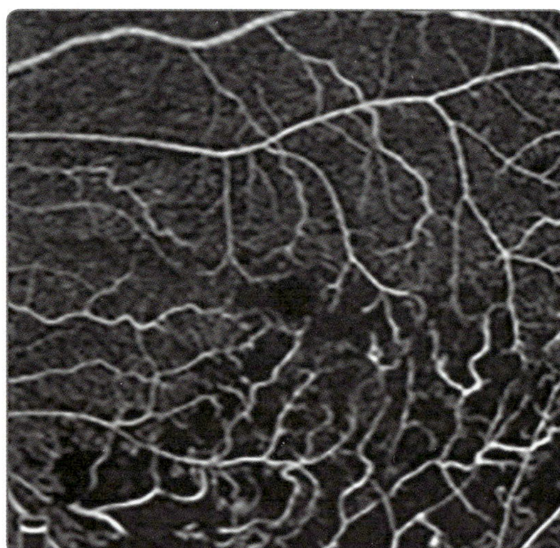

Figure 4 Branch venous occlusion with vascular dropout in the superficial vascular plexus. (Optovue)

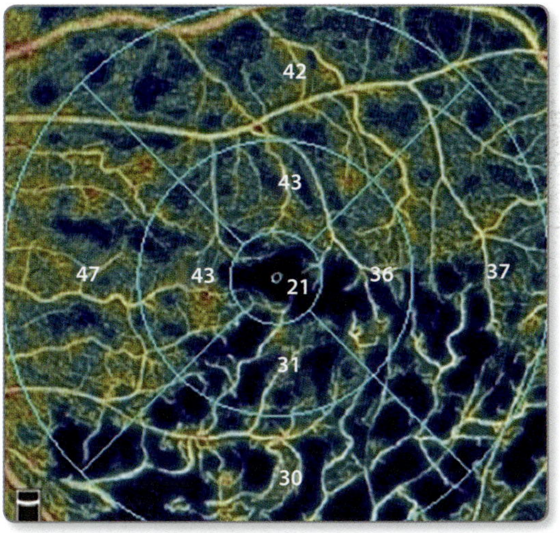

Figure 5 Branch venous occlusion. Same case. Vascular density map at the superficial vascular plexus level. The numerical values expressed in the upper right table refer to the circular grid superimposed onto the angioflow image. (Optovue)

to high density vascular areas, and the cold colors show low flow or no flow density. An average vascular density value is obtained for each sector of the map.

Vascular density may be calculated separately for the superficial and the deep vascular networks.

Box 1: OCT angiography quantitative parameters today

- Flow area
- Nonflow area
- Vessel density map

Box 2: OCT angiography quantitative parameters in future

- Flow speed
- Vessel diameter
- Vessel perimeter index
- Blood vessel tortuosity
- Area of foveal avascular zone
- Contour irregularity
- Parafoveal avascular density

Flow speed

The flow speed measurement software is not yet clinically available. It will be expressed numerically and shown on a scale of false colors. The warm colors are given to high speed vascular areas, and the cold colors show low flow speed (**Boxes 1** and **2**).

5 Normal retinal anatomy and OCT angiography

Bruno Lumbroso, Maria Cristina Savastano

Pathophysiology

The blood-retina barrier: Tight junctions and barrier variation

The blood-retinal barrier regulates the flow of substances entering and leaving the eye. It is essential to prevent, in the retinal tissues, the variations that occur constantly in the body circulation. Blood-retinal barrier also drains waste from tissues. The diffusion of nutrients and waste is determined by the blood-retinal barrier of both the retinal and choroidal vessels. Diffusion is the movement of molecules in liquids or gases from regions of high concentration to regions of low concentration.

Alteration of the blood-retinal barrier is the base for most ocular disorders, diabetic retinopathy, inflammation, and macular degeneration.

The blood-retinal barrier is formed by cells, tightly bound together, to prevent certain fluids and substances from entering or leaving the retinal tissue. It is composed of the nonfenestrated retinal circulation capillaries and the tight junction between the retinal epithelial cells that prevent the passage of large molecules from the choroid vessels into the retina. It plays an essential role in the preservation and maintenance of the ocular setting. It prevents the free diffusion of materials between blood and retina, supplies nutrients and removes waste from the retina to maintain a constant retina.

The hemato-retinal barrier involves two components: the endothelium of the retinal vessels and the retinal pigment epithelium. The blood-retina barrier is composed of both an inner and an outer barrier.

Inner blood-ocular barrier

Retinal blood vessels are similar to cerebral blood vessels in maintaining the inner blood-ocular barrier. The barrier comprises the microvascular endothelium which line the vessels. This physiological barrier consists of a single layer of nonfenestrated endothelial cells, which have occluding junctions. The tight junctions located between these cells arbitrate diffusion of molecules from the blood to the retina, regulating the fluids and shielding the ocular tissues from the variations that arise continuously in the whole body. The inner blood-retinal barrier (BRB) is created by complex tight junctions of retinal capillary endothelial cells.

Outer blood-ocular barrier

The pigment epithelium sustains the external blood-ocular barrier. The outer BRB refers to the barrier formed at the retinal pigment epithelial (RPE) cell layer. This barrier regulates the movement of protein, nutrients and fluid from the choroid to the subretinal space. It is formed of tight junctions between pigment epithelial cells.

Retina and choroid are composed of cells and intercellular spaces. Intercellular spaces represent the regular pathways for the fluid and substances circulation. There are two exceptions: the capillary pores; and zonulae occludentes. Capillary pores are part of endothelial cells and covered by portions of the cytoplasmic membrane; they allow the diffusion of substances. Zonulae occludentes are intercellular junctions: the cell membranes of the neighboring cells are tightly attached, thus preventing diffusion.

Normal retinal vessels are "tight". Retinal capillaries do not carry pores and intercellular spaces are closed by zonulae occludentes.

In many disorders, retinal vessels may become permeable. Retinal vessels leak when zonulae occludentes open, when endothelial cells are lost, rendering the endothelial lining incomplete. Opening of zonulae occludentes is typically the case in inflammatory conditions. Leakage out of diabetic microaneurysms is usually caused by a loss of endothelial cells. Leakage from proliferated retinal vessels is very pronounced. It is caused by both the occurrence of pores and an incomplete endothelial lining.

Normal choroidal vessels have pores and are permeable to diffusion. The pigment epithelial zonulae occludentes are tight. The zonulae occludentes of the retinal pigment epithelium forms the BRB for substances circulating through the pore-bearing, porous choroidal vessels, while for the retinal vessels the barrier is located in the vascular wall itself.

OCT, OCT angiography, basic normal anatomy and histology

OCT and OCT angiography allowed us to visualize in vivo, the retinal structure and vasculariation (**Figure 1**). To understand OCT images, it is necessary to compare with retina and choroid histology, even if a perfect parallelism is lacking. In fact, some structures (photoreceptor

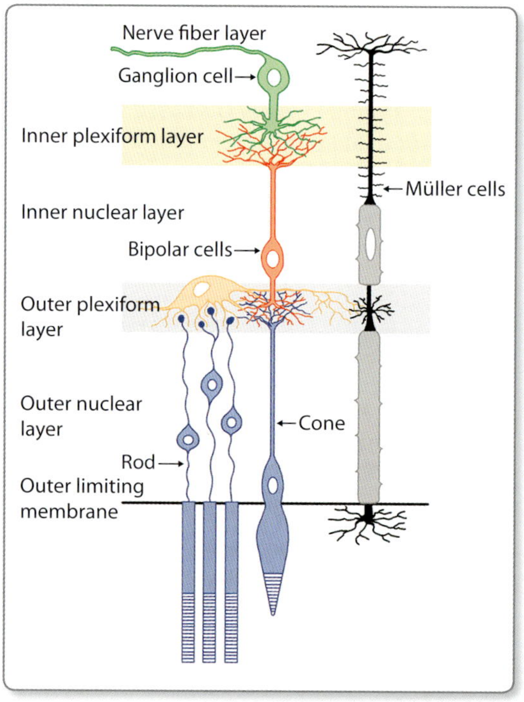

Figure 1 Retinal layers. From top to bottom, we notice optic nerve fiber layer, with the inner limiting membrane formed by Müller's cell fibrillae.

Ganglion cell layer. These cells have a big nucleus and their axons form the optic fiber layer.

Inner plexiform layer, connecting bipolar and ganglion cells. It includes horizontal structures, consisting in part of Müller's cell fibrillae. Inner nuclear layer of bipolar cells.

Outer plexiform layer, connecting photoreceptors and bipolar cells. It includes horizontal structures made of horizontal cells and Müller's cell fibrillae.

Photoreceptor nucleus layer. The outer limiting membrane, formed by fibrillae from Müller's fibers, generates a net surrounding cones and rods.

Ellipsoid zone: Inner/outer photoreceptor segment junction Cone and rod inner segment interdigitation between the cone and rod external tips and the epithelial cell fibrillae.

Visual cells chains are formed by photoreceptors (cones and rods) linked to bipolar cells that are linked in turn to ganglion cells, whose axons form the optic fibers.

The Müller cells are vertical fibrous elements that participate in the formation of the internal and external limiting membranes. Their nucleus is located in the inner nuclear layer beside the bipolar cells. Fibrils project from the Müller fibers, participating to the formation of the inner and outer plexiform layers.

Each of the cones and rods are composed of an inner and outer part. The inner part or cell body has a slightly elongated shape. The nucleus almost entirely fills the cell body and is in contact with the outer limiting membrane.

The outer portion of the photoreceptor consists of two parts: an inner and outer segment. The outer segment is fairly short, roughly conical for the cone in shape and consists of a succession of superimposed disks. For the rods, the outer segment is a thin cylindrical formation, consisting of numerous disks overlying each other. The inner segment is , in turn, formed by two parts, an internal myoid zone and an external filamentous zone or ellipsoid zone.

Till now we thought that the sharply hyper-reflective strip, at a short distance from the retinal pigment epithelium-choriocapillaris unit is formed by the connection between inner and outer segment. Some authors suppose that is the ellipsoid portion of the inner segment that is hyper-reflective and forms the hyper-reflective strand.

inner/outer segment junction, photoreceptor outer segment junction, and pigment epithelium cell villosities) are visible on OCTs because of their optical density and quality, independent of their thickness, although they are not visible on histological sections.

Retina is formed by a complex framework of fibers, capillaries and cells organized in vertical and horizontal structures that create efficient anatomical and functional barriers (**Figures 2a** and **2b**). Framework of intersecting supporting horizontal and vertical structures explains localization, dimensions and shape of exudates, hemorrhages, cystoid cavities that we can analyze with OCT and OCTA.

Retinal scaffold: Vertical and horizontal structures

In the extramacular area, the retinal scaffold is quite simple. Müller cells unite the inner limiting membrane to the outer limiting membrane crossing the two plexiform layers.

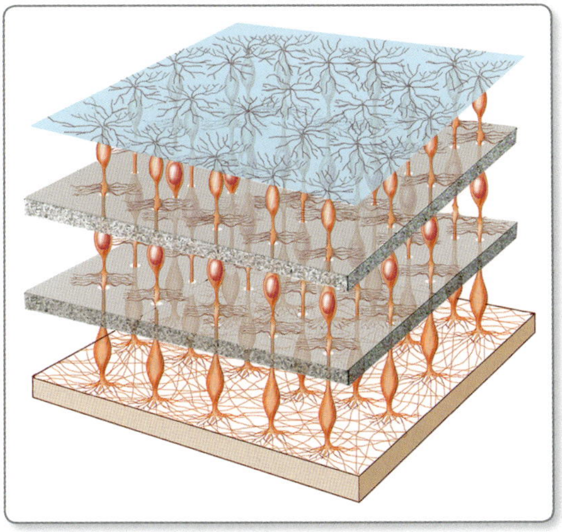

Figure 2a Retina framework. In the extramacular area, the retinal framework is quite simple. Müller cells unite the inner limiting membrane to the outer limiting membrane crossing the two plexiform layers. Retina horizontal structures are formed by inner and outer plexiform layers (green), inner and outer limiting membranes (blue). Pigment epithelium is another horizontal structure (red). Vertical structures are Müller fibers and cell chains consisting of photoreceptors linked to bipolar and ganglion cells.

Macula presents a higher degree of complexity and its structure is less resilient than retina extra-macular framework. Müller cells and Henle fibers are diagonally placed (**Figures 3, 4, 5a** and **5b**). Macular Müller cell body is slanted. Seen frontally, the macular structure is radial.

The anatomy of the macula explains why cystoid edema is flower or honeycomb shaped. Pathological processes extension in the macular area is blocked vertically and horizontally by these barriers.

At the fovea cystoid edema cavities find little obstacles to their stretching. The weakness of Müller cell framework in the macular area explains the large dimensions reached at the fovea by cavities.

Vertical scaffold

Müller cells are fibrous elements that provide support to retina. Their physiological function is very complex. They unite the inner and outer limiting membranes. Their nuclei are located in the bipolar cell layer. From Müller cell body originate horizontal fibrils that take an important part in the meshwork forming the inner and outer plexiform layers frame.

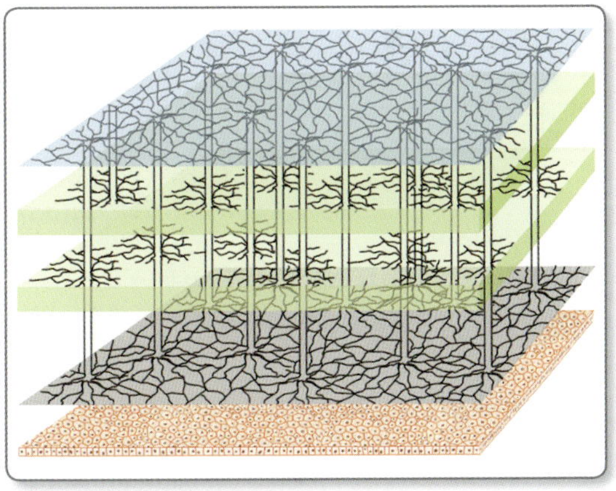

Figure 2b Retina framework. From Müller cells have origin fibrils that take part in the structure of the two plexiform layers. Vertical and horizontal structures limit the expansion of pathologic lesions, exudates, hemorrhages and edema.

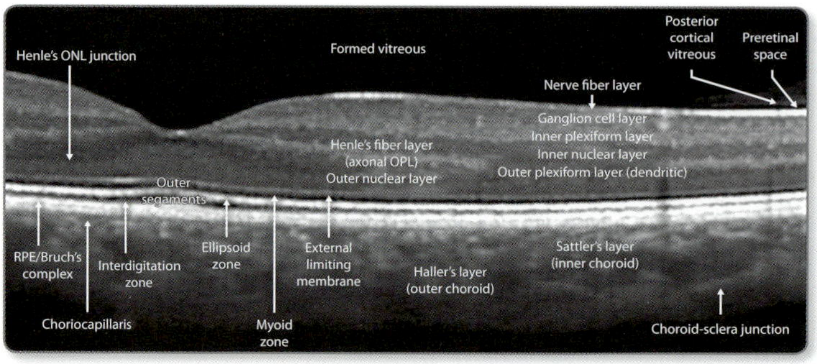

Figure 3 A panel of retina specialists developed this nomenclature of the retinal layers examined on structural OCT. This nomenclature is universally accepted.
Courtesy: Giovanni Staurenghi.

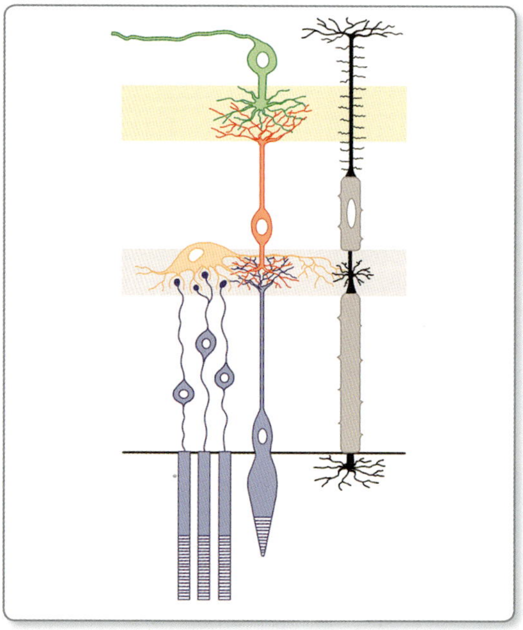

Figure 4 Cellular chains and Müller's cells: Retinal cells form chains of photoreceptors (cones or rods), linked to bipolar cells, which in turn are connected to ganglion cells, whose axons constitute the optic fibers. Parallel to the cellular chains are Müller's cells.

The Müller's cells are vertical fibrous elements that join the internal and external limiting membranes. Müller cells provide support to retina. Their physiological function is very complex. They unite the inner and outer limiting membranes. Their nuclei are located in the bipolar cell layer. From Müller cell body originate horizontal fibrils that take an important part in the meshwork forming the inner and outer plexiform layers frame. The chains formed by photoreceptors cells linked to the bipolar cells and to ganglion cells are other important vertical structures. At the macula, Müller cells and Henle fibers are not vertical but oblique and macula structure is less solid.

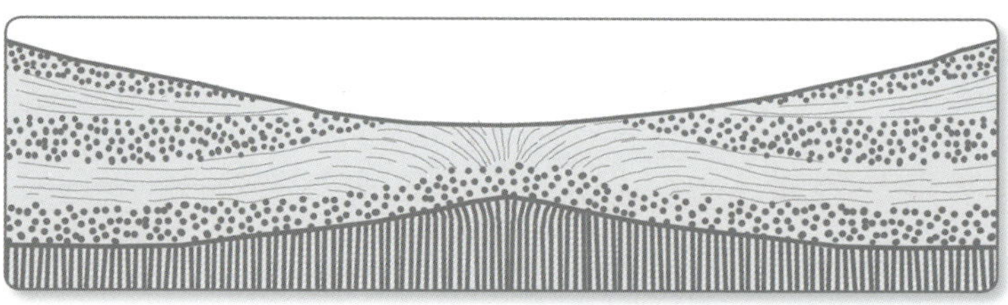

Figure 5a Henle's fiber cross section structure. At the fovea level, the photoreceptor nuclei are organized in the fovea. From those nuclei spread out the Henle's fibers, connecting photoreceptors and bipolar cells. Macula presents a higher degree of complexity and its structure is weaker than retina extra macular framework. Müller cells and Henle fibers are diagonally placed.

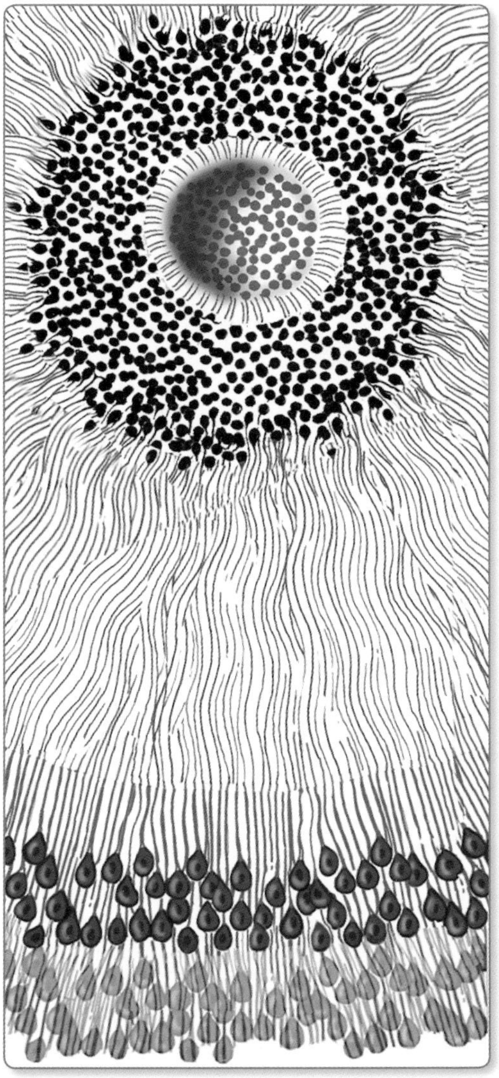

Figure 5b Henle's fiber radial "en face" structure. At the fovea level, the photoreceptor nuclei (seen as a ring shaped aggregation of black dots) are organized around the fovea. From those nuclei extend the Henle's fibers, radially organized at 360 degrees, connecting photoreceptors and bipolar cells. Thus, a radial structure is formed, the infrastructure of which will decide the pseudocyst shape and layout within the cystoid edema ('flower' or 'beehive' shaped). Macula presents a higher degree of complexity and its structure is weaker than retina extramacular framework. Seen frontally the macular structure is radial. The anatomy of the macula explains why cystoid edema is flower or honeycomb shaped.

The chains formed by photoreceptors cells linked to the bipolar cells and to ganglion cells are other important vertical structures.

At the macula, Müller cells and Henle fibers are not vertical but oblique and macula structure is less strong (**Figure 6**).

Seen frontally the macular structure appears radiating outward from the fovea.

Horizontal scaffold

We can divide retina layers in two main sections: Inner retina and outer retina.

Inner retina

The inner limiting membrane is a thin membrane that adheres to nerve fibers and is formed by Müller's fiber end ramifications. It is the basement membrane of the Müller cells.

Ganglion cell complex. Inner Plexiform Layer

Inner plexiform layer, ganglion or multipolar cell layer and optic fiber layer forms the ganglion cell complex or inner retina (**Figure 7**).

Originating from the ganglion cells, the nerve fibers head for the optic nerve along an arcuate path. Being formed by horizontal structures this layer is clearly hyper-reflective.

The ganglion cell layer consists of bulky cells, the axons of which head for the optic disk forming the optic fiber layer.

Inner plexiform layer: This layer connects bipolar and ganglion cells. It is slightly hyper-reflective, due to its horizontal structures and, in terms of OCT segmentation, delimits inner and outer retina. Inner retina forms an important functional unit. The ganglion cell complex is composed by the inner plexiform layer, the ganglion cells layer and the nerve fiber layer.

Outer retina

It houses the vertical bipolar cells nuclei whose axons are located within the outer plexiform layer, and the Müller's cell nuclei. On OCT scan, it is slightly hyporeflective.

The outer plexiform layer connects photoreceptors and bipolar cells. It includes the horizontal axons of the horizontal cells. Bipolar cells connect ganglion cells with photoreceptors.

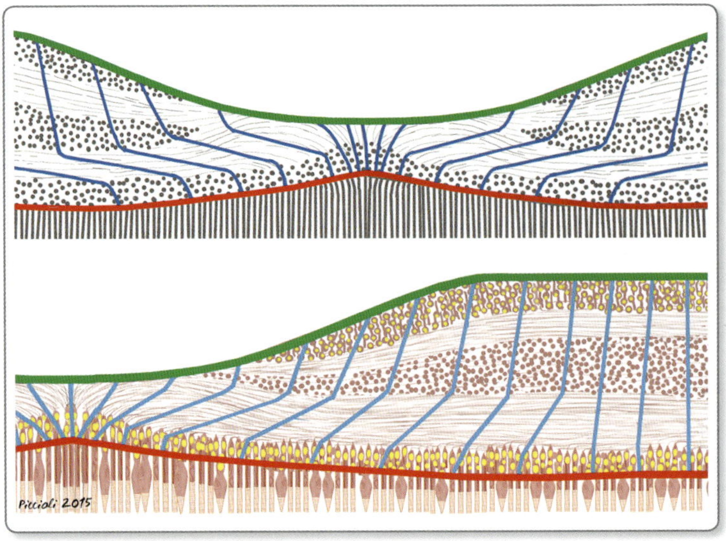

Figure 6 Macular framework and Müller cells. Macular framework presents a high degree of complexity and its structure is weaker than retina extramacular framework.

Müller cells and Henle fibers are diagonally placed. Macular Müller cells body is slanted and takes a Z shape. Seen frontally the macular structure is radial. The structure of the macula explains why fluid accumulates in the spaces between Müller cells. Cystoid edema is flower or honeycomb shaped due to Müller cells disposition. Fluid extension in the macular area is blocked vertically and horizontally. At the fovea cystoid edema cavities find little obstacle to their stretching. The weakness of Müller cell framework in the macular area explains the large dimensions reached at the fovea by cavities.

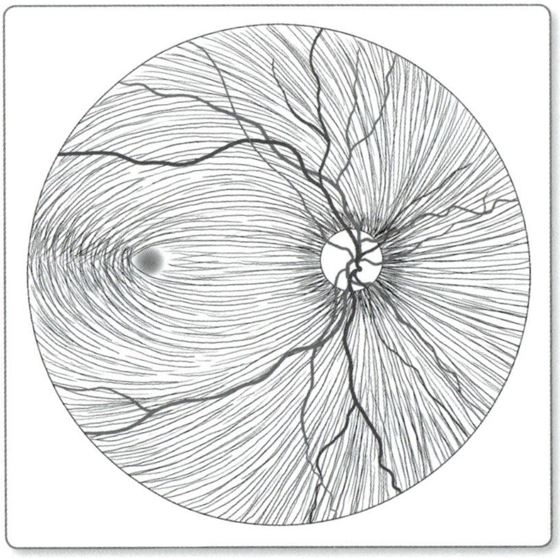

Figure 7 Nerve fiber layer map. Originating from the ganglion cells, the nerve fibers head for the optic nerve along an arcuate path on the temporal side, fan shaped on the nasal side. This morphology will shape the scotomas in visual fields, in glaucoma. Being formed by horizontal structures this layer is clearly hyper-reflective.

On OCT scan, it is hyper-reflective. The horizontal axons of the horizontal cells are located here and their nuclei are in the layer of the bipolar cells or internal nuclear layer.

Photoreceptors, cones and rods

The photoreceptor layer is part of outer retina and includes the outer nuclear layer, consisting of visual cell nuclei. This layer forms a hypo-reflective band, and is much thicker at the fovea level (**Figures 8a** and **8b**).

The photoreceptor cell body is elongated and the nucleus fills the cell body. The protoplasm forms a projecting foot on top, contacting the bipolar cells. The outer portion is divided in two: inner segment and outer segment. The latter is short and conical and is formed by a stacked succession series of disks. The inner portion is also divided in two: the inner myoid and the outer filamentous areas. The connection between the inner and outer segments appears on OCTs as a hyper-reflective horizontal band, currently called ellipsoid zone.

The outer limiting membrane is very thin and forms a dense net surrounding the cone and rod base. It is formed by fibrillae originating from the Müller's fibers; the outer limiting membrane is parallel to the ellipsoid.

The ellipsoid line is parallel to the pigment epithelium band. Due to the longer dimension of the cones at the fovea, this line is clearly distanced, at the foveola level, from the hyper-reflective band constituted by the pigmented epithelium.

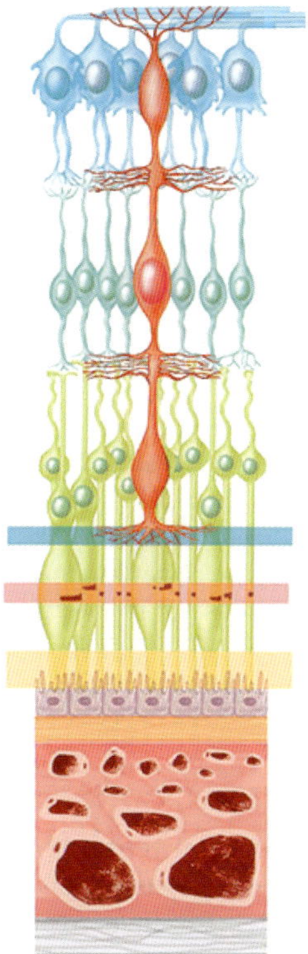

Figure 8a Vertical Müller cell outside the macular area.

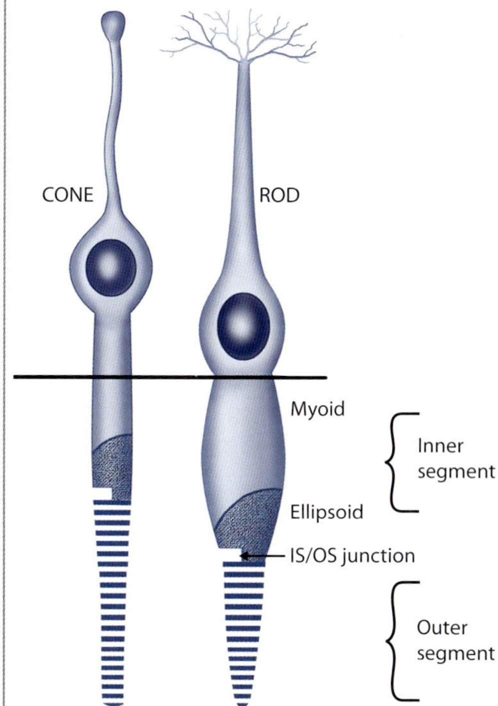

Figure 8b Cones and rods. The photoreceptor layer is part of outer retina and includes the outer nuclear layer, consisting of visual cell nuclei. The photoreceptor cell body is slightly elongated. The nucleus fills the cell body. The protoplasm forms a projecting foot on top, contacting the bipolar cells. The outer portion is divided in two: inner segment and outer segment. The latter is short and conical and is formed by a stacked succession series of disks. The inner portion is also divided in two: the inner myoid and the outer filamentous areas. The connection between the inner and outer segments appears on OCTs as a hyper-reflective horizontal band (called ellipsoid zone).

Retinal pigment epithelium

The pigment epithelium consists of a layer of polygonal cells. The polygonal cell inner part is cup-shaped and forms villosities that receive the cone and rod tips. The nucleus is located in the outer cell area. Externally, the pigment cell is in close contact with Bruch's membrane. On OCT scans, the pigment epithelium seems to be constituted of 3 parallel bands: two relatively thick, hyper-reflective bands, separated by a hyporeflective thin line. The first hyper-reflective layer is an interface between pigment epithelium and the photoreceptor outer segment, while the second, more external layer comprises the pigment epithelium cell bodies, together with their respective nuclei.

Bruch's membrane

Strong adhesions unite pigment epithelium cells, Bruch's membrane and choriocapillaris. Usually, the Bruch's membrane in not visible on OCT, but when there are drusen or small pigmented epithelium elevations, it appears as a fine horizontal line.

Choroid

The choriocapillaris is thin and hyper-reflective. It consists of a single layer of polygonal vascular lobules which independently receive blood from the short posterior ciliary arteries.

The larger vessels form the Sattler (medium sized vessels) and Haller (large vessels) layers of the choroid (**Figure 9**). The connective tissue between vessels has a low to high reflectivity depending on age and vascular sclerosis and pigment deposits.

The large vessel layer is in contact with the lamina fusca and the suprachoroidal space.

The lamina fusca is a heavily pigmented structure separated from the sclera by the suprachoroidal space. The suprachoroidal space is normally virtual and seen only when filled with fluid. It is in contact with sclera.

The venous blood is drained from the smaller veins into the vortex veins, of which there are one or two per quadrant. In young people, the choroid has a thickness of about 320 microns. Thickness decreases with aging after 25 years. Choroid thickness decreases also with myopia. It increases in hypermetropia.

Sclera

OCT can reach sclera showing the oblique channels for short posterior ciliary arteries and short posterior ciliary nerves that cross it (**Figure 10**). It is frequently possible to observe one or more posterior ciliary arteries. They appear like oblique hyporeflective channels in the scleral thickness.

Optic disk

The horizontal cross section scan shows the physiological cup into which the nerve fibers enter displaying continuity with the optic disk fibers.

The retina is sharply truncated at the limits of the papilla. The pigment epithelium and the choriocapillaris layer stop abruptly, while the superficial nerve fibers continue their course becoming the fibers of the optic nerve. The scleral ring can be seen.

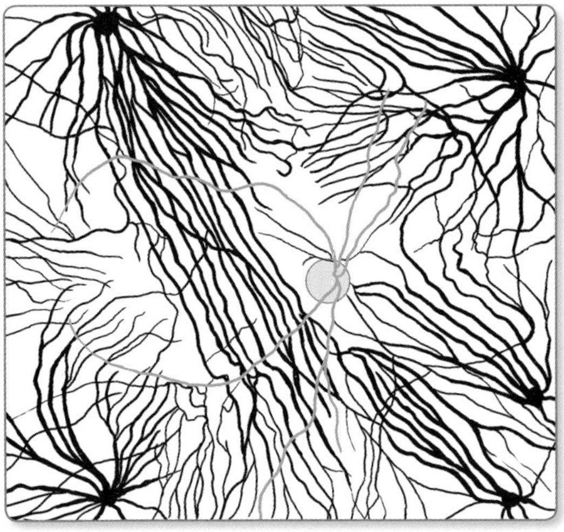

Figure 9 Choroid venous network map. The larger vessels form the Sattler (medium sized vessels) and Haller (large vessels) layers of the choroid. The larger vessels cross diagonally the posterior pole. The connective tissue between vessels has a low to high reflectivity. The venous blood is drained from the smaller veins into the vortex veins, of which there are one or two per quadrant.

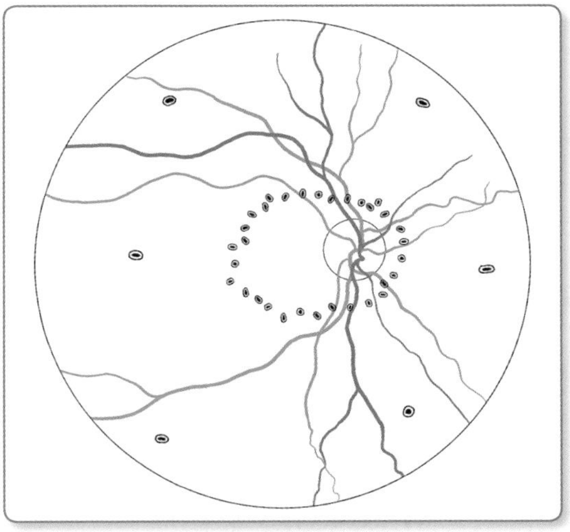

Figure 10 Sclera, posterior ciliary arteries. OCT can show the oblique channels for short posterior ciliary arteries and short posterior ciliary nerves that cross sclera. It is frequently possible to observe one or more posterior ciliary arteries. They appear like oblique hyporeflective channels in the scleral thickness.

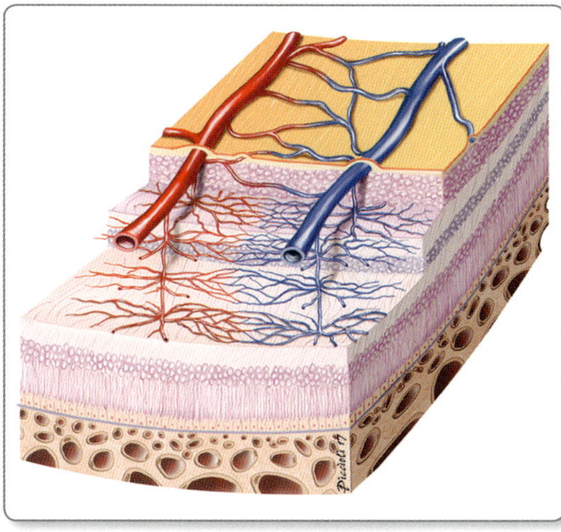

Figure 11 Normal retinal vasculature anatomy. David Huang has described four retinal vascular networks. However for clinical use, we will study the two major networks: Clinically the retinal vasculature is formed by at least two separate parallel vascular layers in the inner retina. The superficial and deep networks are connected by vertical vessels. The superficial network, the superficial vessels form multiple white linear structures (flow) that converge towards the fovea. They originate from the large upper and lower vascular arcades. Secondary vessels leave the main vessels, forming a spider web. Around the avascular area, the capillaries form continuous perifoveal arcades with regular meshes. The deep vascular network which is formed by 2 layers of capillaries organized in vortex and drained into the veins of the intermediate capillary network and the deep capillary network. Connections between superficial and deep networks. They consist in vertical vessels forming anastomoses between the superficial and deeper vessels of the deep plexus. It is highly likely that deep network is the primary venous drainage site for retinal vascularization. The deep network forms a dense meshwork of fan shaped capillaries with numerous horizontal and radial interconnections. The farthest point of vessels fan out and interconnect to form a complex pattern.

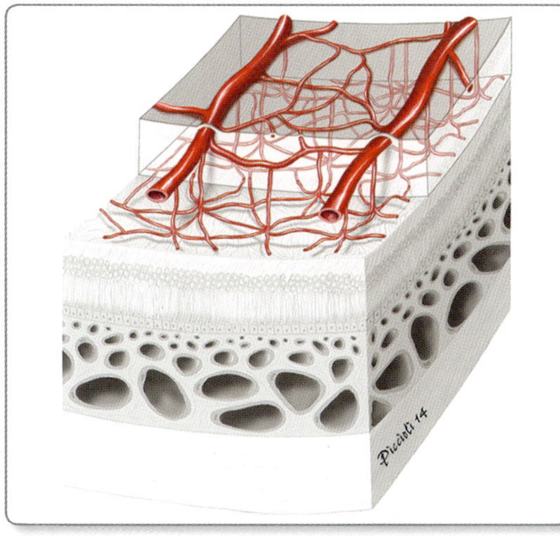

Figure 12 Normal retinal vasculature anatomy and OCT angiography. David Huang has shown that four different layers can be observed.

Normal retinal vasculature anatomy and OCT angiography

David Huang has shown that four different layers can be observed. Clinically the retinal vasculature is formed by at least two separate parallel vascular layers in the inner retina. For clinical everyday routine, we will study the two major networks:

The superficial and deep networks are connected by vertical vessels (**Figures 11** to **14**).

The superficial network

The superficial vessels form multiple white structures (flow) that converge towards the fovea, giving origin to the avascular foveal zone. Vessels originate from the large upper and lower vascular arcades. Secondary vessels leave the main vessels, forming a spider web. Around the avascular area, the capillaries form continuous perifoveal arcades with regular meshes. The superficial capillary network is composed of terminal arterioles, small veins and capillaries.

The deep vascular network

This is formed by 2 layers of capillaries organized in vortex and drained into the veins of the intermediate capillary network and the deep capillary network.

Connections between superficial and deep networks

They consist of slanted vertical short vessels forming anastomoses between the superficial and deeper vessels of the same deep plexus. The interconnecting vascular branches originate from the superficial net, go deeper and deeper, and finally open as a fan in the deep plexus.

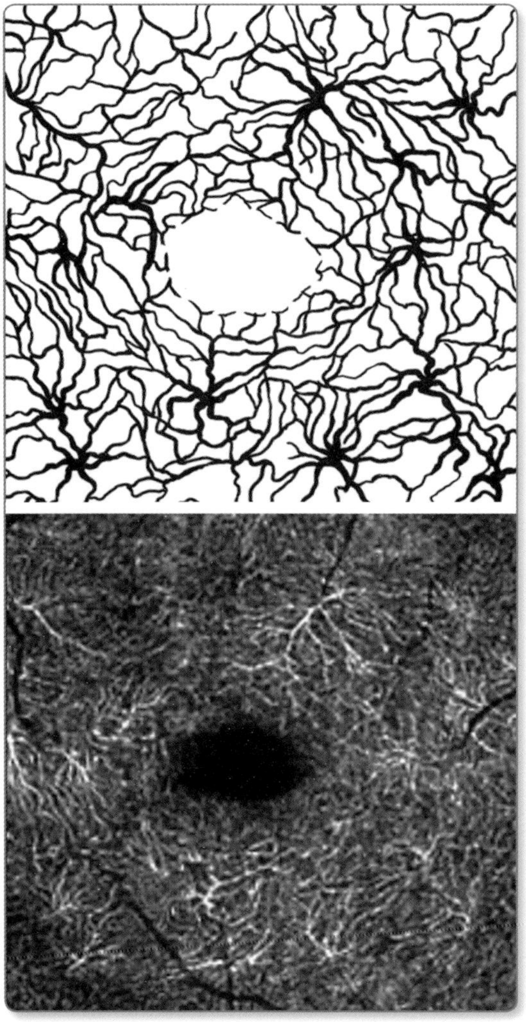

Figure 13 Normal retinal vasculature anatomy and OCT angiography. Deep vascular network.

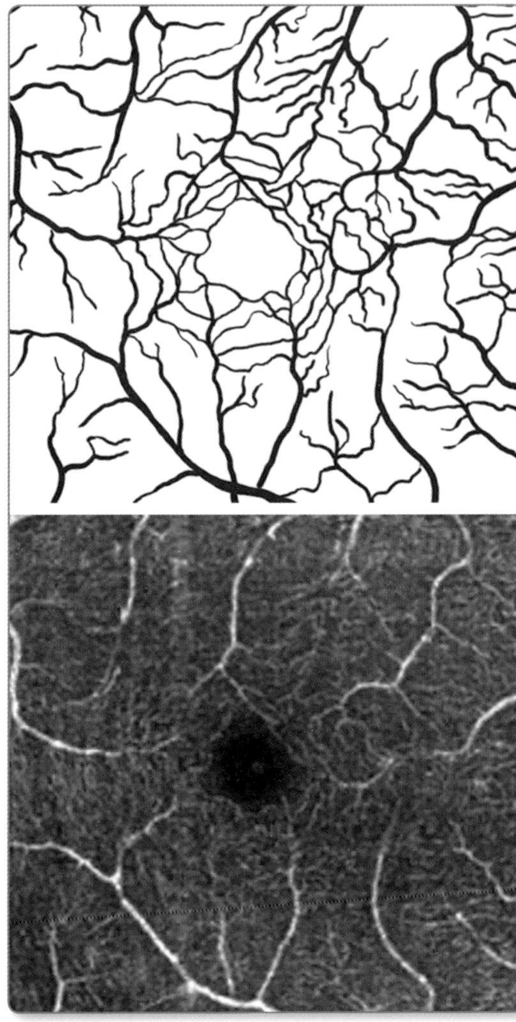

Figure 14 Normal retinal vasculature anatomy and OCT angiography. Superficial vascular network.

From each lower extremity of the vertical anastomoses, horizontal vessels fan out that interconnect to form a complex pattern**.**

It is highly likely that the deep network is the primary venous drainage site for retinal vascularization. The deep network forms a dense meshwork of fan shaped capillaries with numerous horizontal and radial interconnections. This close-knit pattern is organized around the avascular foveal zone. The farthest vessels fan out and interconnect to create a complex pattern (**Figures 15** and **16**).

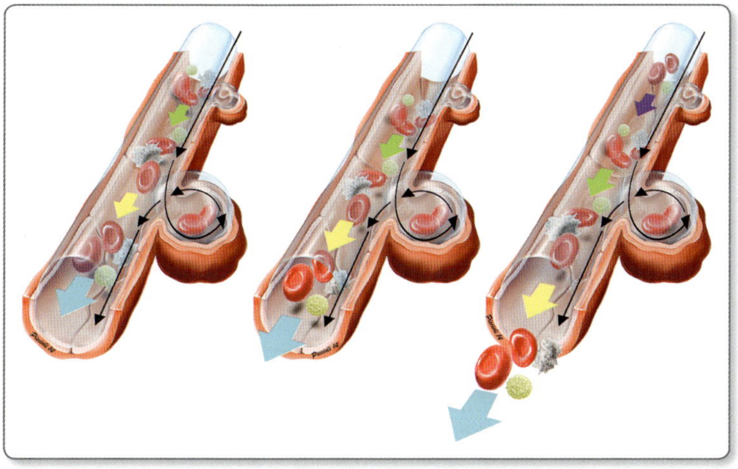

Figure 15 Angio-OCT technology uses blood cells movement (Flow) in vessels instead of dye to record vascular network. The device records only elements that move.

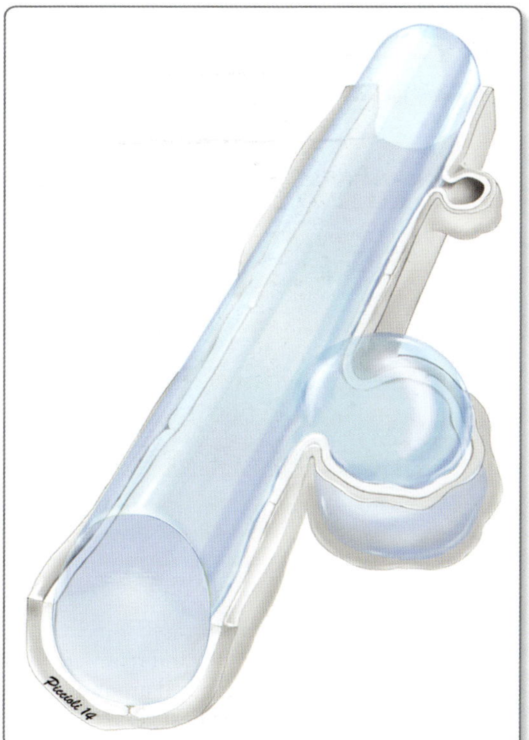

Figure 16 The device records only elements that move inside the vessel walls (flow). What we see in the angio-OCT is a cast of the vessels contents. We do not see the walls themselves.

6 Pathophysiology of age-related macular degeneration

Bruno Lumbroso

Introduction

Age-related macular degeneration (AMD) is a multifactorial disorder, a complex interplay of factors, with both genetic and environmental risk influences. It progresses from an early to a late form. AMD definitions are numerous and differ from each other. Furthermore, they must be revised every time new mechanisms and new factors emerge. AMD is not the result of a simple mechanism but is a much more complex interaction of environmental and genomic aspects.

Early stages

Drusen characterize the early stages. They can be hard, few, small, distinct or soft confluent. A high number of drusen is a risk factor for the progression to late stages of AMD. Pigment deposits in the retinal pigment epithelium (RPE) are also risk factors for late stage AMD.

Many risk factors for AMD development and progression have been identified. Deregulation of complement cascade and deregulation of lipid metabolism have an important part in AMD beginning and progress. Different biochemical pathways leading to geographic atrophy and/or choroidal new vessels may operate simultaneously. These factors connect to develop and evolve in two late stages—(1) atrophy or (2) neovascular form. Deregulation of complement cascade and deregulation of lipid metabolism have an important part in AMD onset and progress.

Late stages

One late stage of AMD, is atrophy, frequently known as geographic atrophy, is characterized by dispersed or confluent areas of degeneration of RPE cells and the overlying photoreceptors, which rely on the RPE for trophic support (**Figure 1**).

The other late stage of AMD, neovascular or wet form of AMD, shows the growth of exudative or nonexudative clusters of blood vessels from the choroid, first below Bruch's membrane and then into the retina causing retinal edema and photoreceptor damage. The term choroidal neovascularization (CNV) brings together different phenotypes and probably several pathologies.

Atrophy and neovascular forms may occur in the same eye or in different eyes at the same time or in succession.

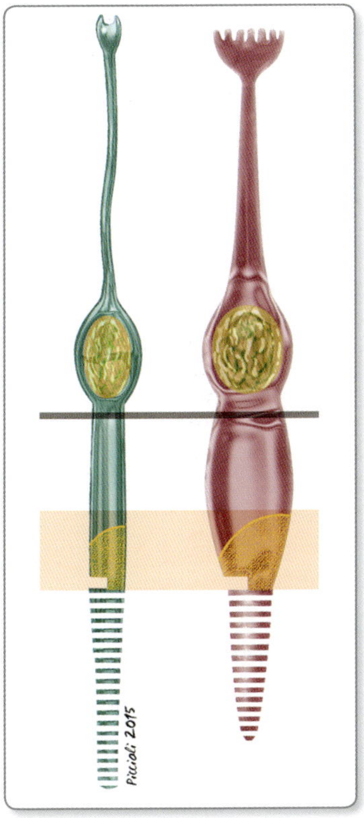

Figure 1
Photoreceptors: rod and cone. The black line is the outer limiting membrane, the yellow stripe shows the Ellipsoid Zone.

Pathogenesis of AMD successive phases (Zarbin)

Aging is the major factor for AMD. However, it is not only an aging alteration (**Box 1**).

Other major factor is oxidative stress that causes retinal pigment epithelial and choriocapillaris damage leading to drusen formation.

Aging, RPE and choriocapillaris damage bring a chronic inflammatory response in the Bruch's membrane and the choroid and deregulation of complement cascade and deregulation of lipid metabolism.

These factors lead to formation of an abnormal extracellular matrix, which blocks diffusion of nutrients to the retina and RPE, producing further damage. This results in defective RPE-choriocapillaris interactions leading to atrophy of the retina, RPE, and choriocapillaris or choroidal new vessel growth.

In this sequence of processes, environment and genetics can modify a patient's susceptibility to AMD.

Box 1: Pathogenesis of AMD successive phases (Zarbin)

Aging is the major factor

Oxidative stress causes:

- Retinal pigment epithelial (RPE) and choriocapillaris damage leading to drusen formation
- Chronic inflammatory response in the Bruch's membrane and the choroid deregulation of complement cascade
- Deregulation of lipid metabolism.

These factors lead to formation of an abnormal extracellular matrix

This results in defective RPE-choriocapillaris interactions leading to atrophy of the retina, RPE, and choriocapillaris or choroidal new vessel growth.

Progression is not linear from one phase to the next.

Progression is not linear from one phase to the next. Better understanding of cell biology, multiple animal models are needed to make progress in AMD pathophysiology knowledge and consequent treatment.

Classification of AMD

A committee of experts[1] in 2013 achieved consensus on a basic clinical classification system based on fundus lesions assessed within 2-disk diameters of the fovea in persons older than 55 years.[1-3]

The committee agreed that a single-term, AMD, should be used for the disease.

- *No visible drusen or pigmentary abnormalities:* No signs of AMD
- *Small drusen (<63 μm), also termed drupelets:* Normal aging changes with no clinically relevant increased risk of late AMD developing
- *Early AMD*: Persons with medium drusen (≥63 to <125 μm), but without pigmentary abnormalities thought to be related to AMD, should be considered to have early AMD
- *Intermediate AMD:* Persons with large drusen or with pigmentary abnormalities associated with at least medium drusen should be considered to have intermediate AMD
- *Late AMD:* Persons with lesions associated with neovascular AMD or geographic atrophy should be considered to have late AMD

Five-year risks of progressing to late AMD are estimated to increase approximately 100-fold, ranging from a 0.5% 5-year risk for normal aging changes to a 50% risk for the highest intermediate AMD risk group (**Box 2**).

Box 2: Basic mechanism of choroidal neovascularization (CNV): three factors

- Bruch's membrane abnormalities
- Retinal pigment epithelium (RPE) cells alteration
- Antiangiogenic factors and angiogenic factors leading to CNV growth

Factors of AMD pathophysiology

Nonmodifiable risk factors

- Age is the main risk factor
- Genetic factors involve a high number of genes that influence the progress of AMD
- Ethnic origin is another important cause. Caucasians are more likely to develop AMD (5.4%) than persons of African origin (2.5%)
- Sunlight, blue or green iris seems to be a factor of higher AMD incidence

Modifiable risk factors

- Smoking is the highest confirmed known risk for AMD, especially for the neovascular form
- Hypertension is an increased risk of AMD
- *Diet:* Many recent studies confirmed that Mediterranean diet is associated to lower AMD incidence. Increased dietary fat is linked with AMD. Obesity is greatly connected with AMD; however, whether there is a causal relationship is uncertain. Antioxidants (green, leafy vegetables), nuts, fish and omega-3 may be associated with reduced risk.

Prevalence of AMD

Prevalence of early AMD varies from 3.5% in those aged 55–59 years to 18% in those aged ≥85 years; for late AMD these figures are 0.1% and 10%. The numbers of affected subjects will increase considerably in the next 50 years. By 2050, the number of individuals in Europe with late AMD will be about 5 million. AMD is a significant public health problem among Europeans and western countries.

References

1. Ferris FL 3rd, Wilkinson CP, Bird A, et al. Clinical classification of age-related macular degeneration. Ophthalmology 2013; 120:844–851.
2. Colijn JM, Buitendijk GHS, Prokofyeva E, et al. Prevalence of Age-Related Macular Degeneration in Europe the Past and the Future. Ophthalmology 2017; 124:1753–1763.
3. Zarbin MA. Current concepts in the pathogenesis of age-related macular degeneration. Arch Ophthalmol 2004; 122:598–614.

7 AMD drusen and pseudodrusen

Bruno Lumbroso, Marco Rispoli

Pathophysiology: Drusen and pseudodrusen

Drusen are deposits located below retinal pigment epithelium (RPE), reticular pseudodrusen are located on the apical surface of the RPE, above the RPE. Drusen are the outcome of waste material accumulation from subretinal tissues and form at sites of decreased choriocapillaris perfusion. Histologically, they contain basal laminar deposits (lipid-rich granules) and basal linear deposits. Drusen are composed of lipids, immune- and inflammatory-related proteins, amyloid-associated proteins, as well as other substances.

Small drusen grow to form soft large drusen. Drusen can grow by incessant accumulation of sub-RPE material or regress by macrophages removal of debris. Very large drusen or drusenoid pigment epithelium detachments are confluent large drusen that merge to form pigment epithelium detachments (> 350 μ in diameter): the inner part of the Bruch's membrane together with the RPE, may split from the outer part of Bruch's membrane, forming a drusenoid pigment epithelial detachment.[1,2] Drusen are usually a thickening of Bruch's membrane with basal linear deposit.

Deposits coming from the RPE constitute a block to water-soluble elements in the plasma, and create a cleavage plane between the RPE basement membrane and the inner layer of Bruch's membrane. The accumulation is also due to the presence of inflammation in the subretinal space.

Optical coherence tomography (OCT) angiography can show the presence of subclinical, silent neovascularization in inside drusenoid elevations (vascularized drusen) (Box 1).

Box 1: Drusen and pseudodrusen

- Hard and soft drusen:
  - Drusen located below RPE, small or large, hard or soft
  - Small, less than 63 μ, intermediate (from 63 μ to 124 μ), and large (> 125 μ)
  - Hard (sharp margins), soft (ill-defined margins), or confluent (adjacent drusen merging together)
- Vascularized drusen
- Pachydrusen
- Cuticular drusen, young subject, asymptomatic, starry-sky appearance in FA (Yannuzzi), small-to-intermediate drusen
- Subretinal drusenoid deposits (reticular pseudodrusen)
- Ghost drusen
- Rare atypical drusen:
  - Doyne honeycomb dystrophy (malattia leventinese)
  - Type II membranoproliferative glomerulonephritis (C3 glomerulopathy)

Hard and soft drusen

Drusen are rounded, white-yellowish lesions located below RPE, mainly at the posterior pole. OCT angiography studies show that the site of drusen formation is influenced by choriocapillaris dysfunction, with drusen more likely to form at sites of decreased choriocapillaris perfusion, secondary to vascular endothelial cell loss.

Drusen are classified according to their size (small or large) and aspect (hard or soft):

They can be small, less than 63 μ, intermediate (from 63 μ to 124 μ) or large (> 125 μ). They form the first elements of the Age-related Eye Disease Study (AREDS) classification.

Apart from their size, drusen can be categorized as: hard (sharp margins), soft (ill-defined margins), or confluent (adjacent drusen merging together) (**Figures 1** and **2**). Hard drusen are sharp areas of hyalinization. Soft drusen are related with basal linear deposits (**Figure 3**).

During age-related macular degeneration (AMD) evolution, drusen increase in size and number, and they can merge. They evolve to wet AMD or geographic atrophy (GA), which the AREDS classify as advanced stage of AMD, stage 4.

Pachydrusen

The term 'pachydrusen' has recently appeared, following RF Spaide's observations on patients with a pachychoroid (**Figure 4**). He highlighted in these eyes the presence of deposits under the EPR having characteristics different from those of serous drusen. While the latter are rather round, with fuzzy outlines and tend to confluence, pachydrusen are often well-defined, isolated, and have a more complex form (oval, or more spiculate contorted).

Cheung et al. found that pachydrusen was significantly associated with choroidal polypoid vasculopathy (PCV). Moreover, in Caucasian patients, it appears that the pachychoroid could be associated with type I neovascularization.

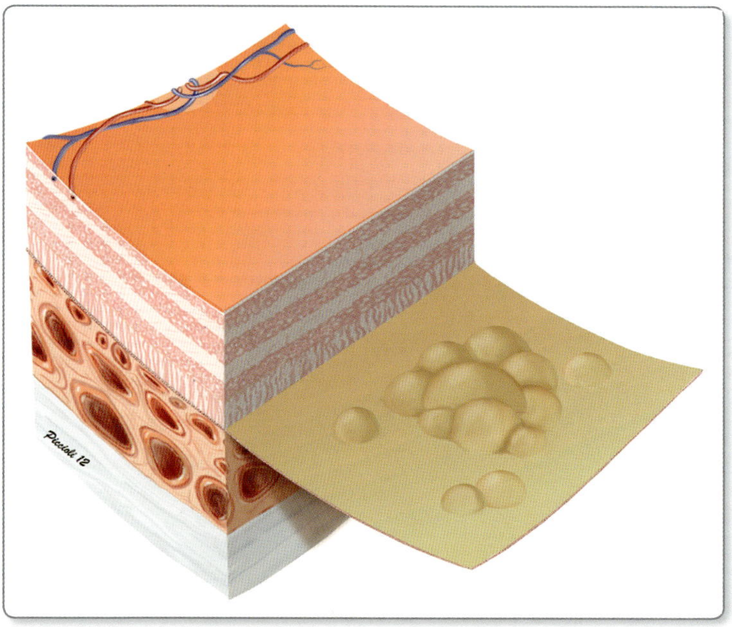

Figure 1 Drusen are rounded, white-yellowish lesions located below RPE, mainly at the posterior pole. OCT angiography studies show that the site of drusen formation is influenced by choriocapillaris dysfunction, with drusen more likely to form at sites of decreased choriocapillaris perfusion. Drusen are classified according to their size (small or large) and aspect (hard or soft): They can be small, < 63 μ, intermediate (from 63 μ to 124 μ) or large (> 125 μ). This scan shows small hard drusen.

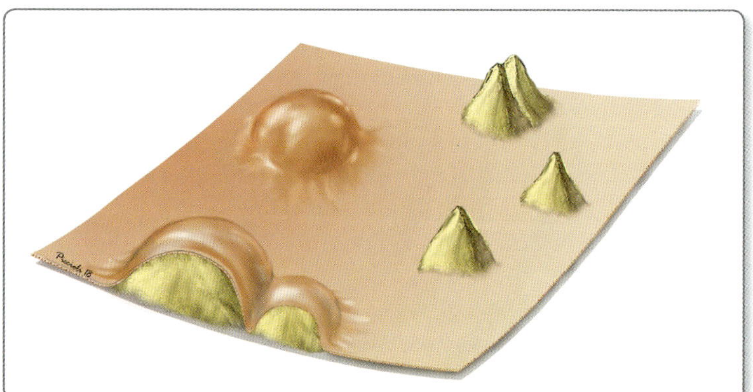

Figure 2 Drusen and pseudodrusen. Drusen are deposits located below RPE, Drusen are composed of lipids, immune and inflammatory related proteins, amyloid associated proteins, as well as other substances. They are the outcome of waste material accumulation from subretinal tissues and form at sites of decreased choriocapillaris perfusion. Reticular pseudodrusen are located on the apical surface of the RPE, above the RPE. Their shape is pyramidal. Histologically, they contain basal laminar deposits (lipid-rich granules) and basal linear deposits.

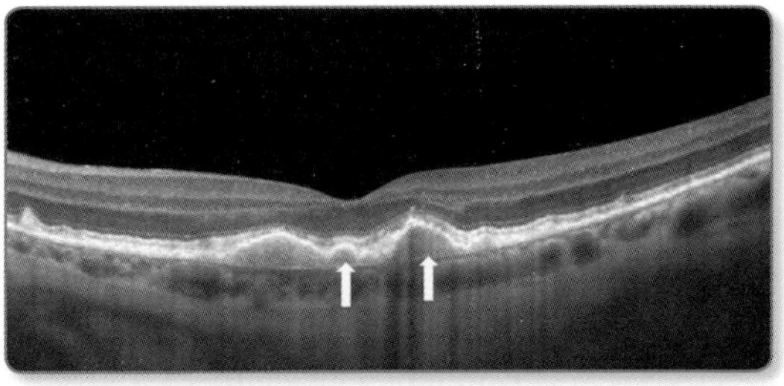

Figure 3 Soft drusen, cross section scan. Apart their size drusen can be categorized as: hard (sharp margins), soft (ill-defined margins), or confluent (adjacent drusen merging together). Hard drusen are sharp areas of hyalinization. This scan shows soft drusen with basal linear deposits.

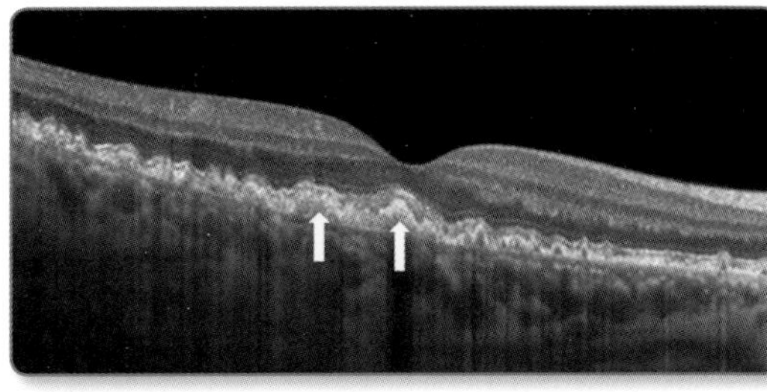

Figure 4 Hard drusen, cross section scan. Drusen are rounded, white- yellowish lesions located below RPE, mainly at the posterior pole. OCT angiography studies show that the site of drusen formation is influenced by choriocapillaris dysfunction, with drusen more likely to form at sites of decreased choriocapillaris perfusion. Drusen are classified according to their size (small or large) and aspect (hard or soft):They can be small, less than 63 µ, intermediate (from 63 µ to 124 µ) or large (>125 µ). This scan shows small hard drusen.

Cuticular drusen

They are drusen of the young subject, often asymptomatic, described many years ago as having a starry-sky appearance in fluorescein angiography (Yannuzzi), and are small-to-intermediate drusen. Countless in number, they are mainly located mainly in peripheral retina outside the vascular arcade and in the midperiphery. Less frequently they are seen at the posterior pole.

They can merge and form larger drusen and develop vitelliform material.

Evolution of vitelliform material leads to resorption and atrophy of the underlying retina, which results in significant visual loss. Choroidal neovascularization may appear and complicate this pathology. Some histologic studies of cuticular drusen state that they are like drusen seen in AMD with age-related macular.

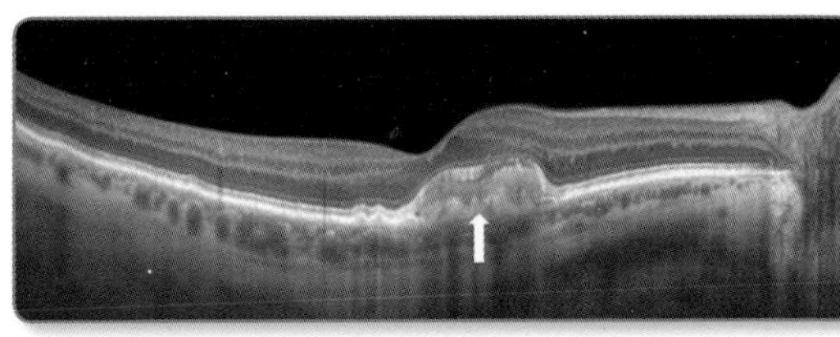

Figure 5 Pachydrusen, cross section scan. The term "pachydrusen" has been proposed by RF Spaide in patients with a thick choroid (>300 µ). He described in these eyes the presence of deposits under the EPR having characteristics different from those of serous drusen. While the latter are rather round, with fuzzy outlines and tend to merge together, pachydrusen (as seen here) are well-defined, isolated, and have a complex shape (oval, or irregular ovoid). Contents are irregularly hyper-reflective. According to Spaide pachydrusen are significantly associated with choroidal polypoid vasculopathy (PCV).

Reticular pseudodrusen

Subretinal drusenoid deposits (reticular pseudodrusen) are multiple rounded, white-yellowish lesions analogous to drusen, arranged in a reticular network pattern. They can be recognized by their reticular-like network, seen best on fundus autofluorescence. They are more prevalent among the advanced age group, more common in women than in men and are typically smaller than soft drusen. Reticular pseudodrusen are located on the apical surface of the RPE, above the *RPE,* and more frequent in the superior macular region (**Figure 5**). On OCT scans, these lesions are shown as granular triangular hyper-reflective deposits placed between the RPE layer and the ellipsoid zone.[3]

Reticular drusen are composed by subretinal drusenoid deposits (SDD) with components somewhat similar to classical AMD drusen, and are located between the RPE and the ellipsoid (photoceptor inner segment/outer segment junction). They differ from drusen in their components that contain lipids different from those found in drusen and do not contain shed disk remnants. They share some proteins with drusen.

The presence of reticular drusen is a risk factor for late AMD, both in the disease eye and in the fellow eye. They are linked with progressive atrophy of the photoreceptor layer, GA, and a greater risk of choroidal neovascularization.

Ghost drusen

Ghost drusen have been described by Querques in patients with GA in 2014 (**Figure 6**). They are pyramidal or cone-shaped structures in atrophic areas below a disorganized pigment epithelium associated with posterior shadowing (**Figure 7**). They appeared on infrared images as hyporeflective lesions capped by a hyporeflective halo with or without hyper-reflective spots inside. On fundus autofluorescence imaging they are either hypo-autofluorescent or mildly hyperautofluorescent.

On structural OCT, the surface of this pyramidal structure is always hyper-reflective, whereas the center appears hyporeflective. The physiopathological mechanism of ghost drusen formation is uncertain.

Vascularized drusen

Querques and Souied have shown that OCT angiography can confirm the presence of subclinical, silent neovascularization in inside drusenoid elevations (vascularized drusen). See chapter on vascularized drusen.[4,5]

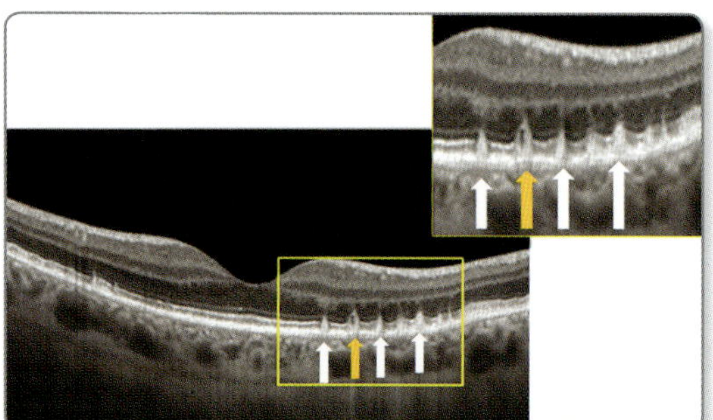

Figure 6 Pseudo drusen. Reticular pseudodrusen cross section scan. Reticular pseudodrusen are located on the apical surface of the RPE, above the RPE. They are more prevalent among the advanced age group, more common in women than in men and are typically smaller than soft drusen. On structural cross section OCT scans, these lesions are shown as granular triangular (pyramidal, cone shaped) hyper-reflective deposits placed between the RPE layer and the ellipsoid zone, reaching the outer retinal membrane. They are seen in the fundus examination as yellowish lesions set in reticular network pattern. In this scan one pseudo drusen appears void and in transforming in ghost drusen (yellow arrow).

Rare atypical drusen

Doyne honeycomb dystrophy

Doyne honeycomb dystrophy (malattia leventinese, autosomal dominant drusen)

Small, yellowish rounded formations under RPE, with honeycomb pattern. Inherited autosomal dominant familial disorder (**Figure 8**).

Type II membranoproliferative glomerulonephritis (C3 glomerulopathy)

ROUNDED, multiple white-yellowish lesions, small-to-medium size drusen surrounded by pigment, present at the posterior pole and in midperiphery (**Figure 9**). Some close to the optic disk, vessels normal. They appear associated with

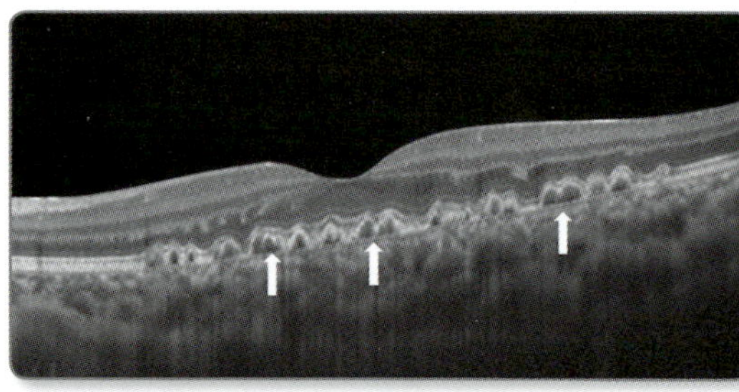

Figure 7 Ghost drusen have been described by Querques in patients with geographic atrophy. They are pyramidal or cone-shaped structures in atrophic areas below a disorganized pigment epithelium associated with posterior shadowing. On structural OCT, the surface of this pyramidal structure is always hyper-reflective, whereas the center appears hyporeflective.

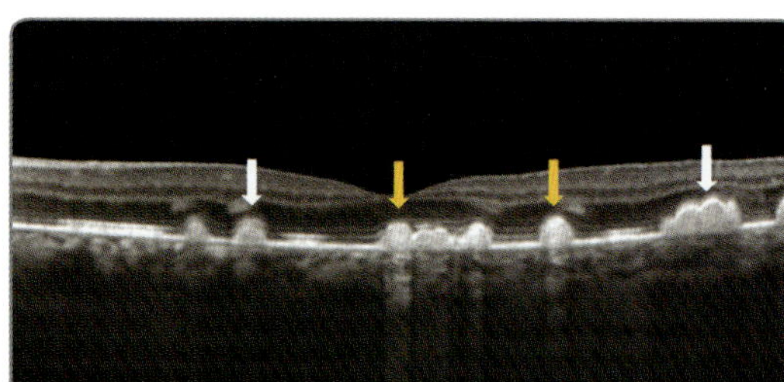

Figure 8 Doyne honeycomb dystrophy (malattia leventinese) Rounded drusen with RPE atrophy. Yellow Arrows show light penetration where RPE is atrophic.

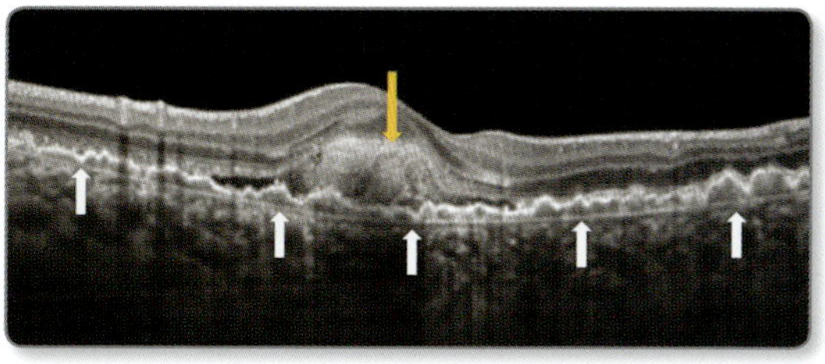

Figure 9 Drusen in type II membranoproliferative glomerulonephritis (MPGN II) cross section scan. Drusen associated with MPGN II, in young patients after a few years' evolution. Rounded, multiple white- yellowish lesions small to medium size drusen surrounded by pigment, present at the posterior pole and in midperiphery. Some are close to the optic disk, vessels appear normal. Sometimes in the follow-up, a pigment epithelium detachment appears followed by choroidal neovascularization (yellow arrow). In this young woman affected by MPGN II, we observe numerous drusen and a choroidal neovascularization that regressed after anti-VEGF injection.

membranoproliferative glomerulonephritis type II (MPGN II), in young patients after a few years' evolution. Sometimes in evolution a pigment epithelium detachment appears followed by choroidal neovascularization.[6]

Early AMD grading

The clinical definition of early AMD varies according to the authors referred. When drusen in the posterior pole are greater than 5 in number and at least 63 μm in size, they seem to indicate an incipient AMD. Later, drusen enlarge and merge resulting in drusenoid elevations. These formations are frequently associated with pigment deposits.

The AREDS grading system offers a simple useful method of determining evolution risk: (1) presence of large drusen (> 125 μm in size) and (2) the presence of pigment abnormalities. With this simple method, one eye having both large drusen and pigment abnormalities has a score of 2 (1 for each criterion), and if both eyes have each risk factor, the score is 4. Using these easy criteria, the AREDS showed that over 5 years, eyes with a risk factor score of 0 had only a 0.4% move to advanced AMD, while those with 1 risk factor had a 3.1% move to advanced AMD. However, when eyes had 2, 3, or 4 risk factors, the rate of advanced AMD conversion to GA or CNV increased to 12%, 26%, and 47% respectively.

Classification proposed by Spaide

The proposed classification has predictive capabilities. Spaide writes:

- Eyes with SDD can go on to atrophy, particularly associated with confluent SDD, whereas macular neovascularization, typically type III macular neovascularization, can develop associated with the dot form of SDD. Regression of SDD can lead to outer retinal atrophy
- Later, outer retinal atrophy can lead to complete outer retina and RPE atrophy
- Pachydrusen are associated with thick choroids, which in turn are associated with progression to type I macular neovascularization or polypoidal choroidal vasculopathy. Eyes with thick choroids, in the absence of central serous chorioretinopathy, do not typically develop GA
- Conventional drusen can go to GA through regression or to type I macular neovascularization. A more typical path is to form focal hyperpigmentation, and in addition to GA, type I, type II, and type III macular neovascularization can develop. The above description is for the pure forms of expression. The progression, if it occurs, has probabilities of producing the forms of late AMD listed, but these are not certainties
- Subretinal drusenoid deposits can occur together and lead to a hybrid of outcomes.
- Subretinal drusenoid deposits and pachydrusen typically are not found together

References

1. Russell SR, Mullins RF, Schneider BL, et al. Location, substructure, and composition of basal laminar drusen compared with drusen associated with aging and age-related macular degeneration. Am J Ophthalmol 2000; 129:205–214.
2. Duvvari MR, van de Ven JP, Geerlings MJ, et al. Whole exome sequencing in patients with the cuticular drusen subtype of agerelated macular degeneration. PLoS One 2016; 11:e0152047.

3. Bonnet C, Querques G, Zerbib J. Hyperreflective pyramidal structures on optical coherence tomography in geographic atrophy areas. Retina 2014; 34:1524–1530.
4. Spaide RF. Disease expression in nonexudative age-related macular degeneration varies with choroidal thickness. Retina 2018; 38:708–716.
5. Querques G, Souied EH. Vascularized drusen: Slowly progressive type 1 neovascularization mimicking drusenoid retinal pigment epithelium elevation. Retina 2015; 35:2433–2439.
6. Kheir V, Dirani A, Halfon M, et al. Multimodal imaging of retinal pigment epithelial detachments in patients with C3 glomerulopathy: case report and review of the literature. BMC Ophthalmol 2017; 17:207.

8 Dry AMD and geographic atrophy

Bruno Lumbroso, Marco Rispoli

Introduction

Atrophic age-related macular degeneration (AMD) is characterized by the deterioration of the retina and the choroid in the posterior pole due to retinal pigment epithelium (RPE) and choriocapillaris atrophy or degeneration. Retinal atrophy is generally preceded by extracellular deposits contiguous to the RPE, soft drusen, cuticular drusen or pseudodrusen. There is a progressive deterioration and loss of RPE, photoreceptor cells, and choriocapillaris layer in the posterior pole. The choroid thickness is greatly reduced to 70 μ or less: normal thickness ranges from 320 μ to 200 μ depending on age. In geographic atrophy (GA) of AMD, the atrophic progression involves all the retinal layers, the pigment epithelium, and choroid.

Atrophy may also develop slowly during repeated CNV treatment by anti-VEGF. Vision loss and scotoma occur when the pigment epithelium atrophy leads to secondary loss of the overlying photoreceptors.

Optical coherence tomographic angiography (OCTA) has shown that *silent* CNV occurs in at least 10% of the cases.

Physiopathogenesis of geographic atrophy

Dry AMD is an inherited disease that is influenced by nutrition and environmental factors. It is a multifactorial disorder. Aging, oxidative stress, and sunlight damage have a central part. However, inflammation and the local activation of the complement system have certainly a role in its pathogenesis. Drusen appear generally at sites of low choriocapillaris perfusion, and their location is predisposed by choriocapillaris suffering. Drusen and pseudodrusen are main risk factors. RPE, Bruch's membrane, and the choriocapillaris are equally involved in the development of dry AMD. RPE dysfunction leads to RPE damage and secondary loss of photoreceptors.

Two main hypotheses may be taken in consideration:

1. An initial RPE breakdown causes a secondary choriocapillaris loss. The choriocapillaris under RPE atrophic area is rarely complete. Thin vessels persist.
2. Choriocapillaris breakdown is the initial cause of secondary RPE atrophy, leading to the alteration and death of the photoreceptors.

These mechanisms of the pathogenesis of AMD, do not exclude reciprocally (**Figure 1**).

Risk factors of AMD

The most commonly recognized risk factors of AMD are age, smoking, diet, and sunlight exposure. The genetic factor is well established by familial studies, and by genome studies.

New classification of atrophy based on OCT and multimodal imaging

The term atrophy brings together different phenotypes and probably various pathologies (atrophy associated with drusen, pseudodrusen or atrophy associated with new vessels). A clear definition of atrophy is necessary given the many phenotypes and the need for early intervention. Classification of Atrophy Meeting (CAM 2018 by the International Expert Group on Atrophy) presents a consensus definition of atrophy.

This classification system is based on OCT for atrophy secondary to AMD. OCT was proposed as the reference standard or base imaging method to diagnose and stage atrophy. Other methods, including fundus autofluorescence, near-infrared reflectance, and color imaging, provided

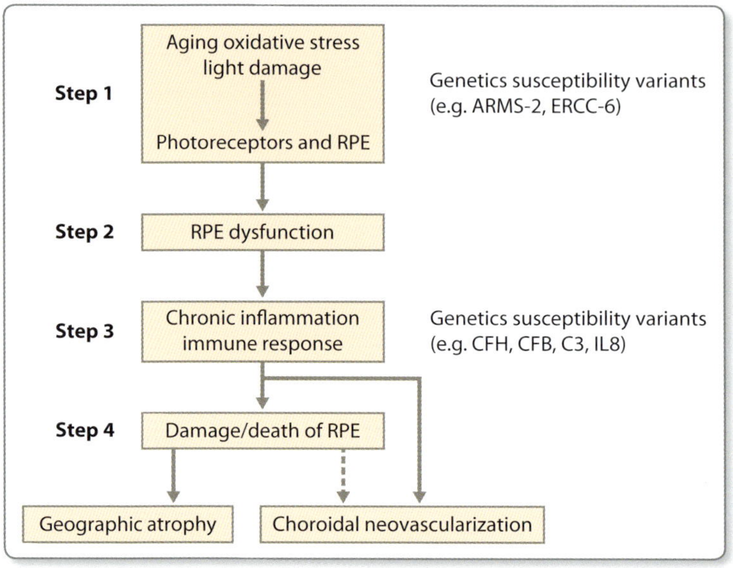

Figure 1 AMD pathophysiology.

complementary and confirmatory information. Specific criteria were defined to establish the presence of atrophy.

It was recognized that photoreceptor atrophy can occur without retinal pigment epithelium (RPE) atrophy and that atrophy can undergo an evolution of different stages.

The group of experts defined four stages of atrophy: four terms and histologic phases were proposed:

1. Complete RPE and outer retinal atrophy (cRORA)
2. Incomplete RPE and outer retinal atrophy (iRORA)
3. Complete outer retinal atrophy (cORA)
4. Incomplete outer retinal atrophy (iORA)

The consensus helped to define a new terminology for atrophy.

Complete atrophy of pigment epithelium and outer retina

Phase (c)RORA (complete RPE + outer retinal atrophy)

Phase (c) RORA (complete RPE + outer retinal atrophy) is the form of complete atrophy with total loss of the EP and the external retina. The four clinical signs are:

1. Hyper-reflectivity of the choroid by window effect with hypertransmission of the light of more than 250 μ; Window effect should have at least 250 μ in diameter to be classified atrophic
2. Zone of attenuation or disappearance of the pigment epithelium and Bruch's membrane of more than 250 μ
3. Evidence of photoreceptor degeneration (damage to the outer nuclear layer, loss of limiting membrane, loss of the ellipsoid line). Loss of function measured by microperimetry.
4. No scrolled RPE or RPE tear

Phase (i)RORA (incomplete RPE + outer retinal atrophy)

It is the model of incomplete atrophy. This is an incomplete form of atrophy that does not meet the three criteria of cRORA but must meet three other criteria:

1. Window effect (hypertransmission) must be present but incomplete or discontinuous
2. Some irregularities of the Pigment Epithelium and Bruch's membrane
3. Degeneration of photoreceptors

There is a correlation between histological sections and OCT for both phases of RORA. Part of the pigment epithelium may persist; however, it will progress to complete atrophy.

At risk of atrophy with incomplete or complete atrophy of the outer retina, but good pigment epithelium (cORA and iORA)

- Drusen bigger than 0.03 μ
- Pigment migration; hyper-reflective RPE

- Interruption of continuity between RPE and Bruch's membrane
- Vitelliform deposit

In conclusion, International experts of CAM report #3 state that it is essential to have a clear and precise nomenclature to define atrophy. Report #3 addresses this need. Multimodal imaging, and mainly OCT remain the reference for the recognition and classification of atrophy. This classification will be useful to assess GA evolution when dry AMD treatment will be available. Multimodal imaging remains the reference for the recognition and classification of atrophy.[1]

Geographic atrophy clinical features

At onset, fundus examination shows drusen and pigment deposits. Later some small yellow atrophic areas appear. Slowly, in a few years the disseminated areas merge, resulting in an atrophic area that is seen as large irregular yellowish space with sharp edges. Drusen are disseminated around it. Fluorescein angiography is not useful in GA. The atrophic area is seen as a window defect with sharp edges.[2]

Cross-section structural OCT in geographic or atrophic macular degeneration

Alterations of retinal outline are seen with sharp demarcation between atrophic and normal retina. OCT scans detect in atrophic macular degeneration a reduction in retinal and of the choroidal thickness and increased penetration of the light in the choroid.

Atrophy is also seen in the outer retinal layers, with thinning in the ellipsoid (IS/OS junction), even outside the main area. There is atrophy of the pigment epithelium, clear increase in the pigment epithelium reflectivity, hyper-reflective clumps at different levels, pigment deposits, backscattering due to reduced absorption of light by the altered retinal tissues. Bruch's membrane is resilient for a long time to atrophy and is seen as a thin line. We observe pigment deposits,

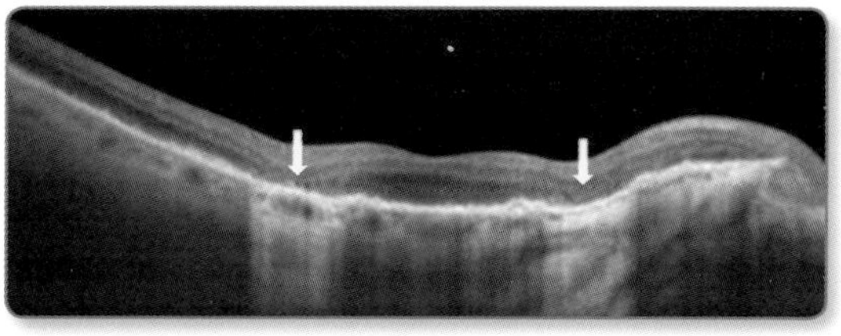

Figure 2 Cross-section scan atrophic age-related macular degeneration (AMD) cross-section scan. OCT scans detect in atrophic macular degeneration a decrease in retinal and choroidal thickness and an increased depth penetration of the light. In this case, central atrophy is seen in the outer retinal layers, with thinning in the ellipsoid (IS/OS junction) around a central area almost normal. There is atrophy of the pigment epithelium, clear increase in the pigment epithelium reflectivity, hyper-reflective clumps at different levels, pigment deposits, atrophy with backscattering (arrows) due to reduced absorption of light by the altered retinal tissues, deeper hyper-reflectivity due to loss of outer layers including photoreceptors. Macular area is less affected by atrophy. Choriocapillaris and the choroid are very thin. Choroid connective tissue shows increased reflectivity and obvious sclerosis of the main choroid blood vessels.

granulations, deeper hyper-reflectivity due to loss of outer layers including photoreceptors, choriocapillaris atrophy.

Choriocapillaris and the choroid are very thin choroid connective tissue shows increased reflectivity and obvious sclerosis of the main choroid blood vessels. The retinal map makes it possible to determine the extent of the atrophic area and to monitor its evolution (**Figures 2** and **3**).

OCT structural hyper-reflective dots have been described by Coscas. These dots, located in the outer retina, (only 10% are in the inner retina) are markers of the suffering of photoreceptors. These hyper-reflective dots converge on the edges of future areas of atrophy.

OCTA in geographic or atrophic macular degeneration

In early GA, OCTA shows a diffuse choriocapillaris flow impairment that most probably plays a role in the advance of GA. Querques has shown there is also reduction in the superficial vascular retinal plexus, associated

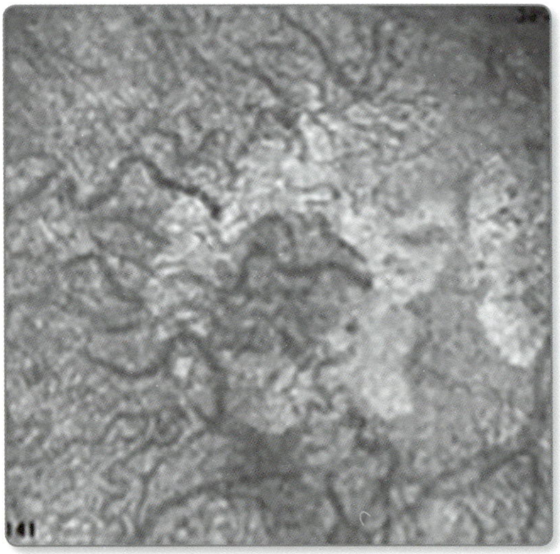

Figure 3 C-scan atrophic AMD '*en face* OCT': There is atrophy of the pigment epithelium, showing a large irregular roundish, geographic area of atrophy. The main choroidal vessels are manifest, dark, sclerosed.

with inner and outer retina thinning, suggesting the damage is not confined to the outer segments (**Figure 4**).

When extensive GA appears, OCTA reveals the participation of photoreceptors and RPE, but also of the central vascular supply. The foveal avascular zone is enlarged. Choriocapillaris shows widespread alteration in the seat of atrophy, and flow is impaired also in the junctional zone surrounding the atrophic center (i.e. areas with preserved RPE Querques G). Total choroidal thickness in GA is decreased well beyond the lesion margins.

Neovascular membranes in atrophic AMD: Silent nonexudative neovascular membranes

OCTA detects the silent CNV present in 10% or more of the cases (**Figure 5**). Philip Rosenfeld considers the ability of OCTA to identify eyes with 'nonexudative neovascular AMD' as its greatest utility. These eyes are defined by the presence of nonexudative AMD with subclinical neovascularization. These cases retain good

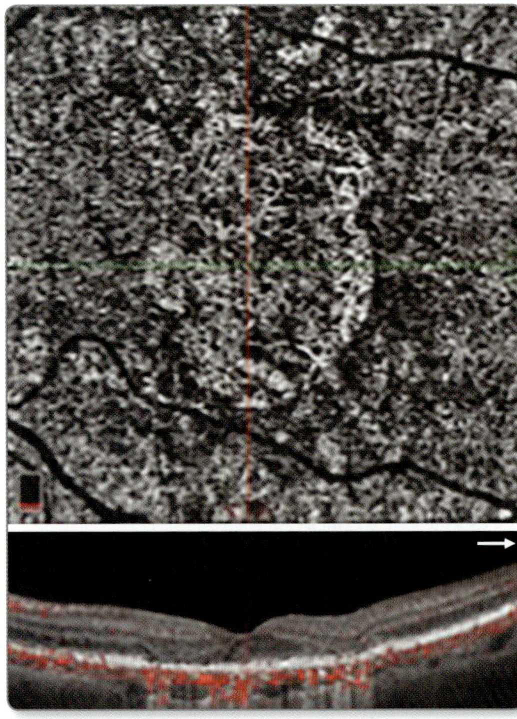

Figure 4 Optical coherence tomographic angiography (OCTA) of choriocapillaris in atrophic AMD. In geographic atrophy (GA), OCTA shows a choriocapillaris flow impairment that most probably plays a role in the advance of GA. When extensive GA appears, OCTA reveals the loss of photoreceptors and RPE, but also of the central vascular supply. The foveal avascular zone is enlarged. Angio B scan, seen below shows choriocapillaris widespread alteration in the center of atrophic zone. Flow is impaired also in the junctional zone surrounding the atrophic center. Total choroidal thickness in GA is decreased well beyond the lesion margins.

vision, they are at increased risk for developing active exudation when compared with eyes without these subclinical lesions.

Although anti-VEGF treatment for this subclinical neovascularization is not recommended, by detecting the neovascularization, OCTA identifies patients who should have close clinical follow-up and daily home monitoring to allow early detection of exudation.

OCTA to anticipate exudation

David Huang et al. presented in 2018 a study of 63 patients with dry AMD in one eye and wet AMD

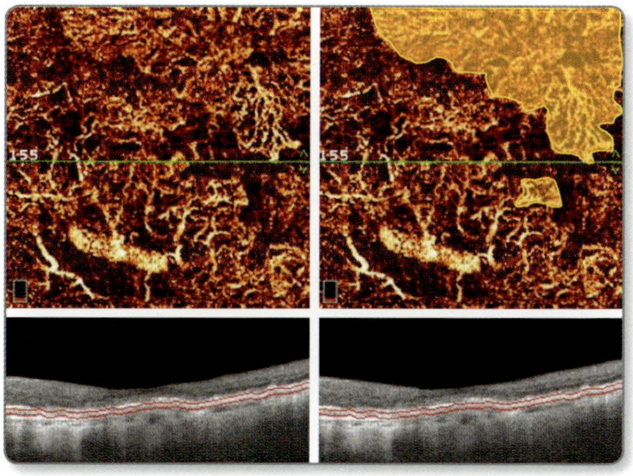

Figure 5 Silent nonexudative subclinical CNV in Atrophic AMD (OCT angiography). Optical coherence tomographic angiography (OCTA) detects the silent fan-shaped CNV above the atrophic area where choroidal vessels are evident. CNV is outlined in yellow. Philip Rosenfeld considers the ability of OCTA to identify eyes with 'nonexudative neovascular AMD' as its greatest utility. These eyes are defined by the presence of nonexudative AMD with subclinical neovascularization. These cases may retain good vision for a long time; however, they are at increased risk for developing active exudation when compared with eyes without these subclinical lesions. Anti-VEGF treatment for this subclinical neovascularization is not, now, recommended. OCTA identifies patients who should have close clinical follow-up and daily home monitoring to allow early detection of exudation. Silent CNV present in 10% or 15% or more of the geographic atrophy cases.

in the other eye. Every 6 months, they scanned nonexuding eyes with OCT-A and found that they were 18 times more likely to become exudative if quiescent choroidal neovascularization (CNV) was detected at OCTA only in the opposite case.

Similarly, Querques found a progression to exudation at 1 year in 21% of adelphic eyes with NVC quiescent compared to a rate of 4% of eyes without NVC quiescent.

David Huang recommends accurate monitoring of these eyes with OCTA to detect a possible rapid progression of quiescent NVC.

Evolution of geographic atrophy

Older age, pseudophakia, smoking, hypertension, diet, and ARMS-2 genotype are associated with faster progression of geographical atrophy.

Factors favoring the progression of GA are:

- Size of the initial lesion (lesions <2.0 mm^2 have a lower progression)
- The presence of multiple atrophy areas
- The presence of atrophy on the other eye and
- Perilesional anomalies on fundus autofluorescence

The development of GA usually begins around the parafoveal region, then evolves into a 'horseshoe' sparing the fovea in early evolution. There is often a bilateral, multifocal distribution. The average progression of atrophy varies from 1.0 mm^2/year to 3.0 mm^2/year with marked individual differences. It takes an average time of 2–3 years for extrafoveal atrophy to reach the fovea. CNV can develop on atrophy margins, with an estimated risk of 10% at 4 years.

During GA progression, along with the EPR lesions, there is a loss of autofluorescent lipofuscin. Lipofuscin accumulates at the periphery of the atrophic area and can be used as a marker of progression of atrophy in form a hyperautofluorescent margin on the FAF. Some perilesional anomalies on the FAF imaging are predictive of atrophy progression. Hypo-autofluorescent areas indicate complete pigment epithelium loss.

Prevention and treatment of atrophic AMD: Diet, alimentation

Smoking is the highest confirmed known risk for AMD. Hypertension is an increased risk of AMD. Increased nutritional fat and obesity are significantly associated with AMD. Sunlight seems to be notably associated with early and late AMD.

Currently, atrophic AMD has no effective treatment. To prevent GA progression, we use the results of the AREDS studies to prevent damage from oxidative stress.

Mediterranean diet seems to be associated to lower AMD incidence. Antioxidants (green, leafy vegetables), nuts, fish, and omega-3 may be associated with reduced risk.

Finally, it is essential to inform patients diagnosed with atrophic AMD, that management solutions exist. Clinicians should advise to treat adequately hypertension, not to smoke, wear sunglasses when outdoors, dieting and physical exercise. Low vision rehabilitation, occupational therapy, psychological care, and access to social benefits undeniably allow patients to be supported and help them cope with the disease.[3-5]

Future treatments of atrophic AMD

The pathophysiology of atrophic AMD is complex and multifactorial, offering many therapeutic targets to explore (Francesco Bandello).

First possibility is chronic inflammation, and several anti-inflammatory treatments are being evaluated: Fluocinolone acetonide implants currently being evaluated in a phase II study in patients with geographic atrophy.

The second opportunity is that of neuroprotective treatments: neuroprotection is being evaluated with brimonidine. In early results efficacy was evaluated at 12 months and showed a reduction in the progression of atrophy from 18.8% to 27.5%.

Another line of research is to prevent toxic accumulation; lipofuscin has a phototoxic and proinflammatory effect. Emixustat reduces lipofuscin accumulation.

Another recently explored pathway is the restoration of choroidal blood flow, particularly with the study of vasodilator treatment.

The complement pathway was evaluated with lampalizumab that inhibits the alternative pathway of complement. It showed no efficacy. However, the complement pathway is not discarded.

Finally, the stem cells represent an auspicious path for the treatment of atrophy.[6]

In conclusion, we do not have yet effective treatments in atrophic AMD. By identifying systemic biomarkers for AMD, such as in plasma or urine, ophthalmologists could potentially identify patients with AMD, correlate with disease progression, and provide personalized treatments. Final objective will be personalized medicine for patients.

References

1. Sadda SR, Guymer R, Holz FG, et al. Consensus Definition for Atrophy Associated with Age-Related Macular Degeneration on OCT: Classification of Atrophy Report 3. Ophthalmology 2018; 125:537–548.
2. Russell SR, Mullins RF, Schneider BL, et al. Location, substructure, and composition of basal laminar drusen compared with drusen associated with aging and age-related macular degeneration. Am J Ophthalmol 2000; 129:205–214.
3. Duvvari MR, van de Ven JP, Geerlings MJ, et al. Whole exome sequencing in patients with the cuticular drusen subtype of agerelated macular degeneration. PLoS One 2016; 11:e0152047.
4. Gopinath B, Liew G, Kifley A, et al. Dietary flavonoids and the prevalence and incidence of age-related macular degeneration. Am J Clin Nutr 2018; 108:381–387.
5. Merle BMJ, Colijn JM, Cougnard-Grégoire A, et al. Mediterranean Diet and Incidence of Advanced Age-Related Macular Degeneration: The EYE-RISK Consortium. Ophthalmology 2019; 126:381–390.
6. Miller JW. Treating AMD: Back to the future. Presented at: American Society of Retina Specialists annual meeting; July 20-25; Vancouver, British Columbia, 2018.

9 Vascularized drusen

Vittorio Capuano, Eric H Souied

Early age-related macular degeneration (AMD) is characterized by the presence of macular drusen and retinal pigment epithelium (RPE) alterations. Drusen are formed by extracellular debris between the basal lamina of the RPE and the inner collagenous layer of the Bruch's membrane.[1-3] Drusen have also been classified in size as small (< 63 µm), intermediate (<63 µm but <125 µm) or large (>125 µm), and in biomicroscopic aspect as soft or hard. Soft drusen are mound-like elevations, typically 63 µm to >1,000 µm.[4,5]

Soft and large drusen are actually considered as the main factor associated with a greater risk for developing advanced (exudative or atrophic) AMD.[4,5]

In clinical practice, early AMD is diagnosticated using clinical examination in scheduled consultation (as frequently is an asymptomatic condition) in 'elderly patients'. Optical coherence tomography (OCT) is the most common ancillary examination for staging and follow these patients. On OCT, soft drusen show the deposition of material under the RPE[3] (**Table 1** and **Figure 1**). Drusen can grow by continuous deposition of sub-RPE material or regress by macrophages elimination of deposition of debris. Regressing drusen[6] appearing as multilaminar sub-RPE hyper-reflectivity (un-phagocitated debris developing calcifications). However, as suggested by Spaide,[7] differential diagnosis between subclinical (nonexudative) neovessels and layers of lipid mineralization is not easy using only OCT examination. The presence of subclinical neovascularization in the context of drusenoid elevations [also referred as vascularized drusen[8] (**Table 1** and **Figure 2**)] is confirmed using combined noninvasive: OCT and invasive: fluorescein and indocyanine green angiography (FA and ICGA). In these cases, FA shows un-hyperfluorescent lesion without leakage while early and late ICGA frames clearly show a well definite hyperfluorescence suggesting the neovascular tissue in the context of hyporfluorescent RPE elevation.

Table 1: Drusen features

	Soft drusen	Vascularized drusen	Quiescent choroidal neovascularization
FA	Minimally hyperfluorescence in late stages (this finding can be variable) without leakage	Hyperfluorescence without leakage	Hyperfluorescence without leakage
ICGA	Hypofluorescence due to masking of fluorescence	Early frames show well definite hyperfluorescent network, late frames show a "plaque"	Early frames show well definite hyperfluorescent network, late frames show a "plaque"
OCT	Sub-RPE Hyperfluorescent homogeneous deposit	Multilaminar sub-RPE hyperreflectivity, suggesting the neovascular tissue in the context of hyperfluorescent RPE elevation	Irregularly slightly elevated RPE without hyporeflective fluid accumulation in the intra-/subretinal space showing a major axis in the horizontal plane.
OCTA	No hypersignal	Neovascular network	Neovascular network

(FA: fluorescein angiography; ICGA: indocyanine green angiography; OCT: optical coherence tomography; OCTA: optical coherence tomographic angiography; RPE: retinal pigment epithelium)

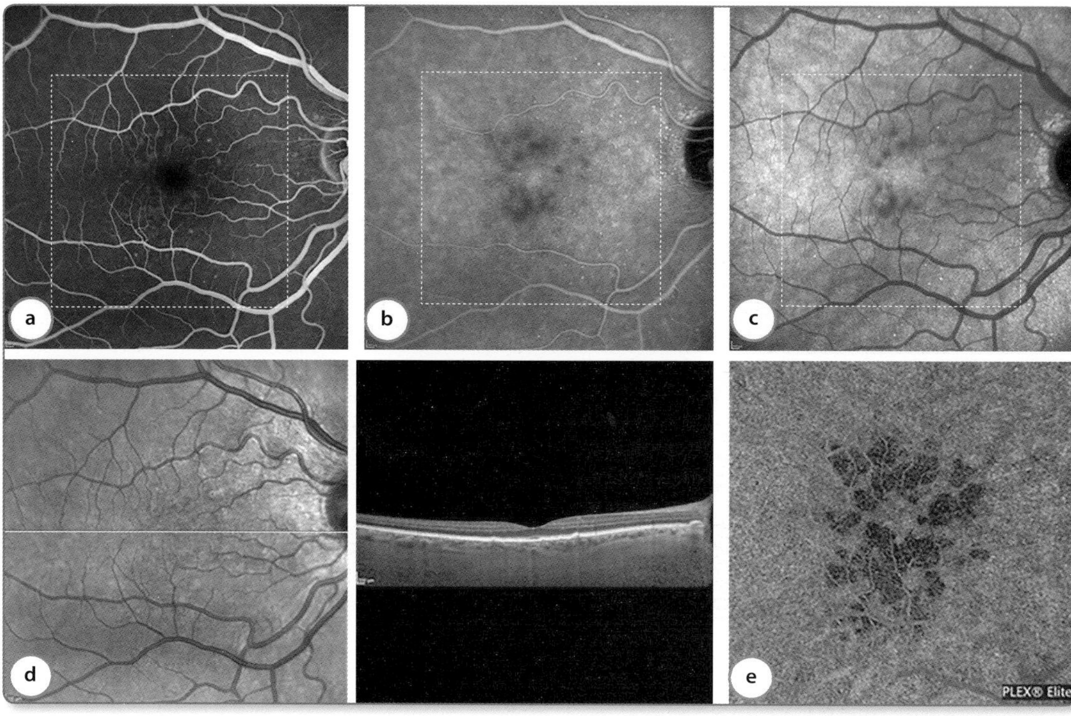

Figure 1 Multimodal imaging of soft drusen: fluorescein angiography (FA) shows hyperfluorescent lesion without leakage (a), early indocyanine green angiography (ICGA) frames show hypofluorescence due to masking of fluorescence (b) up to late ICGA frames (c). Optical coherence tomography (OCT) shows subretinal pigment epithelium (RPE) hyperfluorescent homogeneous deposit (d). Optical coherence tomographic angiography (OCTA) shows no hypersignal (e).

More recently, a new noninvasive tool called optical coherence tomographic angiography (OCTA) has been available changing the clinical practice in these cases. OCTA shows better and faster presence of neovascular (sub-RPE) tissue in the context of drusenoid deposit (**Figure 2**).

In 2015, Querques and Souied also defined the differences and the resemblance between vascularized drusen (**Table 1** and **Figure 2**) and quiescent choroidal neovascularization (CNV)[9] (**Table 1** and **Figure 3**).

Vascularized drusen presenting on OCT multilaminar hyper-reflectivity and collections of moderately reflective material in the sub-RPE space may indeed represent subclinical type 1 CNV. Quiescent CNV was described as stable irregularly slightly elevated RPE without hyporeflective fluid accumulation in the intra-/ subretinal space showing a major axis in the horizontal plane.[9] Natural history of these two entities finally defined their difference: while vascularized drusen developed multilaminar

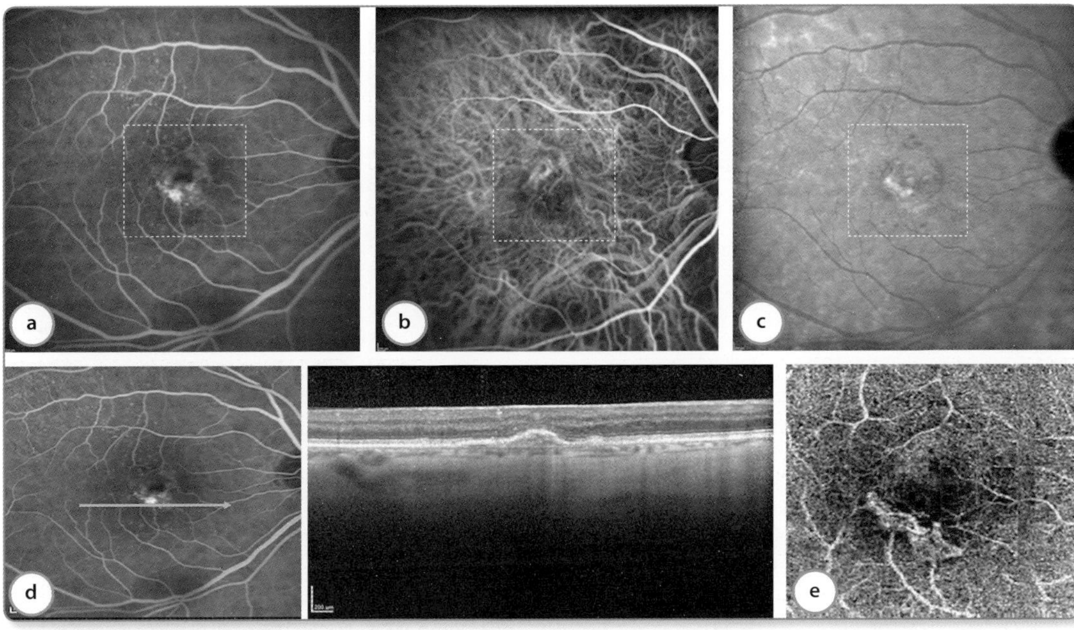

Figure 2 Multimodal imaging of vascularized drusen: fluorescein angiography (FA) shows un hyperfluorescent lesion without leakage (a), early indocyanine green angiography (ICGA) frames clearly show a well definite hyperfluorescent network (b), late ICGA frames show a 'plaque' (c). Optical coherence tomography (OCT) shows a drusenoid elevations characterized by a multilaminar subretinal pigment epithelium (RPE) hyperreflectivity, suggesting the neovascular tissue in the context of hyperfluorescent RPE elevation (d). Optical coherence tomography angiography (OCTA) shows a neovascular network localized in the upper part of drusen in correspondence of the hyper-reflective dome-shaped RPE elevation mimicking drusenoid RPE elevation on OCT (e).

(vertical) hyper-reflectivity, quiescent CNV enlarge in (horizontal) size. On the other hand, both of them can develop fluid.

In conclusion, vascularized tissue can be found in the context of a drusenoid deposit and his identification is not easy using only OCT examination. Ophthalmologist should be aware that what looks like a drusenoid RPE elevation on OCT, may indeed represent a vascularized tissue, which could be investigated using multimodal retinal imaging including FA and ICGA. In this context, OCTA (safe and noninvasive examination) can be considered as a useful tool also in early AMD patients.

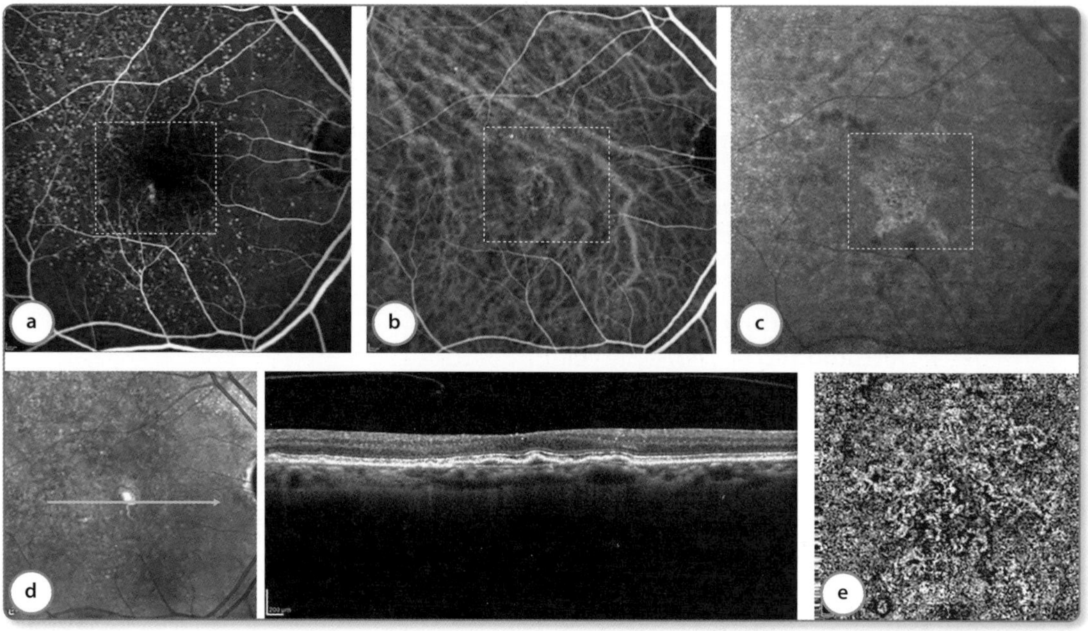

Figure 3 Multimodal imaging of quiescent choroidal neovascularization: Fluorescein angiography (FA) shows un hyperfluorescent lesion without leakage (a), early indocyanine green angiography (ICGA) frames clearly show a well definite hyperfluorescent network (b), late ICGA frames show a 'plaque' (c). Optical coherence tomography (OCT) shows irregularly slightly elevated RPE without hyporeflective fluid accumulation in the intra-/subretinal space showing a major axis in the horizontal plane (d). Optical coherence tomographic angiography (OCTA) shows a neovascular network (e).

References

1. Hageman GS, Mullins RF. Molecular composition of drusen as related to substructural phenotype. Mol Vis 1999; 5:28.
2. Bressler NM, Silva JC, Bressler SB, et al. Clinicopathologic correlation of drusen and retinal pigment epithelial abnormalities in age-related macular degeneration. Retina 1994; 14:130–142.
3. Spaide RF, Curcio CA. Drusen characterization with multimodal imaging. Retina 2010; 30:1441–1454.
4. Ferris FL, Davis MD, Clemons TE, et al. A simplified severity scale for age-related macular degeneration: AREDS Report No. 18. Arch Ophthalmol 2005; 123:15704.
5. Seddon JM, Sharma S, Adelman RA. Evaluation of the clinical age-related maculopathy staging system. Ophthalmology 2006; 113:260–266.
6. Querques G, Georges A, Ben Moussa N, et al. Appearance of regressing drusen on optical coherence tomography in age-related macular degeneration. Ophthalmology 2014; 121:173–179.
7. Spaide RF. Enhanced depth imaging optical coherence tomography of retinal pigment epithelial detachment in age-related macular degeneration. Am J Ophthalmol 2009; 147:644–652.
8. Querques G, Souied EH. Vascularized Drusen: Slowly Progressive Type 1 Neovascularization Mimicking Drusenoid Retinal Pigment Epithelium Elevation. Retina 2015; 35:2433–2439.
9. Querques G, Srour M, Massamba N, et al. Functional characterization and multimodal imaging of treatment-naive "quiescent" choroidal neovascularization. Invest Ophthalmol Vis Sci 2013; 54:6886–6892.

10 OCT angiography in fibrocellular and fibrovascular phenotypes of neovascular age-related macular degeneration in remission

Lea Querques, Mariacristina Parravano, Enrico Borrelli, Adele Chiaravalloti, Massimiliano Tedeschi, Riccardo Sacconi, Ilaria Zucchiatti, Francesco Bandello, Giuseppe Querques

Age-related macular degeneration (AMD) is the leading cause of irreversible central vision loss among older individuals in developed countries.[1] While early and intermediate AMD are clinically characterized by the accumulation of drusen, the late form of AMD is recognized for the development of macular choroidal (type 1 and 2) or retinal neovascularization (type 3), or geographic atrophy (GA).[2] The presence of an exudative neovascular lesion characterizes the exudative or neovascular form of AMD.[2] It should be noted, however, that macular neovascularization (MNV) can be present without features of exudation, an entity referred to as 'nonexudative neovascular AMD'.[3-5]

Most cases of severe vision loss in AMD are the result of MNV (85%).[1] Indeed, while the widespread use of intravitreal antivascular endothelial growth factor (anti-VEGF) treatment has considerably improved the prognosis in neovascular AMD, the vision is still substantially affected in these eyes, even in those cases treated with anti-VEGF therapies and with resolved exudation. Macular scar formation has been identified as one of the main predictors of visual function.[6] Since a fibrous component is typically present within neovascular lesion, neovascularizations are also known as fibrovascular lesions.[7] However, in some eyes, this increase in the fibrous component within neovascular lesion results in the development of a macular scar, which is accompanied by a regression and/or condensation of the pathological vessels.[8] Therefore, during anti-VEGF therapy, some neovascular AMD eyes may reach remission (no subretinal hemorrhage, sign of fluid in or under the retina, and treatment for at least 6 months). Remission may be achieved because of an absence of neovascular leakage (fibrovascular phenotype) or alternatively for the development of a macular scar (fibrocellular phenotype). Macular scar, also called fibrocellular lesion,[9] is identifiable as a well-demarcated white or yellow lesion that is characteristically hyper-reflective on infrared (IR) and optical coherence tomography (OCT) images. MultiColor (MC) images (Heidelberg Engineering, Heidelberg, Germany) were demonstrated to be useful in the identification of fibrosis with a detection sensitivity of 100%.[10]

Several studies employing OCT angiography (OCTA) have tried to expand our knowledge on neovascular AMD.[11] Using OCTA, a study in eyes with type 1 MNV demonstrated that in 75% of the eyes, a highly organized vascular complex may be identified (**Figure 1**).[12] Furthermore, a large main central vessel trunk or feeder vessel was noted in 72% of these eyes, with two different patterns identified: (1) a branching pattern in all directions from the center of the lesion ('medusa' pattern), and (2) a branching pattern from one side of the lesion ('sea-fan' pattern). Importantly, the type 1 lesion size was compared between OCTA and ICGA,[13] and the latter study illustrated that type 1 MNV measured smaller on OCTA images compared to both intermediate and late phase ICGA images, suggesting that dye leakage may reduce the

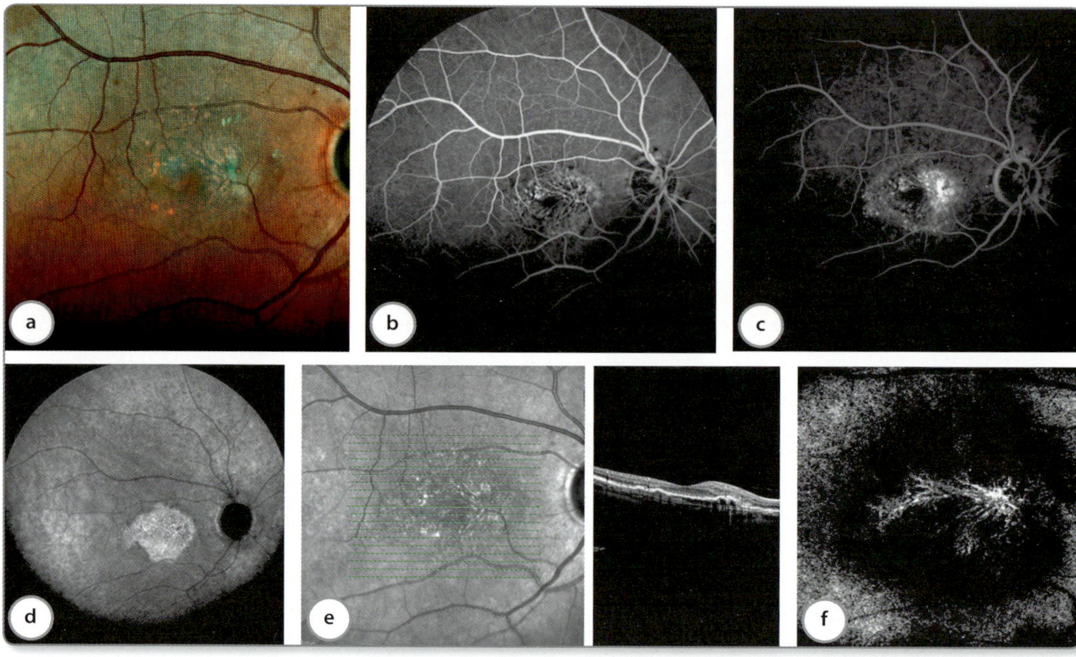

Figure 1 Multimodal imaging of a type 1 macular neovascularization associated with age-related macular degeneration (AMD). (a) Multicolor image shows areas of retinal pigment epithelium (RPE) alteration and mottling in the macula. (b and c) Early- and late-phase fluorescein angiography (FA) shows several irregular areas of stippled hyperfluorescence with leakage. (d) Late-phase indocyanine green angiography (ICGA) reveals a hyperfluorescent subfoveal lesion. (e) The structural optical coherence tomography B-scan shows the presence of a fibrovascular pigment epithelial detachment. (f) Flow within a neovascular lesion is seen on the corresponding *en face* optical coherence tomographic angiography (OCTA) image.

accurate assessment of the dimensions of type 1 MNV with ICGA. Using OCTA, type 2 MNV is visualized below the outer retina and appears either as a glomerulus-shaped lesion or as a medusa-shaped complex (**Figure 2**).[14] The lesion visualized on OCTA corresponds topographically to a well-demarcated hyperfluorescent area in the early frames of FA images.[14] Subretinal hyper-reflective material or SHRM[15] by spectral domain structural OCT may represent various tissue forms, including type 2 MNV; and OCTA may be an important tool to elucidate the composition of SHRM.[16]

Using a multimodal imaging approach, our group recently investigated quantitative and qualitative imaging characteristics of treated neovascular AMD eyes in remission (no subretinal hemorrhage, sign of fluid in or under the retina, and no treatment for at least 6 months). The aim of our study was to evaluate whether an extensive fibrosis may impair macular function, this investigated using microperimetry, and the multimodal imaging may differentiate the fibrocellular and fibrovascular phenotypes. To do so, we prospectively collected data from 41 eyes with neovascular AMD in remission. The neovascular AMD cohort was divided into two subgroups according to the presence of extensive fibrosis (macular scar) yielding a group of 19 eyes showing evidence of macular scar on MC images (fibrocellular group), while 22 eyes were characterized by absence of fibrosis (fibrovascular group) (**Figures 3** to **5**).

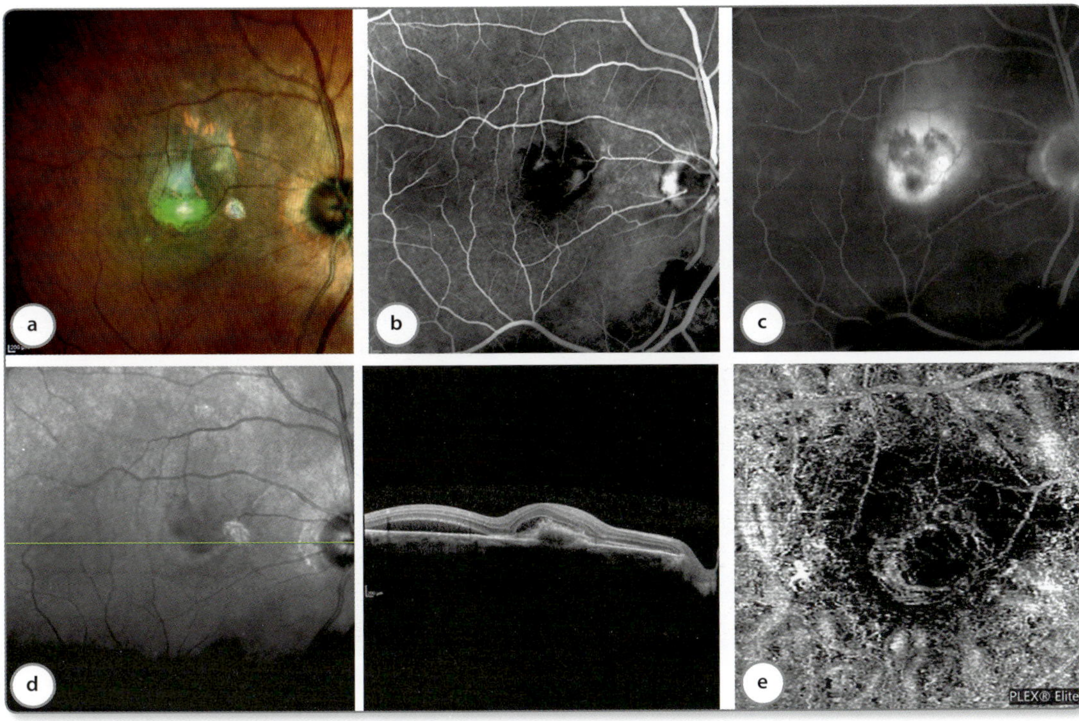

Figure 2 Multimodal imaging of mature type 2 macular neovascularization associated with age-related macular degeneration (AMD). (a) Multicolor image shows areas of a yellowish lesion in the macula. (b and c) Early- and late-phase fluorescein angiography (FA) shows an area of well-demarcated hyperfluorescence in the early phase with leakage in the late phase. (c) The green arrow on the near-infrared reflectance image (d) shows the location and direction of the structural OCT B-scan (e) illustrating a thin area of subretinal hyper-reflective material, as well as subretinal fluid. A neovascular lesion is identified with corresponding optical coherence tomographic angiography (OCTA).

Our results showed that neovascular AMD eyes with fibrocellular lesions are more likely associated with damage of the retinal pigment epithelium (RPE). Importantly, we observed a direct relationship between RPE atrophy and the presence of fibrocellular scar (but not fibrovascular lesion), even after accounting for confounding factors, such as type of NV and number of previous anti-VEGF injections, which may be associated with an increase in occurrence of RPE atrophy.[17] Furthermore, using OCTA, our study demonstrated the presence of residual vessels into the fibrocellular lesions. Notably, we displayed that the fibrocellular phenotype is characterized by a reduced perfusion of the pathological vessels in comparison with the fibrovascular phenotype and that the presence of fibrocellular scar is the factor most impacting the NV perfusion density, which furnishes strong evidence corroborating the hypothesis that an increase in the fibrous component is accompanied by a regression and/or condensation of the pathologic vessels.[18,19] In addition, we observed that the eyes with the fibrocellular phenotype had a significant worse visual acuity and macular sensitivity, the latter quantified using microperimetry.

Given that NV may be even considered as an attempt at recapitulating the impaired perfusion from the choriocapillaris, results of this study may

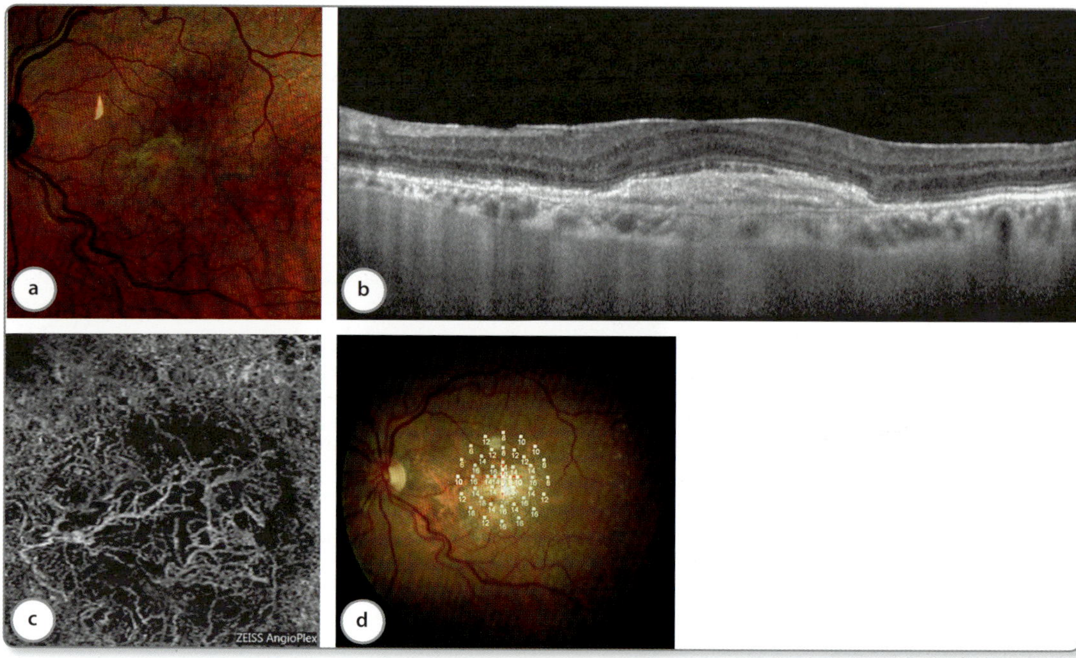

Figure 3 Multimodal imaging and microperimetry from a patient with age-related macular degeneration (AMD)-associated type 1 macular neovascularization and no fibrosis. (a) Multicolor image shows areas of retinal pigment epithelium (RPE) alteration and mottling in the macula. (b) The structural optical coherence tomography B-scan shows the presence of a fibrovascular pigment epithelial detachment with nonhomogeneous reflectivity. (c) Flow within a neovascular lesion is seen on the corresponding *en face* optical coherence tomographic angiography (OCTA) image. (d) Retinal sensitivity values on fundus photography image demonstrate a moderate reduction of the retinal sensitivity in the macula.

offer new important insights related to disease mechanisms. We may speculate that, on reaching a state of remission, the neovascular lesion may be thus important to nourish the RPE and outer retinal layers. On contrary, a neovascular regression and fibrocellular replacement may reduce this nourishment and consequently cause their atrophy. This process may ultimately lead to a reduction in macular function. Since efforts to minimize neovascular fibrosis have met with limited success and might represent a therapeutic intervention occurring too late to rescue vision, therapeutic approaches to induce maturation of vessels in fibrosis rather than their abolishment should be considered as a better target in neovascular AMD treatments.

References

1. Jager RD, Mieler WF, Miller JW. Age-Related Macular Degeneration. N Engl J Med 2008; 358:2606–2617.
2. Ferris FL, Wilkinson CP, Bird A, et al. Clinical classification of age-related macular degeneration. Ophthalmology 2013; 120:844–851.
3. Roisman L, Zhang Q, Wang RK, et al. Optical Coherence Tomography Angiography of Asymptomatic Neovascularization in Intermediate Age-Related Macular Degeneration. Ophthalmology 2016; 123:1309–1319.
4. de Oliveira Dias JR, Zhang Q, Garcia JMB, et al. Natural History of Subclinical Neovascularization in Nonexudative Age-Related Macular Degeneration Using Swept-Source OCT Angiography. Ophthalmology 2018; 125:255–266.
5. Carnevali A, Cicinelli MV, Capuano V, et al. Optical Coherence Tomography Angiography: A Useful Tool for Diagnosis of Treatment-Naïve Quiescent Choroidal Neovascularization. Am J Ophthalmol 2016; 169:189–198.

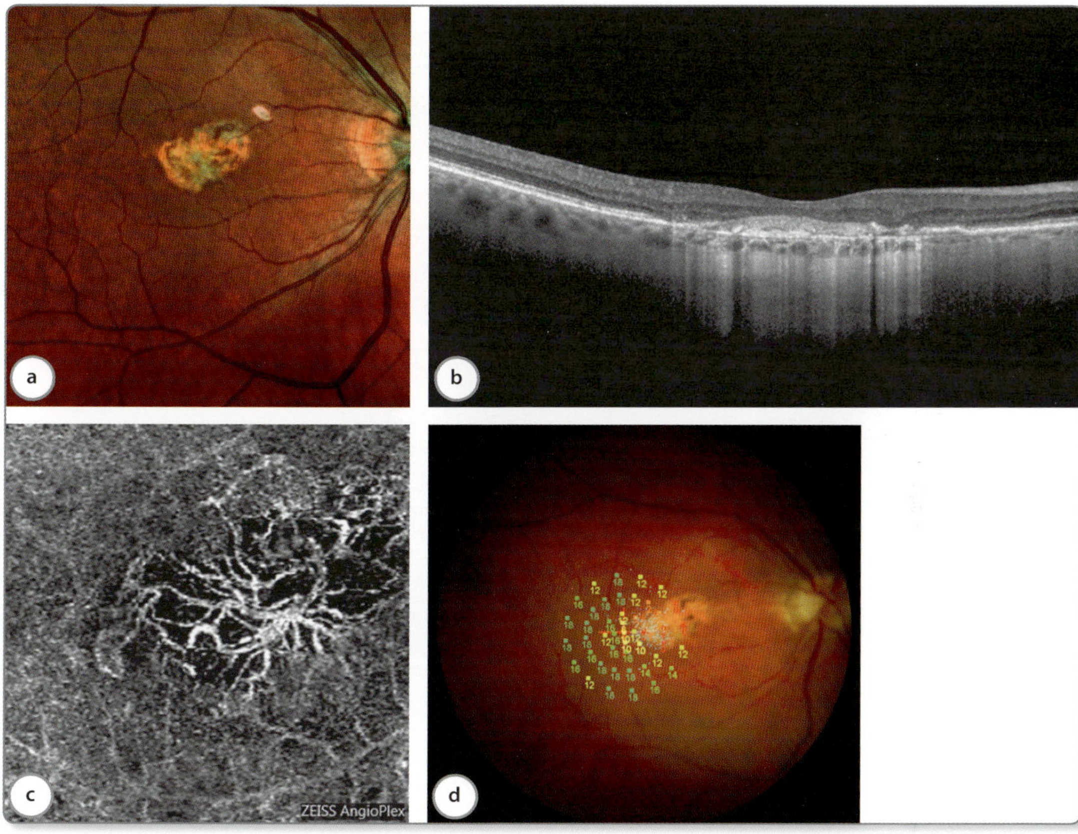

Figure 4 Multimodal imaging and microperimetry from a patient with age-related macular degeneration (AMD)-associated type 1 macular neovascularization and localized fibrosis. (a) Multicolor image shows bright lime-green regions in the macula corresponding to a localized area of macular scar. (b) The structural optical coherence tomography B-scan confirms the presence of a hyper-reflective fibrocellular pigment epithelial detachment with retinal pigment epithelium (RPE) atrophy. (c) Optical coherence tomography angiography (OCTA) imaging shows the presence of flow into the fibrocellular lesion. (d) A localized impairment of the retinal sensitivity is evident from the microperimetric examination, which is overlapped to the fundus photography image.

6. Hogg R, Curry E, Muldrew A, et al. Identification of lesion components that influence visual function in age-related macular degeneration. Br J Ophthalmol. 2003; 87:609–614.
7. Friedlander M. Fibrosis and diseases of the eye. J Clin Invest 2007; 117:576–586.
8. Schmidt-Erfurth U, Waldstein SM. A paradigm shift in imaging biomarkers in neovascular age-related macular degeneration. Prog Retin Eye Res 2016; 50:1–24.
9. Grossniklaus H. Histopathologic and ultrastructural findings of surgically excised choroidal neovascularization. Submacular Surgery Trials Research Group. Arch Ophthalmol 1998; 116:745–749.
10. Graham KW, Chakravarthy U, Hogg RE, et al. Identifying features of early and late age-related macular degeneration: A Comparison of Multicolor Versus Traditional Color Fundus Photography. Retina 2018: 38:1751–1758.
11. Borrelli E, Sarraf D, Freund KB, et al. OCT angiography and evaluation of the choroid and choroidal vascular disorders. Prog Retin Eye Res 2018; 67:30–55.
12. Kuehlewein L, Bansal M, Lenis TL, et al. Optical Coherence Tomography Angiography of Type 1 Neovascularization in Age-Related Macular Degeneration. Am J Ophthalmol 2015; 160:739–748.e2.
13. Costanzo E, Miere A, Querques G, et al. Type 1 Choroidal Neovascularization Lesion Size: Indocyanine Green Angiography versus Optical Coherence Tomography Angiography. Invest Ophthalmol Vis Sci 2016; 57:307–313.

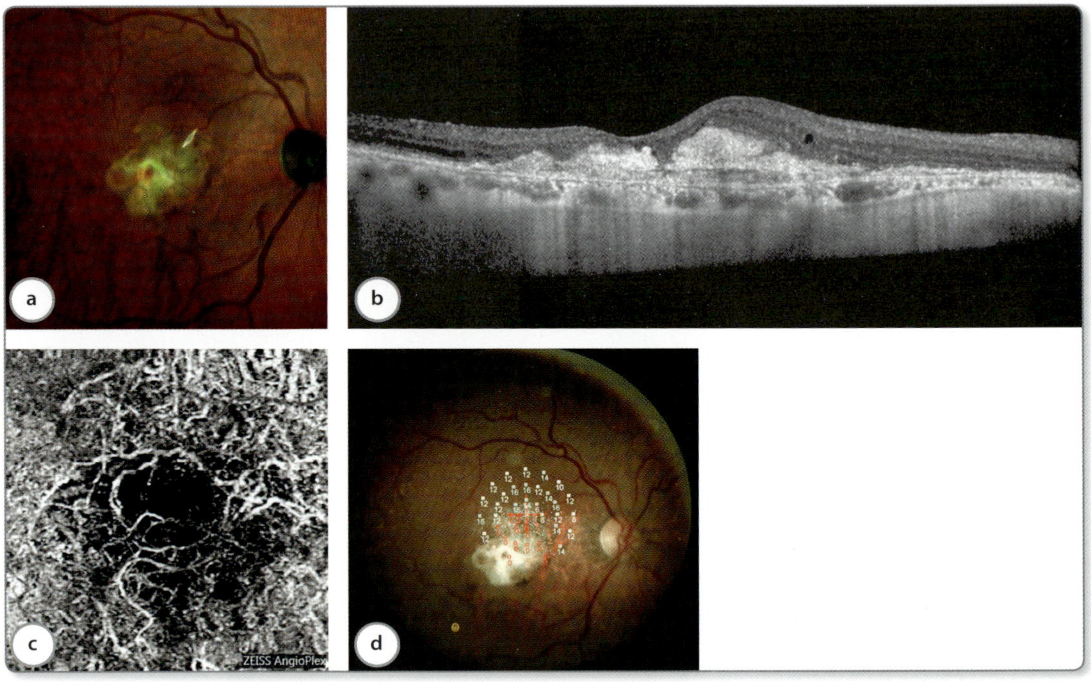

Figure 5 Multimodal imaging and microperimetry from a patient with age-related macular degeneration (AMD)-associated type 2 macular neovascularisation and diffuse fibrosis. (a) Multicolour image shows a yellowish region in the macula corresponding to an extensive area of macular scar. (b) The structural optical coherence tomography B-scan shows the presence of a subretinal hyper-reflective material. (c) Flow within the fibrocellular lesion is seen on the corresponding *en face* optical coherence tomographic angiography (OCTA) image. (d) Retinal sensitivity values in decibel over the fundus photography image show a diffuse impairment of the retinal sensitivity in the macula.

14. El Ameen A, Cohen SY, Semoun O, et al. Type 2 neovascularization secondary to age-related macular degeneration imaged by optical coherence tomography angiography. Retina 2015; 35:2212–2218.
15. Willoughby AS, Ying GS, Toth CA, et al. Subretinal Hyperreflective Material in the Comparison of Age-Related Macular Degeneration Treatments Trials. Ophthalmology 2015; 122:1846–1853.e5.
16. Dansingani KK, Tan ACS, Gilani F, et al. Subretinal hyperreflective material imaged with optical coherence tomography angiography. Am J Ophthalmol 2016; 169:235–248.
17. Kaszubski P, Ben Ami T, Saade C, et al. Geographic Atrophy and Choroidal Neovascularization in the Same Eye: A Review. Ophthalmic Res 2016; 55: 185–193.
18. Hinton DR, He S, Lopez PF. Apoptosis in surgically excised choroidal neovascular membranes in age-related macular degeneration. Arch Ophthalmol 1998; 116:203–209.
19. Ishikawa K, Kannan R, Hinton DR. Molecular mechanisms of subretinal fibrosis in age-related macular degeneration. Exp Eye Res 2014; 142:19–25.

11 CNV pathophysiology, definition and classification

Bruno Lumbroso

CNV physiopathology

Choroidal neovascularization (CNV) is the first step of a choroidal scar or a wound healing response to a lesion of the retinal pigment epithelium (RPE). CNV looks like a misdirected wound healing process.

Globally, CNV development is due to abnormalities in or around Bruch's membrane that leads to alteration in RPE cells, which later determines development of CNV. New vessels appear at choriocapillaris level and will grow through Bruch's membrane under the RPE first and then perforate it and emerge in the outer retina.

Basic mechanism of CNV involves three factors:

1. Bruch's membrane abnormalities
2. RPE cells alteration
3. Antiangiogenic factors and angiogenic factors leading to CNV growth.

Alteration in pigment epithelium cells

A localized RPE deterioration and dysfunction is a decisive event leading to macular degeneration, and then CNV. After its onset, the degeneration process is progressive and inexorable. From degeneration, there is no return. The basic tissue lesion in macular degeneration is a fault in the RPE and choriocapillaris. Causes are diverse and wide ranging.

Bruch's membrane lesion

Waste material from pigment epithelium accumulate in Bruch's membrane and aggregate in the form of drusen and basal laminar deposits. This change blocks the normal transit of metabolites and fluids. The route of waste out from the neurosensory retina is reduced. Abnormalities in or around Bruch's membrane, always present in case of CNV, suggest that Bruch's membrane lesion associated with alteration of the RPE predisposes the development of CNV. Vascular endothelial growth factor is present during this initial phase and is then released by RPE. Bruch's membrane localized damage is necessary for the neovascularization to cross the membrane barrier from the choroid to the retina.

Antiangiogenic and angiogenic factors

The balance between antiangiogenic factors (PEDF and other) and angiogenic factors (VEGF and other) determines the formation of a network of new vessels. Vascular endothelial growth factor (VEGF) is an important ocular angiogenic factor correlated with the development of CNV. VEGF induces vascular permeability, endothelial cell proliferation, and cell migration and is a key stimulation for retinal neovascularization. The pigment epithelium-derived factor (PEDF) has an inhibitory effect on neovascularization (**Boxes 1** and **2**).

Development of CNV

Angiogenesis

Angiogenesis is the mechanism through which new blood vessels form from preexisting vessels. It is a normal process in vessel growth and development, as well as in wound healing.

Box 1: Choroidal neovascularization (CNV) classification

Jung Freund AJO 2014:

- Type 1: 40% underneath the pigmented epithelium
- Type 2: 9% subretinal
- Type 3: 24% intraretinal
- Type 4: 17% mixed

Angiogenesis can be modified by treatment, but the key cause is not affected.

Spaide (2015) described clearly and brilliantly angiogenesis and arteriogenesis processes. The sprouting of vascular endothelial cells to form new vessels from preexisting vessels is chiefly stimulated by VEGF, with some less important factors. Vascular endothelial cells and their mural cells have a common basement membrane that collapses under metalloproteinases influence. Some of the endothelial cells become tip cells, which lead the neovascular development. Neighboring endothelial cells become stalk cells. The tip cells lead the proliferating stalk cells growth. The stalk cells then create a lumen, generate a basement membrane, and perfusion begins.

Vessel maturation is marked by reduced proliferation of endothelial cells, pericyte recruitment, pericyte maturation, and increased formation of cell junctions. Angiogenesis is an incessant process that is produced when necessary and until the incentives for proliferation decline (**Figures 1 to 6**).

Box 2: Choroidal neovascularization (CNV) classification

Exudative:

- Type 1: 40% underneath the pigmented epithelium
- Type 2: 9% subretinal
- Type 3: 24% intraretinal
- Type 1 + 2: 17% mixed

Other types:

- Myopic
- CRSC CNV
- Residual new vessels in fibrous scars.

Nonexudative

Biomarkers of neovascularization activity in AMD in OCT angiography

Biomarkers of CNV activity in exudative age-related macular degeneration (AMD) are well recognized in optical coherence tomography (OCT) where they are characterized by subretinal and intraretinal fluid. Biomarkers in OCT angiography (OCTA) are less well codified.

David Sarraf, Xu et al. identified two types of biomarkers:

1. *Short-term biomarkers*: Short-term biomarkers are correlated with disease activity at a given time. They are vascular arcade, and peripheral loops, 'sea-fan' appearance, peripheral arborization, dark halo. These criteria do not consider the area of the lesion or the neovascular diameter.
2. *Long-term biomarkers*: These provide better information on CNV activity and its evolutionary potential. David Sarraf, Xu et al. classified CNVs in three categories according to their evolutionary profile:

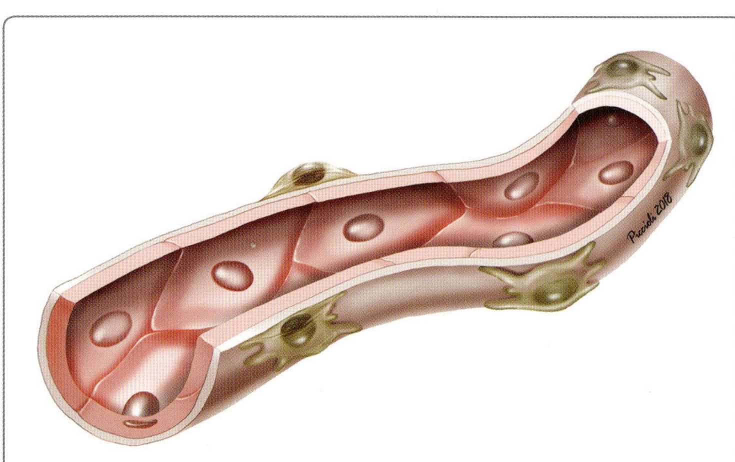

Figure 1 *Angiogenesis* is the mechanism through which new blood vessels form from pre-existing vessels. It is a normal process in vessel growth and development, as well as in wound healing. Angiogenesis can be modified by treatment, but the key cause is not affected. Here you can see normal vessel before angiogenesis.

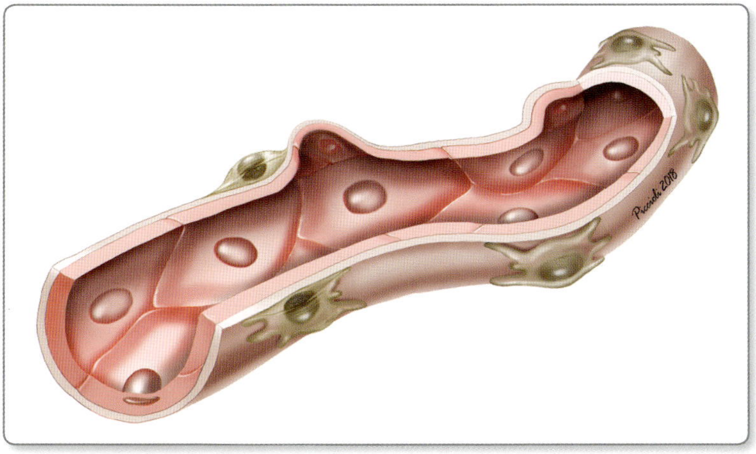

Figure 2 Angiogenesis: Collapse of the vessel wall leading to stalk formation. The sprouting of vascular endothelial cells to form new vessels from preexisting vessels is chiefly stimulated by vascular endothelial growth factor (VEGF), with some less important factors. Vascular endothelial cells and their mural cells have a common basement membrane that collapses under metalloproteinases influence.

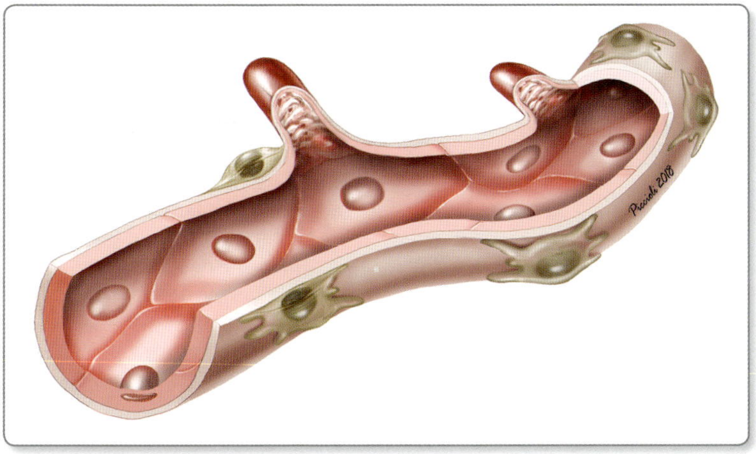

Figure 3 Angiogenesis: Tip cells and stalks. Some of the endothelial cells become tip cells, which lead the neovascular development. Neighboring endothelial cells become stalk cells. The tip cells lead the proliferating stalk cells growth.

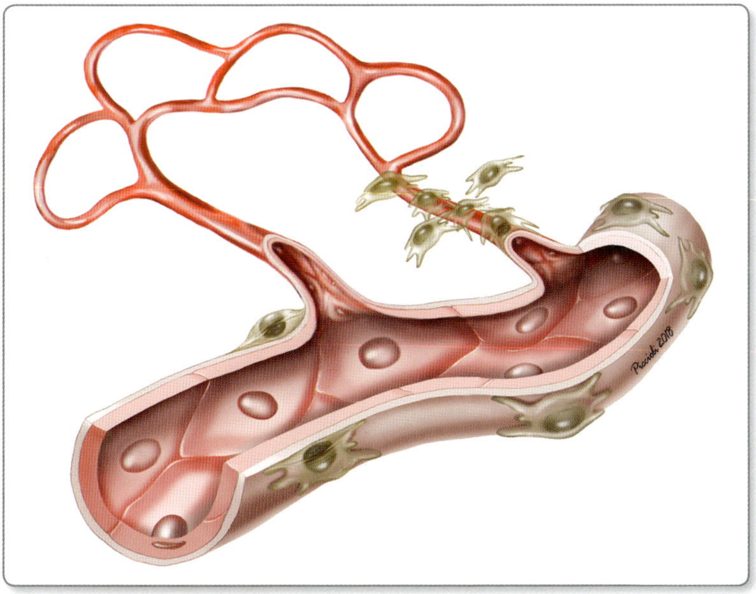

Figure 4 Angiogenesis: Lumen formation. The stalk cells then create a lumen, generate a basement membrane, and perfusion begins. Pericytes begin to proliferate.

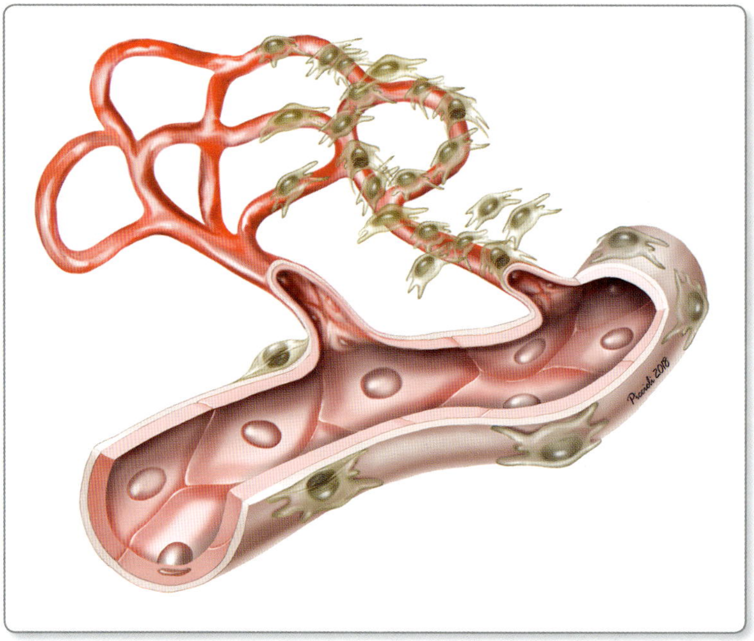

Figure 5 *Angiogenesis*, maturation, and pericytes proliferation. Vessel maturation is marked by reduced proliferation of endothelial cells, pericyte recruitment, pericyte proliferation, pericyte maturation, and increased formation of cell junctions.

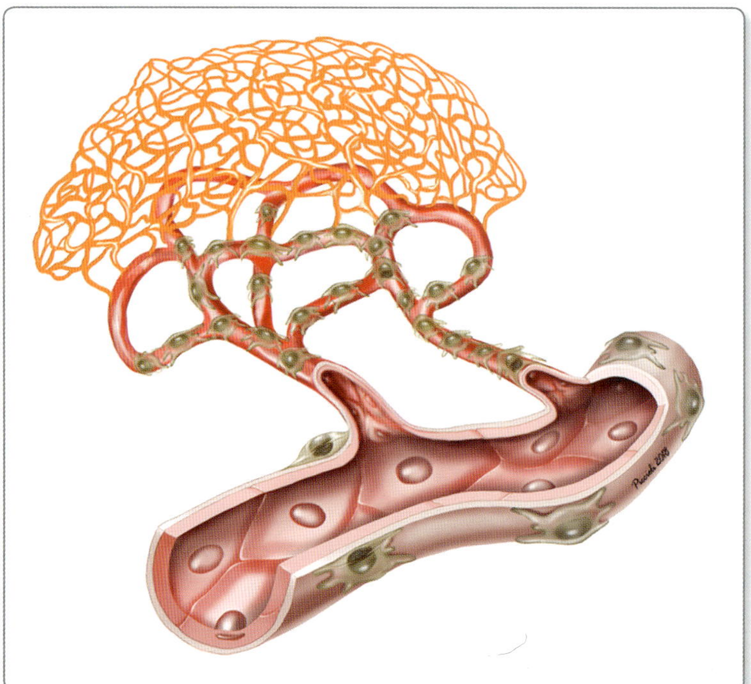

Figure 6 *Angiogenesis*: Angiogenesis is an incessant process that is produced when necessary and until the incentives for proliferation decline. Here you can see a recurrence with fringe proliferation of small active capillaries.

- *Immature CNV*: They are formed of many tangled new vessels associated with a form of peripheral 'fringe'. These CNVs have significant growth potential.
- *Mature CNV*: They are composed of large vessels in sea-fan shape. They have a moderate rate of progression and are generally more resistant to anti-VEGF.
- *Hypermature CNV*: They are composed of large thick straight vessels, with a 'tree in winter' appearance. Their progression rate is usually zero.

These OCTA biomarkers allow understanding of the evolutionary profile of CNV and the potential for long-term progression of the disease. David Sarraf has categorized the CNV progression as symmetrical, asymmetrical, or having a fingertip extension.

David Sarraf gave us a good vision on the importance of OCTA biomarkers in the long run. To know if one must treat again, the exudative signs at the OCT-B are enough. The evolution of CNV is interesting to understand to forecast visual prognosis. The artificial intelligence will help us to confirm our intuitions.

CNV growth

Growth may vary largely immature, mature, or hypermature.

There are fast growths (with doubling of surface from one examination to another), slow growth, and regression.

Arteriogenesis

The dilation of vessels in response to high-flow states occurs as a normal process in new vessel growth and is called arteriogenesis. As stated by Spaide 'angiogenesis is the sprouting of new capillaries, while arteriogenesis is the dilation of preexisting channels by active proliferation and remodeling of the vessel wall'.

Early and intermediate AMD are categorized by drusen and pigment deposits. The late stages of AMD are documented by the neovascularization, or geographic atrophy. Since OCTA is used in ophthalmology, we know that neovascularization can be present without exudation, a new entity denoted as nonexudative, silent, quiescent, subclinical neovascular NV.

CNV definition

One or more disorders?

Choroidal neovascularization may be considered as a repair response to a lesion of the RPE. CNV can be observed in many totally different disorders. In a normal process of wound healing, angiogenesis is the mechanism through which new blood vessels form from preexisting vessels.

Things were easier at the times of fluorescein angiography; we had only classic and occult CNVs. Now we struggle about with types 1, 2, 3 and may be type 4 CNVs, CNV exudative, and nonexudative, active, silent, asymptomatic, quiescent or regressive, CNV on normal, thin choroid or thick pachychoroid, immature, mature, or hypermature CNV.

The term CNV covers many different clinical features and certainly a large range of different pathologies. We use only one word to take in many diverse clinical features. These different features could be a single disease, successive stages of the same disease, or group together completely diverse disorders (**Boxes 3** to **19**).

All these CNV phenotypically can look very much alike or may show huge differences, and some have utterly divergent features. Some images share only limited particulars, but disorders may be very close, other images look quite the same but have different genotypes.

Are all CNV a unique malady with many syndromes, are they successive stages of the same disease (as different as a tadpole that will become a frog) or do they group together completely diverse disorders (as different as tuberculosis from rubella)?

The major cause of CNV is age-related macular degeneration. AMD is the most frequent cause of vision loss in the developed countries.

Box 3: Basic mechanism of choroidal neovascularization (CNV)

Three factors:

1. Bruch's membrane abnormalities
2. RPE cells alteration
3. Antiangiogenic factors and angiogenic factors leading to CNV growth

(RPE: retinal pigment epithelium)

Box 4: Choroidal neovascularization (CNV) features

Exudative type 1:
- Pigment epithelium flat detachment
- Fibrous and vascular content.

Exudative type 2:
- Subretinal fluid
- Diffuse edema
- Cystoid edema
- Hemorrhages
- Alterations of the outer retinal layers
- Photoreceptors severe lesions.

Exudative type 3:
- Pigment epithelium detachment
- Intraretinal and subretinal fluid
- Cystoid edema
- Hemorrhages.

Exudative type 4, or mixed type: Type 1 and type 2 CNVs coexist in the same lesion—
- Pigment epithelium fibrovascular flat detachment
- Subretinal fluid
- Cystoid edema
- Hemorrhages
- Alterations in the outer retinal layers.

Nonexudative:
- Pigment epithelium flat detachment frequent
- No subretinal fluid
- No diffuse edema
- No cystoid edema
- No hemorrhages
- No or rare alterations of the outer retinal layers
- No photoreceptors severe lesions.

Box 5: Choroidal neovascularization (CNV) assessment

- Morphology
- Capillary density: Dense or sparse
- Branches dense or sparse subdivision and arborization
- Loops present or lacking
- Vessels thin or thick
- Vessels straight or sinuous
- Flow quantification

Exudative or nonexudative

Box 6: Choroidal neovascularization (CNV) morphology in general

- Coral shaped
- Fan shaped
- Medusa head
- Wheel shaped
- Tangled
- Bare tree shaped
- Filament like
- Star shaped
- Tuft shaped
- Glomerular

Box 7: Choroidal neovascularization (CNV) capillaries density

- Densely packed
- Sparse
- Thin
- Thick
- Numerous
- Rare

It is characterized by progressive deterioration of photoreceptors and pigment epithelium, Bruch's membrane lesions and, in wet AMD, neovascularization. Atrophic lesions lead to a generally slow vision decrease, CNV leads to fast vision deterioration. Most of AMD cases are dry AMD (80%), only 20% of cases are wet AMD (**Boxes 20** to **25**).

Box 8: Choroidal neovascularization (CNV) loops morphology

- Mainly located in the periphery where they can merge forming
- Arcade continuous or interrupted
- Wheel-shaped CNV
- Fan shaped
- Coral bush shaped.

Box 9: Choroidal neovascularization (CNV) loops density

- Frequent
- Rare
- Thin
- Dense inside the arborizations.
- Loops are rarely found in tangled new vessels and in bare tree CNV.

Box 10: Choroidal neovascularization (CNV) morphology: Type 1

- Medusa head
- Coral
- Bicycle wheel
- Fan or sea-fan
- Dead tree
- Tangled
- Filament-like

Box 11: Type 1 new vessels fluorescein angiography

- Early leakage
- Leakage increases slowly, progressively
- Dye oozing
- Margins blurred
- Leakage irregular
- CNV seen as blurred hyperfluorescence area

Box 12: Type 1 new vessels indocyanine green (ICG) features

- In early frames, the feeder vessel and its ramifications
- Late ICG frames, a plaque with sharp margins
- Rarely margins are blurred
- Plaques single or multiple
- Two or three plaques may overlap
- Hyperfluorescent dots (hot spots) present or lacking

Box 13: Type 1 choroidal neovascularization (CNV) structural optical coherence tomography (OCT) features

- Flat, irregular, or undulated pigment epithelium elevation
- Fluid between the pigment epithelium elevation and Bruch's membrane
- Alterations, irregularities, thickening disruption of the ellipsoid zone
- Neuroepithelium partially disrupted
- Fibrous layers under elevated epithelium
- Elevated pigment epithelium tears frequent

Box 14: Type 1 choroidal neovascularization (CNV) morphology

- Coral shaped
- Fan shaped
- Medusa head
- Wheel shaped
- Tangled
- Arborization
- Fractal aspect, small, large
- Bare tree
- Filamentary

Box 15: Perilesional dark halo

Small

Large:

- Halo variation after treatment
- Halo pulsation in time lapse follow-up

Box 16: Possible causes of perilesional dark halo

- Morphological changes in the choriocapillaris
- Screen effect (fluid, pigment, and hemorrhage)
- Choriocapillaris blood flow variations
- Blood sequestering

Box 17: Type 2 choroidal neovascularization (CNV) morphology

- Coral shaped
- Fan shaped
- Medusa head
- Wheel shaped
- Rounded
- Arborization
- Star shaped

Box 18: Type 3 choroidal neovascularization (CNV) morphology

- Tuft shaped
- Star shaped

Box 19: Type 4 choroidal neovascularization (CNV) morphology

Type 4 CNV includes two or more vascular parallel flat stratified formations overlaid at several levels: Type 2 new vessels above the pigment epithelium. Deeper down, underneath the pigment epithelium but above Bruch's membrane, one or more larger and irregular type 1 CNV:

Morphology of type 1 CNV in type 4 mixed CNV:

- Coral shaped
- Fan shaped
- Medusa head
- Wheel shaped
- Tangled
- Arborization
- Bare tree
- Filamentary

Morphology of type 2 CNV in type 4 mixed CNV:

- Coral shaped
- Fan shaped
- Medusa head
- Wheel shaped
- Rounded
- Arborization
- Star shaped

Box 20: Exudative choroidal neovascularization (CNV) evolution: Maturation, arterialization features

- Capillaries become wider, thicker, and straighter
- Thinner capillaries disappear
- Later fibrosis and photoreceptors alterations
- Dark halo around the new vessels

Box 21: Fibrous scar

- Some large vessels
- Thick and straight, with irregular flow
- No thin capillaries
- No fine loops are visible

Box 22: Causes of subretinal neovascular membranes

Frequent:

- AMD
- Idiopathic polypoidal vasculopathy
- Retinal angiomatous proliferations (RAP)
- Myopia
- Idiopathic new vessels in young patients
- Pseudohistoplasmosis
- Traumatic choroidal ruptures
- Complications of laser photocoagulation
- Angioid streaks

Rare:

- Choroiditis
- VKH
- Choroidal nevus
- Osteoma
- Pseudovitelliform macular dystrophy
- Stargardt disease
- Best disease

Box 23: Causes of choroidal neovascularization (CNV) in children

- Myopia
- Stargardt disease
- Best disease
- Inflammatory
- Choroiditis
- VKH
- Presumed histoplasmosis
- Serpiginous
- Idiopathic
- Traumatic choroidal ruptures
- Laser induced

Box 24: Causes of retinal scars

- Advanced macular degeneration
- Diabetic fibrovascular membrane
- Laser scars
- Fibrous scars
- Chorioretinitis
- Myopia
- Traumatic choroidal ruptures
- Complications of laser photocoagulation
- Angioid streaks

Box 25: Exudative and nonexudative choroidal neovascularization (CNV)

- Nonexudative: Inactive or low activity
- Nonexudative: Long-term or short-term remission
- Exudative: Active
- Persistent exudation: Active, refractory

CNV clinical classification

History

Currently, CNVs are assessed and classified based on their localization, morphology, and two new important factors: exudation and choroid thickness.

Fluorescein angiography classification

Exudative CNVs are known since the first days of fluorescein angiography. They were divided in classic and occult CNV before advent of OCTA. Nonexudative CNV could be seen with difficulty using ICG angiography.

Classification by Jung and Freund in 2014

Structural OCT and cross-section OCT allowed choroidal neovascularization classification by Jung and Freund in 2014:

- Type 1: 40% underneath the pigmented epithelium
- Type 2: 9% subretinal
- Type 3: 24% intraretinal
- Type 4: 17% mixed.

Clinical CNV classification based on morphology and OCTA features (Lumbroso, Rispoli, 2019)

Exudative CNV

- Type 1: Underneath the pigment epithelium
- Type 1+2: 17% mixed
- Type 1 CRSC CNV
- Type 1 IPV
- Type 2 subretinal, above pigment epithelium
- Type 2 myopic
- Type 3: Intraretinal
- CNV exudative in other types of Bruch's lesions
- Residual new vessels in fibrous scars.

Nonexudative CNV

- Nonexudative type 1 CNV in AMD, in intermediate AMD, in atrophic AMD
- Nonexudative type 1 CNV in pachychoroid, CRSC
- Nonexudative precursor to exudative type 1 CNV
- Exudative type 1 CNV evolution to nonexudative CNV after treatment
- Arterialized nonexudative CNV after treatment
- Nonexudative residual new vessels in fibrous scars
- Nonexudative separate clinical entity (or entities).

The nonexudative CNV could be subdivided differently as follows:

- Naive, silent, frequent, seen in pachychoroid, AMD
- CNV exudative, before conversion to nonexudative quiescent for more than 6 months after treatment (mainly AMD)
- CNV first nonexudative before conversion into an exudative form
- Complication of atrophic or geographical AMD
- Nonexudative active flow in fibrotic scars (AMD).

CNV clinical classification based on choroid thickness and Bruch's membrane condition (Lumbroso, Rispoli, 2019)

Another clinical approach of classifying CNV is possible and logical. CNV could be classified according to the thickness of choroid.

We categorize CNV in five main categories, according to choroid thickness and Bruch's membrane condition:

Normal choroid thickness and normal Bruch's membrane:

- nAMD type 1, type 2, mixed type 1 + type 2.

Normal choroid thickness and ruptured choroid and Bruch's membrane lesions:

- CNV in abnormalities or breaks in Bruch's membrane and choriocapillaris
- CNV in choroid traumatic rupture
- CNV in complications of laser photocoagulation
- CNV in angioid streaks
- CNV in inflammatory disorders, choroiditis, and chorioretinitis
- CNV on margin of atrophic areas
- CNV in fibrous scars.

Thick choroid and normal Bruch's membrane:

- Pachychoroid complex, CRSC
- Polypoidal neovasculopathy
- Filamentous CNV.

Thick choroid and ruptured Bruch's membrane:

- Some CNV in choroiditis.

Thin choroid and normal Bruch's membrane:

- Myopia
- Atrophic AMD.

Thin choroid and ruptured choroid and Bruch's membrane lesions:

- CNV posterior pole choroiditis of myopic young women
- CNV on margin of atrophic areas.

In each of these five categories, CNV may be exudative or nonexudative.

Clinical classification based on CNV activity (Lumbroso, Rispoli, 2019)

To confirm the complexity of classification, another clinical approach is to classify CNV according to activity or quiescence.

Exudative and Nonexudative CNV

- Exudative: Active
- Persistent exudation: Active, CNV refractory to treatment
- Nonexudative: Inactive or low activity
- Long-term nonexudative CNV
- Nonexudative short-term remission.

12 Exudative choroidal neovascularization

Bruno Lumbroso, Marco Rispoli

New factors for CNV nomenclature: Exudation, activity biomarkers, and choroid thickness

Since optical coherence tomography (OCT) angiography is replacing dye angiography, choroidal neovascularizations (CNVs) are assessed and classified based on their localization, morphology, and three new important factors: wall exudation and choroidal thickness and activity biomarkers. Optical coherence tomographic angiography (OCTA) has revealed the existence and importance of nonexudative choroidal neovascularization.

Many designations have been assigned to CNV according to their feature: medusa head, coral bush, bicycle wheel, dead tree, etc. It is more important to quantify the capillary density. It can be dense or sparse; Branches subdivision and arborization give other useful information on the fractal pattern. Loops display activity and growth. If they are lacking, CNV is quiescent or less active. Vessels can be thin or thick, straight, or sinuous. Peripheral vascular arcade can be complete, broken, or completely lacking.

A specific software allows flow quantification. Future software will show flow speed.

Fluid presence helps to define exudative or nonexudative new vessels. Dark halo around CNV, sign of low vessel density, or flow can be quantified.

Type 1, type 1 + 2 (mixed) CNV, type 2, and type 3 in normal thickness choroid

We observe age-related macular degeneration in normal thickness choroid in most of the CNV types that we study in this chapter (**Boxes 1 to 12**).

Box 1: Choroidal neovascularization (CNV) features

Exudative type 1:

- Pigment epithelium wavy flat detachment
- Fibrous and vascular content
- No retinal edema

Exudative type 2:

- Subretinal fluid
- Diffuse edema
- Cystoid edema
- Hemorrhages
- Alterations of the outer retinal layers
- Photoreceptors severe lesions

Exudative type 3:

- Pigment epithelium detachment
- Intraretinal and subretinal fluid
- Cystoid edema
- Hemorrhages

Exudative mixed type: Type 1 and Type 2 CNVs coexist in the same lesion—

- Pigment epithelium fibrovascular flat detachment
- Subretinal fluid
- Cystoid edema
- Hemorrhages
- Alterations in the outer retinal layers

Nonexudative:

- Pigment epithelium flat detachment frequent
- No subretinal fluid
- No diffuse edema
- No cystoid edema
- No hemorrhages
- No alterations of the outer retinal layers
- No photoreceptors lesion

Box 2: Choroidal neovascularization (CNV) report

- NV morphology
- Capillary density: Dense or sparse
- Branches subdivision and arborization: Dense or sparse
- Fractal aspect, small, large
- Loops: Present or lacking
- Vessels thin or thick
- Vessels straight or sinuous
- Flow: fast, slow, intermittent, irregular, pulsating
- Exudative or nonexudative

Box 3: Choroidal neovascularization (CNV) general morphology

- Coral shaped
- Fan shaped
- Medusa head
- Wheel shaped
- Tangled
- Bare tree shaped
- Filamentary
- Star shaped
- Tuft shaped
- Glomerular

Box 4: Choroidal neovascularization (CNV) capillaries density

- Densely packed
- Sparse
- Thin
- Thick
- Numerous
- Rare

Box 5: Choroidal neovascularization (CNV) arcade morphology

- Arcade is set in CNV periphery where loops merge forming
- Arcade continuous or broken up

Box 6: Choroidal neovascularization (CNV) loops compactness

- Frequent
- Lacking
- Rare
- Thin
- Dense inside the arborizations

Box 7: Type 1 new vessels fluorescein angiography

- Early leakage
- Leakage increasing progressively
- Dye oozing
- Leakage margins blurred

Box 8: Type 1 new vessels indocyanine green (ICG) features

- In early ICG frames, feeder vessel and branches
- Late ICG frames, a plaque with sharp or blurred margins
- Plaques single or multiple
- Plaques may overlap
- Hot spots present

Box 9: Type 1 choroidal neovascularization (CNV) structural optical coherence tomography (OCT) features

- Flat irregular or undulated pigment epithelium elevation
- Fluid between the pigment epithelium elevation and Bruch's membrane
- Irregularities, thickening, disruption of the ellipsoid zone
- Neuroepithelium partially disrupted
- Fibrous layers under elevated epithelium
- Infrequently pigment epithelium tears

Box 10: Type 1 choroidal neovascularization (CNV) morphology 1

- Coral bush shaped
- Fan shaped
- Medusa head
- Wheel shaped
- Tangled
- Arborization
- Bare tree
- Filamentary

Box 11: Type 1 choroidal neovascularization (CNV) morphology 2 fractal aspect

- Small
- Large

Box 12: Perilesional dark halo

- Small
- Large
- Dense

Type 1 new vessels (formerly occult) (Figures 1 to 6)

Localization: Type 1 new vessels (formerly called occult) develop under a pigment epithelium flat or undulated elevation, between the elevated pigment epithelium and Bruch's membrane. The contents of the pigment epithelial detachment (PED) may be fluid or fibrovascular tissue.

Fluorescein angiography features

In early leakage hyperfluorescence, lesion margins are blurred.

Indocyanine green (ICG) features

In the very early frames, the feeder vessel and its ramifications can be seen; in the late frames, a plaque.

Structural OCT features

Type 1 neovascular membranes are located underneath an irregular, elongated detachment

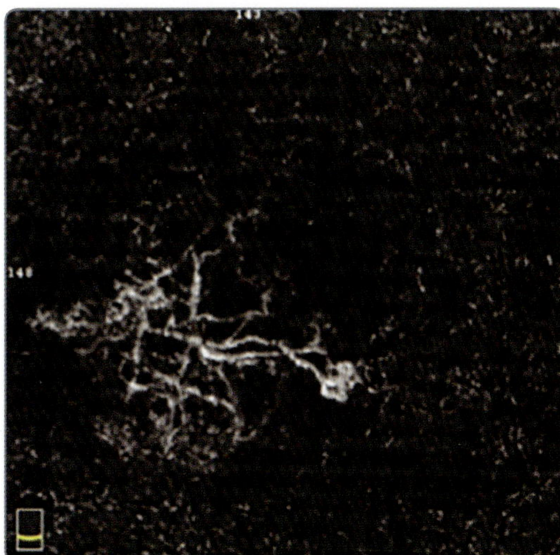

Figure 1A Optical coherence tomography (OCT) angiography and cross-section scan type 1: Choroidal neovascularization (CNV) OCT angiography type 2 new vessels develop under a small pigment epithelium elevation, often between the elevated pigment epithelium and Bruch's membrane: the capillaries are sparse, the vessels are thick. There is a central bundle of feeder vessels. A finger-like projection has developed in the CNV periphery showing that the CNV is active. A dark halo surrounds the CNV. (Optovue)

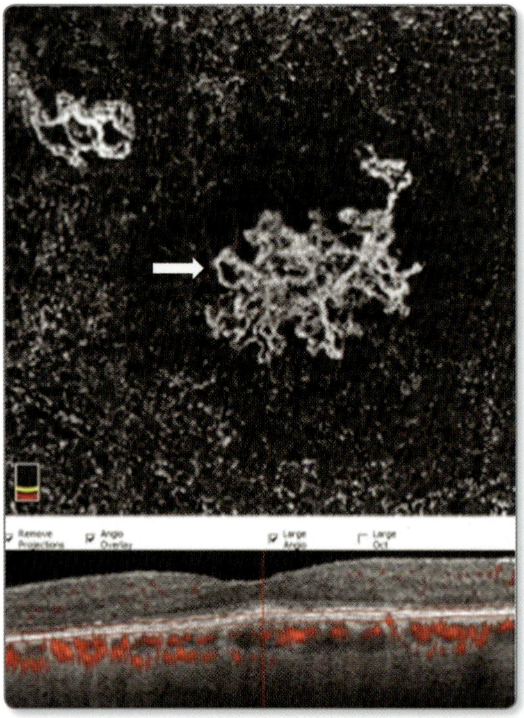

Figure 1B Optical coherence tomography (OCT) angiography and cross-section scan type 1: In this case, two CNVs are seen, two bush-like structures where capillaries are sparse, vessels are thick. In each vessel network, there is a central core of feeder vessels. Some loops (arrow) are seen in the choroidal neovascularization (CNV) periphery and contribute to the formation of the peripheral vascular arcade showing that the CNVs are active. A dark halo surrounds the CNVs. (Optovue)

of the pigment epithelium with disruption and fragmentation of the pigment epithelium. Later in evolution, the new vessels perforate Bruch's membrane and breakthrough pigment epithelium. Retinal pigment epithelium rips or tears may appear.

OCT angiography features

Type 1 new vessels may look like a medusa head, coral bush, bicycle wheel, fan, dead tree, tangled network, filaments, and vascular loop. This loop is mostly seen in the CNV periphery. Loops are rare in the filamentous new vessels and in the bare tree-like new vessels. The capillaries may be dense or sparse, the vessels may be thin and numerous. They may be frequent, rare and thin, or dense, forming complex arborization. There is a feeder trunk or bundle of feeder vessels. Sarraf differentiated immature, mature, and hypermature forms.

During the evolution, arterialization makes vessels become thicker, straighter, and rigid with loss of the thinner capillaries. Evolved CNV takes bare tree features.

Filamentary new vessels are observed in age-related macular degeneration and in pachychoroid. Type 1 new vessels generally have a larger surface than type 2 new vessels.

Growth

Choroidal neovascularization may have a symmetrical, asymmetrical growth, or have a fingertip extension (Sarraf).

Perilesional dark halo

A halo or dark circle around the new vessels is observed in 80% of the cases. It could be due to morphological changes in the choriocapillaris, screen effect, blood sequestering, or choriocapillaris blood flow alterations (**Figures 7** and **8; Boxes 13** and **14**).

Exudation

Dye angiography and structural OCT show, if there is exudation.

Type 1 + 2 new vessels (mixed type—formerly type 4)

Type 1 CNVs perforate pigment epithelium and penetrate under the retina and then into the retinal avascular layer. These CNVs include two or more vascular parallel flat stratified formations overlaid at several levels. They form a flat wavy retinal pigment epithelium (RPE) elevation with stratified contents. There is fluid under the detached epithelium as well as subretinal fluid. Alterations, irregularities, thickening of the ellipsoid zone are normally seen. OCT can show fibrovascular tissue layers under the elevated epithelium. There are always disruption and fragmentation of the pigment epithelium.

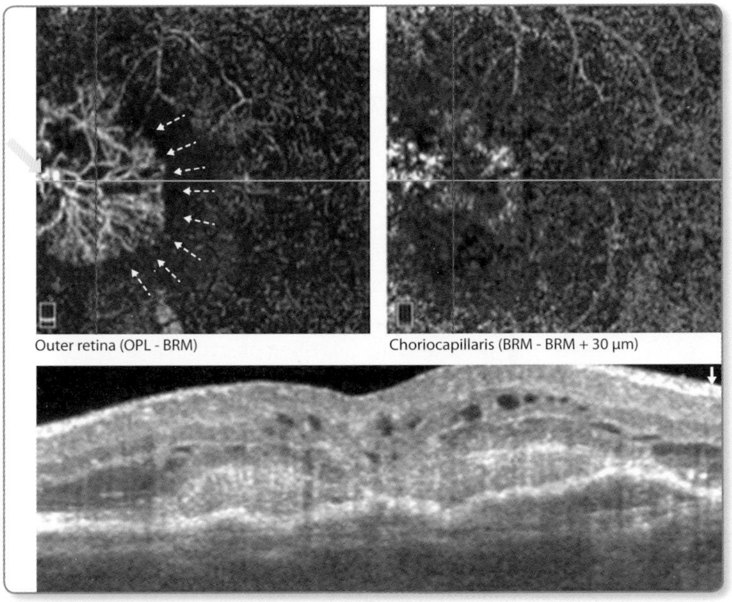

Figure 2 *'En face'* optical coherence tomography (OCT) angiography and cross-section OCT. Type 1 new vessels develop between a pigment epithelium flat elevation and Bruch's membrane. No subretinal fluid detachment is seen, some cystic cavities are present. Capillaries are sparse, the vessels are thick. There is a bundle of feeder vessels (yellow arrow) and a peripheral vascular arcade (dashed arrows). (Optovue)

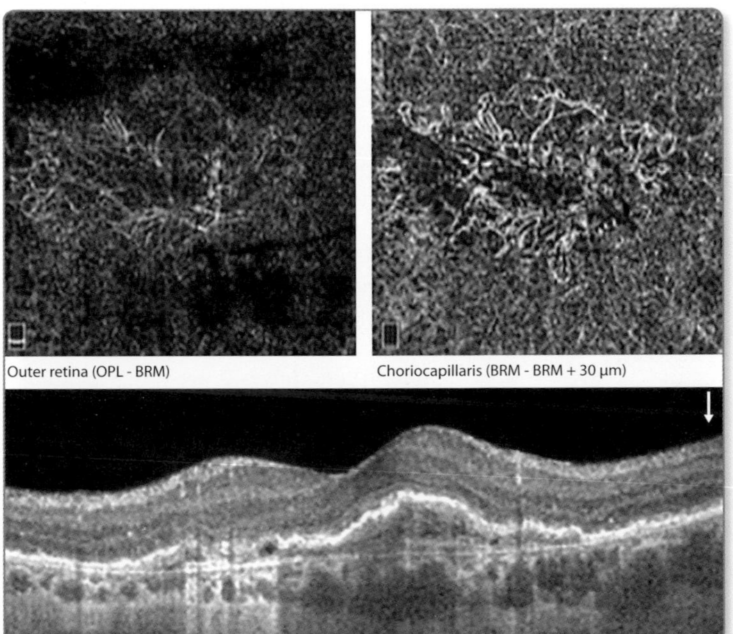

Figure 3 *'En face'* optical coherence tomography (OCT) angiography and cross-section OCT. Type 1 new vessels appearing as an irregularly rounded formation. The loops are mainly located in the periphery showing that the membrane is active. B scan shows a thick fibrovascular formation under an irregular pigment epithelium elevation and no retinal edema. (Optovue)

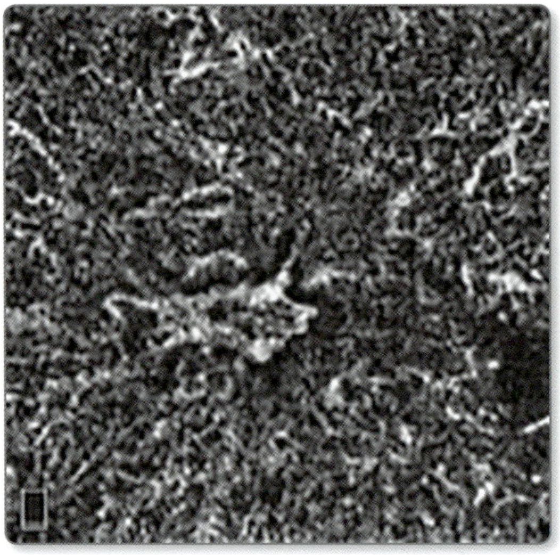

Figure 4 *'En face'* optical coherence tomography (OCT) angiography small irregular type 1 choroidal neovascularization (CNV) net. (Optovue)

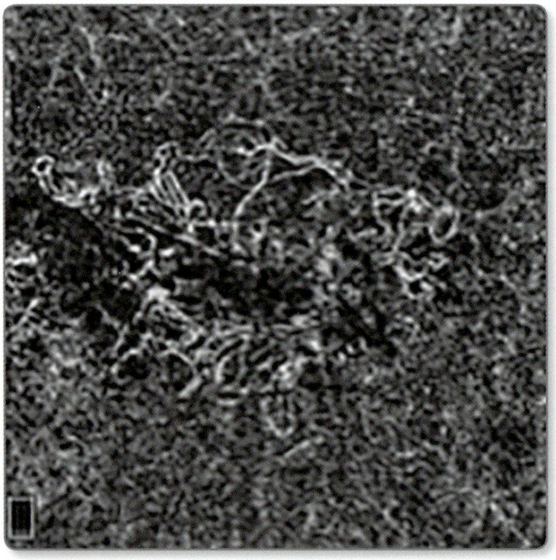

Figure 5A *'En face'* optical coherence tomography (OCT) angiography. Type 1 bush-like new vessels, with thin dense profuse capillaries. Loops are seen at the network periphery. The feeder vessels are difficult to see. A peripheral arcade and dark halo surround the new vessels. The fine capillaries, vessel loops, and the anastomoses show that this choroidal neovascularization (CNV) has high activity. (Optovue)

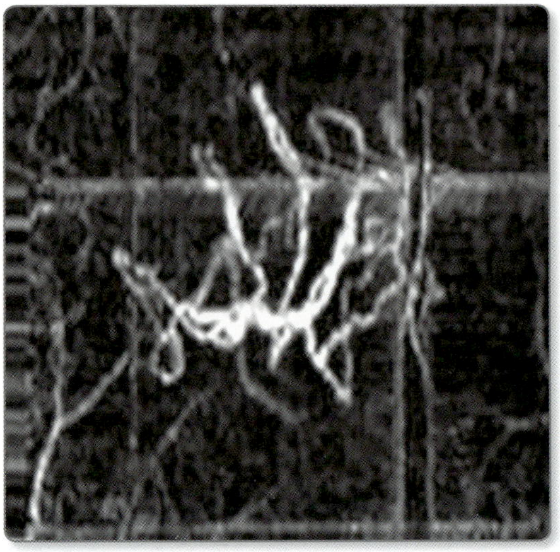

Figure 5B *'En face'* optical coherence tomography (OCT) angiography bare tree. Type 1 choroidal neovascularization (CNV) with bare tree features: very few loops, no peripheral arcade, and no small capillaries. A dark halo surrounds the new vessels. The residual vessels are stiff, thick, and straight. This CNV is quiescent. Bare tree CNVs are frequently the result of adequate CNV treatment. (Optovue)

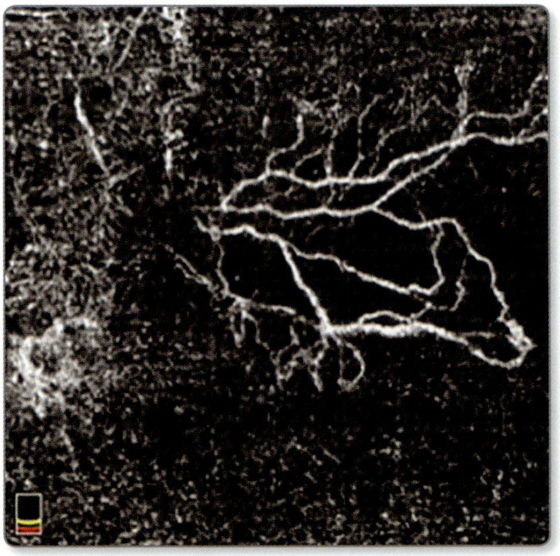

Figure 6 *'En face'* optical coherence tomography (OCT) angiography. Type 1 filament-like choroidal neovascularization (CNV) in central serous chorioretinopathy (CSC). The filament-like tangled new vessels are typically seen in pachychoroid disorders and in chronic epitheliopathy where they are observed in 20/30% of cases. Fine capillaries vessel loops and anastomoses are lacking. (Optovue)

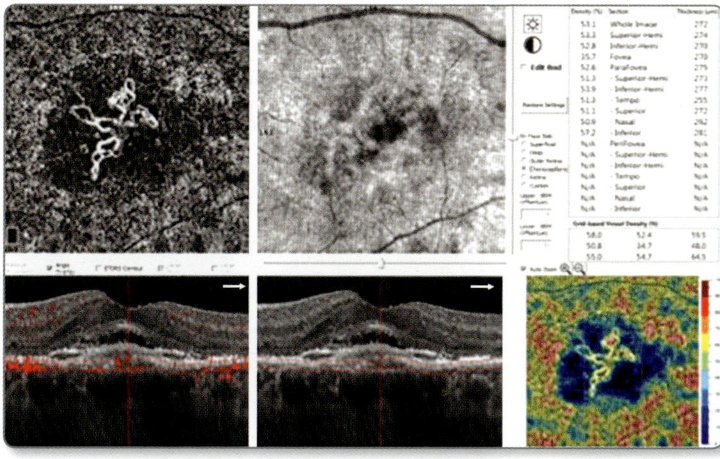

Figure 7 Dark halo around choroidal neovascularization (CNV). Optical coherence tomography (OCT) sheet showing angio *en face* OCT, angio OCT B-scan, *en face* structural OCT, structural OCT B-scan, and vascular Density map. There is a large dark or black halo or dark circle around the new vessels. The halo could be due to morphological changes in the choriocapillaris, screen effect or choriocapillaris blood flow alterations, or blood sequestering. Halo area fluctuates in conjunction with the new vessels area. (Optovue)

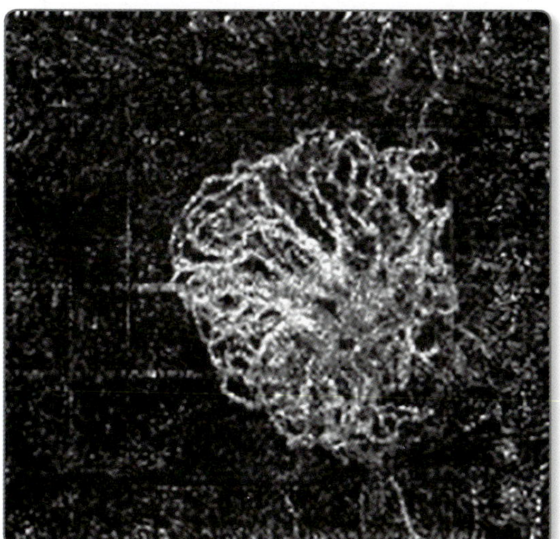

Figure 8 Type 1 new vessels coral bush shaped. *En face* optical coherence tomography (OCT) angiography flow. Capillaries are densely packed, small, and thin. The peripheral vascular arcade is complete, central core feeder vessels are apparent. A dark halo surrounds the new vessels. Halo cause is still discussed: it could be due to morphological changes in the choriocapillaris, screen effect or choriocapillaris blood flow alterations, or blood sequestering. (Optovue)

Box 13: Possible causes of perilesional dark halo

- Morphological changes in the choriocapillaris
- Choriocapillaris blood flow variations
- Slow blood flow
- Pulsating blood flow
- Blood sequestering
- Screen effect (fluid, pigment, and hemorrhage)

Box 14: Type 2 choroidal neovascularization (CNV) morphology

- Coral bush shaped
- Fan shaped
- Medusa head
- Wheel shaped
- Arborization
- Star shaped

Type 2 new vessels (formerly classic CNV) (Figure 9)

Localization

These vessels develop in the subretinal space above the pigment epithelium and penetrate into the outer avascular area. Intraretinal fluid (diffuse edema and cystoid edema) and retinal elevations are constant.

Fluorescein angiography

Type 2 classic new vessels are more easily sharply seen and smaller than type 1 occult new vessels, and hyperfluorescence is more marked.

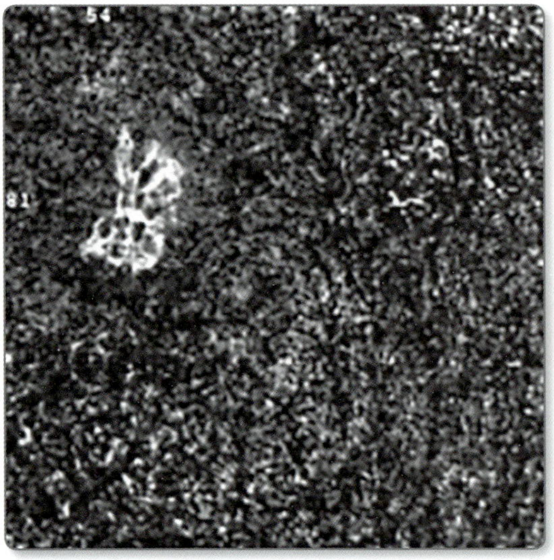

Figure 9 Type 2 small new vessels with irregular shape. A feeder core and a peripheral arcade are evident. A dark halo surrounds the new vessels. Type 2 choroidal neovascularizations (CNVs) are located above retinal pigment epithelium (RPE) and below retina. They are generally smaller than type 1 CNV. (Optovue)

Structural OCT features

The neovascular membrane is seen as a reflective formation. Type 2 membranes may be located directly in front of the retinal pigment epithelium and, at times, they merge with the disorganized pigment epithelium and invade the retina. Cystoid and diffuse edema, hyper-reflective small speckles, and hemorrhages are almost always present.

OCT angiography features

Type 2 new vessels are located above the pigment epithelium. Flow is high. They later spread more deeply into retina. The network area is smaller than in type 1. Capillaries are densely packed. Loops are seen in periphery and contribute to the formation of a continuous arcade, the wheel, and fan-like new vessels. A large feeder trunk or a bundle of feeder vessels are always found. There is always a dark halo around the new vessels. Dye angiography and OCT show exudation (**Boxes 13** to **17**).

Type 3 new vessels, also known as retinal angiomatous proliferations or chorioretinal anastomosis (Figure 10)

Type 3 NVs develop in the neurosensory retina at the deep vascular retinal network level

Box 15: Type 3 choroidal neovascularization (CNV) morphology

- Tuft shaped
- Star shaped

Box 16: Type 1 + 2 choroidal neovascularization (CNV) morphology

Type 1 + 2 CNVs include two or more vascular parallel flat stratified formations overlaid at several levels: Type 2 new vessels above the pigment epithelium. Deeper down, underneath the pigment epithelium but above Bruch's membrane, one or more larger and irregular type 1 CNV:

Morphology of type 1 CNV in mixed CNV:

- Coral shaped
- Fan shaped
- Medusa head
- Wheel shaped
- Tangled
- Arborization
- Bare tree
- Filamentary

Morphology of type 2 CNV in mixed CNV:

- Coral shaped
- Fan shaped
- Medusa head
- Wheel shaped
- Arborization
- Star shaped

Box 17: Exudative choroidal neovascularization (CNV) evolution: maturation, arterialization features

- Capillaries become wider, thicker, and straighter
- Thin capillaries disappear
- Later fibrosis and photoreceptors alterations
- Dark halo around the new vessels

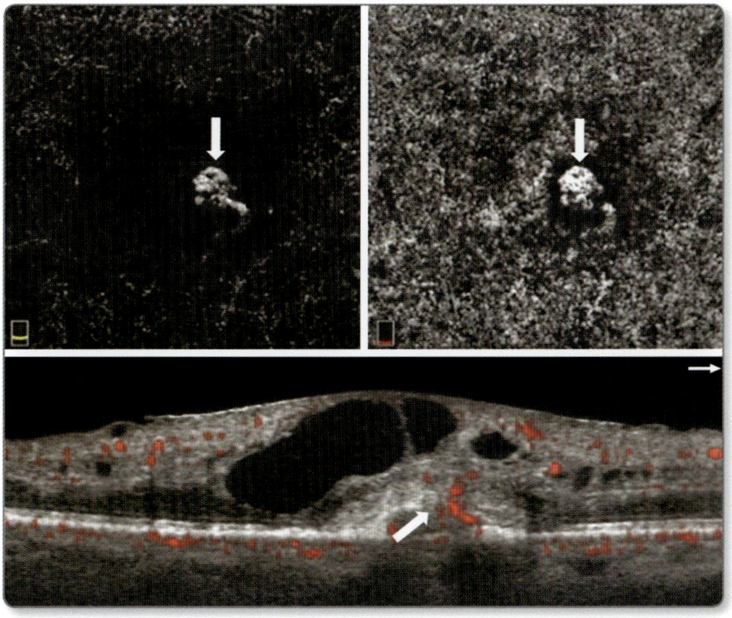

Figure 10 Type 3 choroidal neovascularization (CNV), optical coherence tomography (OCT) angiography. Type 3 new vessels located in the avascular outer retina. In the right-hand side figure, the small tuft-shaped CNV is surrounded by projection artifacts from the inner vascular nets. In the left-hand side image, the projection artifacts from the inner vascular nets have been removed by Optovue software. Cross-section angio scan shows type 3 new vessels located in the deep avascular outer retina, close to a pigment epithelium detachment. Cystoid edema with large irregular cells. Arrows indicate new vessels. (Optovue)

and expand rapidly toward the RPE. Later, neovascularization enlarges and extends deeply towards the pigment epithelium ('kissing' a small RPE detachment) and, superficially towards the retinal surface. Pigment epithelium detachment appears, enclosing vessels that merge with vessels from retina to form anastomosis. It is always associated with widespread diffuse retinal edema. Cystoid cavities appear rapidly. Fluorescein angiography (FA) and indocyanine green angiography (ICGA) of type 3 NVs show a hyperfluorescent intraretinal vascular formation, characterized by retinal–retinal anastomosis, with a hot spot in ICGA frames (**Boxes 18** to **20**).

OCT angiography features

Optical coherence tomographic angiography in type 3 NVs shows a retinal–retinal anastomosis originating from the deep capillary vascular plexus forming a tuft-shaped or glomerular-shaped high-flow network in the outer retina. NVs later will merge with vessels in the sub-RPE space and with vessels from choroid.

Exudative CNV evolution: Disciform scar

After 1 year and numerous intravitreal injections, arterialization features appear: capillaries become wider, thicker, and straighter (**Figure 11**). Outer retinal layer lesions show pigment deposits,

Box 18: Causes of subretinal neovascular membranes

Very frequent:

- Age-related macular degeneration (AMD)
- Idiopathic polypoidal vasculopathy
- Retinal angiomatous proliferations (RAP)
- Myopia

Frequent:

- Idiopathic new vessels in young patients
- Presumed histoplasmosis
- Traumatic choroidal ruptures
- Laser-induced NV
- Angioid streaks
- Choroiditis

Rare:

- Vogt-Koyanagi-Harada (VKH) disease
- Inflammatory
- Serpiginous
- Choroidal nevus
- Osteoma
- Pseudovitelliform macular dystrophy
- Stargardt disease
- Best disease

Box 19: Causes of choroidal neovascularization (CNV) in children

- Myopia
- Stargardt disease
- Best disease
- Inflammatory
- Choroiditis
- Vogt-Koyanagi-Harada (VKH) disease
- Presumed histoplasmosis
- Serpiginous
- Idiopathic
- Traumatic choroidal ruptures
- Laser induced

Box 20: Causes of retinal scars

- Advanced macular degeneration
- Diabetic fibrovascular membrane
- Laser scars
- Chorioretinitis
- Myopia
- Traumatic choroidal ruptures
- Laser photocoagulation
- Angioid streaks

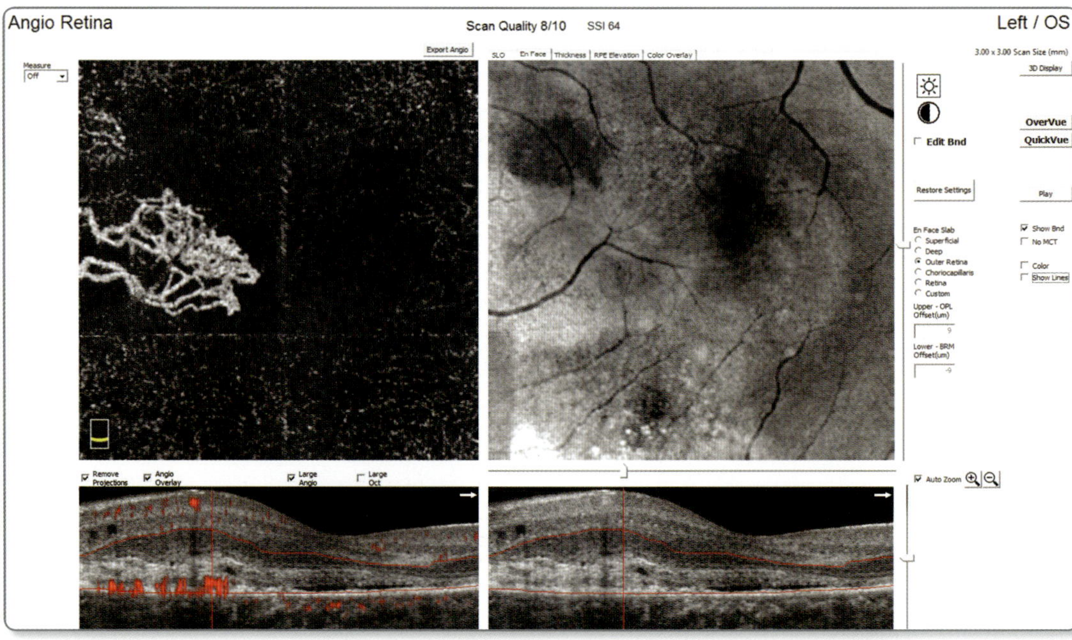

Figure 11 Type 2 choroidal neovascularization (CNV) arterialized vessels, optical coherence tomography (OCT) angiography, and angio B-scan. After repeated numerous intravitreal injections, arterialization features appear. Capillaries become wider, thicker, and straighter while the thinner capillaries disappear. Outer retinal layer lesions are frequent with fibrosis and photoreceptor alterations. There is a dense dark halo around the new vessels. Arterialization features appear approximately after 1 year and half treatment duration. (Optovue)

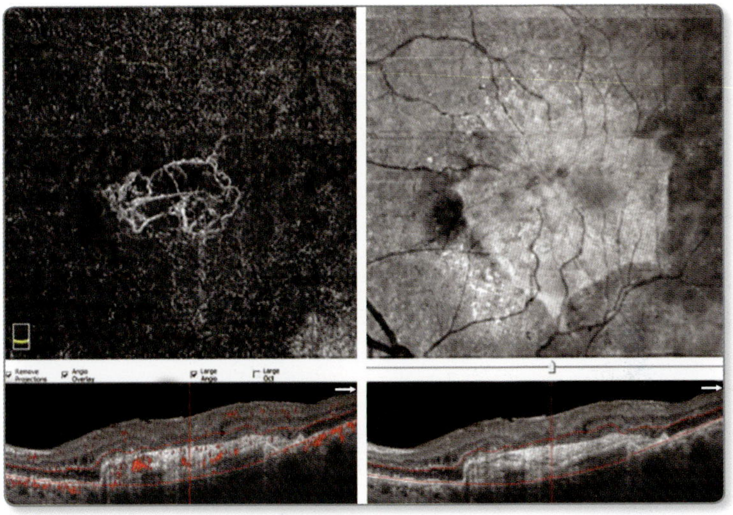

Figure 12 Fibrotic scar with nonexudative vessels. After a long evolution and many anti-vascular endothelial growth factor (VEGF) injections, a fibrovascular scar has formed. Optical coherence tomography (OCT) angiography (left-hand figure): inside the fibrous scar tissue some large vessels thick and straight, with an irregular flow persist. No thin capillaries or fine loops are visible. On the right-hand figure ('*en face*' scan), a large fibrovascular irregular scar is evident. The angio B-scan highlights the still flowing vessels. (Optovue) (Projection Artifact Removal Software on)

fibrosis, and photoreceptors alterations. There is always a dark halo around the new vessels. Later, a fibrovascular scar appears with large nonexudative vessels, thick and straight, with an irregular flow. A fibrous pigmented large disciform scar develops with severe irremediable vision loss. Vessels may be exudative or nonexudative (**Figure 12** and **Box 21**).

Nonexudative choroidal neovascularization (silent, quiescent, and asymptomatic CNV)

Since the advent of OCT angiography, we know that about 10–20% of neovascularizations are not exposed by fluorescein angiography. Quiescent NVs were unknown during the fluorescein era, and have been described in the first days of angio-OCT by Bailey and David Huang. Non-exudative choroidal neovascularization is not rare in patients with normal thickness choroid and frequent in thick choroid. We do not yet know if exudative and nonexudative CNVs are a single disease with many clinical aspects, or successive stages of the same disease or group completely different diseases or different, successive later stages of a single disease (See Chapter 14).

Box 21: Fibrovascular scar

- Vessels, sparse, large, thick, and straight
- Exudative or nonexudative
- Irregular or slow flow
- Lacking thin capillaries
- Lacking loop
- Lacking arcade
- Dense halo due to fibrous tissue screen effect

13 Nonexudative, silent, subclinical, quiescent choroidal neovascularization clinical features and practical implications

Bruno Lumbroso, Marco Rispoli, Maria Cristina Savastano

Introduction

David Huang, Steven Bailey, and Yali Jia, using optical coherence tomographic angiography (OCTA), detected in 2014 for the first time the existence of nonexudative choroidal neovascularization (CNV). These nonexudative CNVs are not rare, but they were impossible to identify with fluorescein angiography and structural OCT. OCT angiography diagnosis of nonexudative CNV is highly sensitive and specific. They do not show leakage on fluorescein angiography nor retinal fluid on OCT, but can be seen as faint new vessels or plaques on ICGA frames. In OCT angiography, they are frequently associated to a flat, irregular retinal pigment epithelium (RPE) detachment, but without visible fluid.

Their significance and natural history are not perfectly known.

We do not yet know all the implications, relevance, and natural evolution of nonexudative CNV. At present, it is uncertain whether one is the predecessor of the other or if they are two separate clinical entities. We are not sure if 'nonexudative choroidal CNV' describes an atypical type 1 CNV, or may be sometimes, a completely different entity.

Nonexudative CNVs are type 1 CNVs. They appear under the pigment epithelium flat detachment: These patients with vascular age-related macular degeneration (AMD) show drusen and pigment deposits around fovea and no evidence of macular fluid on structural OCT imaging.

Pathophysiology

David Huang, Steven Bailey, and Jia state that these vessels have adequate capillary endothelial or RPE barrier function to prevent fluid from exuding into the retinal tissue, and visual function is not affected. They write that relationship between exudative and nonexudative CNV is unknown (see Chapter 14).

Etiology

Nonexudative NVs comprise most probably histologically more mature vessels with competent endothelial cell junctions. They are observed in different and dissimilar occurrences.

- They are frequently seen in pachychoroid group of disorders
- They can also be seen in late evolution of treated type 1 exudative AMD
- Some cases of nonexudative CNV have been described in intermediate AMD
- Other nonexudative choroidal neovascularization cases are seen as residual blood channels in fibrotic scars
- Most of them have been described as stage preceding exudative CNV
- Some could be separate unknown entities (**Boxes 1** to **3**)

Box 1: Classification of nonexudative choroidal neovascularization (CNV)

- Nonexudative type 1 CNV in AMD
- Nonexudative type 1 CNV in pachychoroid
- Nonexudative type 1 CNV intermediate AMD
- Nonexudative precursor to exudative type 1 CNV
- Exudative type 1 CNV evolution to nonexudative CNV after treatment
- Arterialized CNV after treatment
- Nonexudative CNV as residual blood channels in fibrotic scars
- Nonexudative separate clinical entity (or entities)

(AMD: age-related macular degeneration)

Box 2: Nonexudative new vessels management

- Close follow-up without treatment

Box 3: Nature of nonexudative choroidal neovascularization (CNV) (Bailey, Yali, and Huang)

- Precursor to exudative CNV
- More mature vessels with competent endothelial cell junctions
- Separate entity from exudative CNV

Terminology

Nonexudative: Quiescent, subclinical, silent, asymptomatic

Localization

Nonexudative new vessels develop at the posterior pole under a pigment epithelium flat wavy detachment, often between the elevated pigment epithelium and Bruch's membrane: They could represent a different subtype of type 1 CNV. The patients show frequently drusen and pigment deposits around fovea and no evidence of macular fluid on structural OCT imaging.

Dye angiography

It does not allow generally to diagnose non exudative CNV: Fluorescein angiography features: No leakage no hyperfluorescence, indocyanine green (ICG) features: generally, in early frames, the feeder vessel and its ramifications can be seen. In the late ICG frames, a plaque with sharp limits can be observed.

Structural OCT features

A flat irregular or undulated pigment epithelium elevation can be noted. No fluid is observed.

OCT angiography features

Morphology

Shape is mostly irregular, in 20% rounded. The capillaries are generally sparse, the vessels may appear thick. They show generally low-capillary density with rare branches subdivision and arborisation. Sometimes, they are long-tangled filaments with rare small capillaries. Loops are occasional, vessels are thick and twisting. Generally they appear as tangled network or filament like. Nonexudative CNVs have rare small capillaries. Feeder vessels are not or are rarely seen (**Figure 1**).

Arterialized CNV after repeated recurrences and treatments may show similar features with thicker and straighter vessels, rigid in aspect with lack of the thinner capillaries. These arterialized vessels can show little or no leakage at fluorescein angiography, raising the issue if nonexudative CNV may be sometimes a result of treatment.

Size

Most nonexudative membranes are large networks with large vessels and very few or no small capillaries.

Perilesional dark halo

No or little halo is seen around the new vessels. This could be due to minor morphological changes in the choriocapillaris, less screen effect, or less choriocapillaris blood flow alterations.

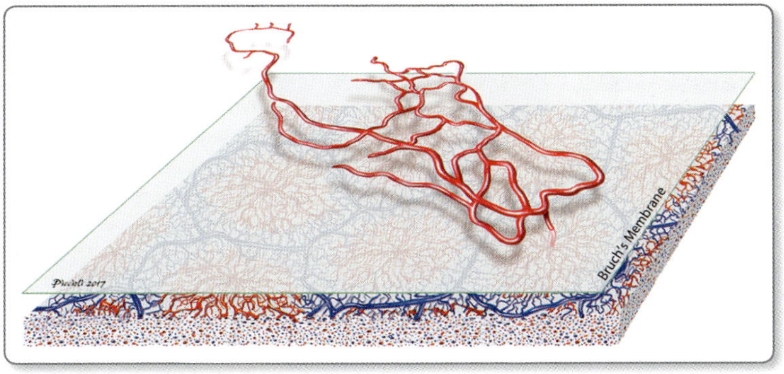

Figure 1 Nonexudative nrew vessels: Shape is mostly irregular, the capillaries are sparse, the vessels show low-capillary density with rare branches. In the case shown here they are long-tangled filaments with rare small capillaries.

Nonexudative CNVs natural history

The evolution of these nonexudative CNVs is very slow. However, they increase slowly in size, sometimes doubling in 3 years. According to David Huang, 80% of them begin to exudate after 1 or 2 years.

In our observation (Lumbroso, Rispoli, Savastano), nonexudative CNVs shape and size may remain unchanged for years. Most grow slowly, without becoming exudative, during follow-up (our personal cases have 4 years follow-up). Vision remains unchanged. The 4-year CNV area curve shows a progressive irregular increase in the CNV area with acute growth spurts. The growth is irregular. However, in half of the cases, the CNV area has more than doubled in 3 years. In the other half of the CNV area, they remain stable with acute growth and regression episodes.

Nonexudative CNV as precursor to exudation

David Huang et al. presented data on a series of eyes with intermediate age-related macular degeneration. They used OCTA to evaluate 63 eyes with intermediate AMD and exudation in the fellow eye. Ten eyes were found to have nonexudative CNV either on the initial scan or a subsequent scan during 24 or more months of follow-up. Of those 10 eyes, eight (80%) progressed to exudation, which occurred within 10 months. In most of the eyes, exudation developed within 6 months. Furthermore, the change from nonexudative CNV to exudative CNV was preceded by rapid growth in lesion size as measured by OCTA. Huang study suggests that nonexudative CNV is a precursor to exudation and should be monitored closely with OCTA. A logical next step would be randomized trials to evaluate whether prophylactic treatment of nonexudative CNV could prevent exudation and save vision in the long-term at reasonable costs. The growth rate of nonexudative lesions as measured by OCTA could be used as the guide for starting and stopping antivascular endothelial growth factor (VEGF) treatment and should be considered in the design of such trials.[1-5]

P Rosenfeld suggests that ability of OCTA to provide noninvasive, fast, detailed, depth-resolved identification of nonexudative neovascular lesions in eyes with AMD suggests the need for a new classification system.

Steven Bailey, Yali Jia, and David Huang conclude that “the real utility will be to observe over time, to learn nonexudative CNVs natural history, which may remain quiescent for long periods of time, regress or wax and wane. It is likely that many quiescent CNVs are precursor to exudative CNV, but a proportion of it potentially also represents more mature vessels with competent endothelial cell junctions or be a separate entity from exudative CNV. Only when features of nonexudative quiescent CNVs are understood the technology be useful to influence prognosis and treatment. Further longitudinal studies are needed to establish what constitute high-risk features. These studies could also shed light on other questions such as the effect of anti-VEGF on nonexudative CNV in the fellow eye.[5-8]

Management

Management of subclinical nonexudative NV is discussed. Close monitoring is advised by most authors, using frequently repeated structural OCT scans and OCT angiography to follow evolution.

David Huang presented data on a series of eyes with intermediate age-related macular degeneration where 80% subclinical CNV progressed to exudation within 10 months. In most of the eyes, exudation developed within 6 months. Furthermore, the change from nonexudative CNV to exudative CNV was preceded by rapid growth in lesion size as measured by OCTA. Huang study suggests that nonexudative CNV is a precursor to exudation.

Randomized trials are necessary to evaluate whether prophylactic treatment of nonexudative CNV could prevent exudation and save vision in the long-term at reasonable costs. David Huang thinks that the growth rate of nonexudative lesions as measured by OCTA could be used as the guide for starting and stopping anti-VEGF treatment and should be considered in the design of such trials (**Boxes 4** to **6**).

Conclusion

1. About 80% quiescent nonexudative, subclinical CNVs are precursors to exudative CNV, observed by David Huang
2. Most probably they are histologically more mature vessels with competent endothelial cell junctions
3. Some may be a separate entity from exudative CNV

Box 4: Etiology of nonexudative choroidal neovascularization (CNV)

- Pachychoroid group of disorders
- AMD
- Late evolution of treated type 1 exudative AMD
- Wet age-related macular degeneration
- Intermediate AMD
- Atrophic AMD
- Stage preceding exudative CNV
- Exudative CNV may evolve to nonexudative CNV after treatment
- Residual blood channels in fibrotic scars
- Separate clinical entities

(AMD: age-related macular degeneration)

Box 5: Detection of nonexudative new vessels

- Slab between outer retina and Bruch's membrane

Box 6: Nonexudative new vessels: What to do?

- Close follow-up without treatment

References

1. Palejwala NV, Jia Y, Gao SS, et al. Detection of nonexudative choroidal neovascularization in age-related macular degeneration with optical coherence tomography angiography. Retina 2015; 35:2204–2211.
2. Querques G, Souied EH. Vascularized drusen: Slowly progressive type 1 neovascularization mimicking drusenoid retinal pigment epithelium elevation. Retina 2015; 35:2433–2439.
3. Roisman L, Zhang Q, Wang RK, et al. Optical coherence tomography angiography of asymptomatic neovascularization in intermediate age-related macular degeneration. Ophthalmology 2016; 123:1309–1319.
4. Sarks SH. New vessel formation beneath the retinal pigment epithelium in senile eyes. Br J Ophthalmol 1973; 57:951–965.
5. Querques G, Srour M, Massamba N, et al. Functional characterization and multimodal imaging of treatment-naive "quiescent" choroidal neovascularization. Invest Ophthalmol Vis Sci 2013; 54:6886–6892.
6. Grunwald JE, Daniel E, Huang J, et al. Risk of geographic atrophy in the comparison of age-related macular degeneration treatments trials. Ophthalmology 2014; 121:150–161.
7. de Oliveira Dias JR, Zhang Q, Garcia JMB, et al. Natural History of Subclinical Neovascularization in Nonexudative Age-Related Macular Degeneration Using Swept-Source OCT Angiography. Ophthalmology 2018; 125:255–266.
8. Yanagi Y, Mohla A, Lee S, et al. Incidence of fellow eye involvement in patients with unilateral exudative age-related macular degeneration. JAMA Ophthalmol 2018; 136:905–11.

14 Nonexudative choroidal neovascularization

David Huang, Yali Jia, Steven T Bailey

Because optical coherence tomographic angiography (OCTA) detects choroidal neovascularization (CNV) with high sensitivity and specificity and is noninvasive and fast, it is introducing us to better ways of diagnosing and monitoring patients with age-related macular degeneration (AMD). Of significant interest is the ability of OCTA to detect and monitor nonexudative CNV.[1] While it is possible to identify nonexudative CNV with indocyanine green angiography (ICGA), the time, expense, and risk associated with ICGA make it impractical for frequent assessment. OCTA eliminates these barriers, making it easy to keep close tabs on nonexudative CNV.

There are several possible variants of nonexudative CNV that can be segregated as either treatment naïve, or previously treated CNV. Treatment-naïve nonexudative CNV occurs when pathologic vessels from the choroid grow through Bruch's membrane (BM) into the subretinal pigment epithelium (RPE) space, however, these vessels have adequate capillary endothelial or RPE barrier function to prevent fluid from exuding into the retinal tissue, and visual function is not affected. Previously treated nonexudative CNV refers to CNV that has responded to anti-vascular endothelial growth factor (VEGF) therapy. Treatment-responsive CNV may include cases that require ongoing intermittent anti-VEGF treatments to prevent exudation and CNV growth. CNV in remission refers to treated CNV that has had no recurrence of exudation for greater than 12 months without treatment.

This chapter focuses on treatment-naïve nonexudative CNV, which has also been called subclinical neovascularization.[1] This entity was rarely discovered prior to the advent of OCTA. But clinicians who routinely screen intermediate AMD patients with OCTA find it to be a common condition.[2-4]

In a prospective longitudinal observational study conducted by our research team at the Casey Eye Institute,[2] we used OCTA to evaluate 63 eyes with intermediate AMD and exudation in the fellow eye at baseline and 6-month intervals for 2 years. Ten eyes were found to have nonexudative CNV either on the initial scan or a subsequent scan during the 24 or more months of follow-up. Of those 10 eyes, eight (80%) progressed to exudation, which occurred within 10 months. In most of the eyes, exudation developed within 6 months. Comparing the rate of occurrence of exudation between the eyes with and without nonexudative CNV, the Cox hazard ratio was 18. Furthermore, the change from nonexudative CNV to exudative CNV was preceded by rapid growth in lesion size as measured by OCTA (an example is shown in **Figure 1**). Nonexudative CNV did not appear in 53 of the eyes during the study. Those eyes had a lower risk of developing exudation.

Our study suggests that nonexudative CNV is a precursor to exudation and should be monitored closely with OCTA. Since exudation could cause irreversible visual loss, the logical next steps would be to evaluate whether prophylactic anti-VEGF treatment of nonexudative CNV could prevent exudation and save vision in the long term at reasonable costs. Prospective randomized trials are needed. The growth rate of nonexudative lesions as measured by OCTA could be used as the guide for starting and stopping such anti-VEGF treatment and should be considered in the design of such trials.

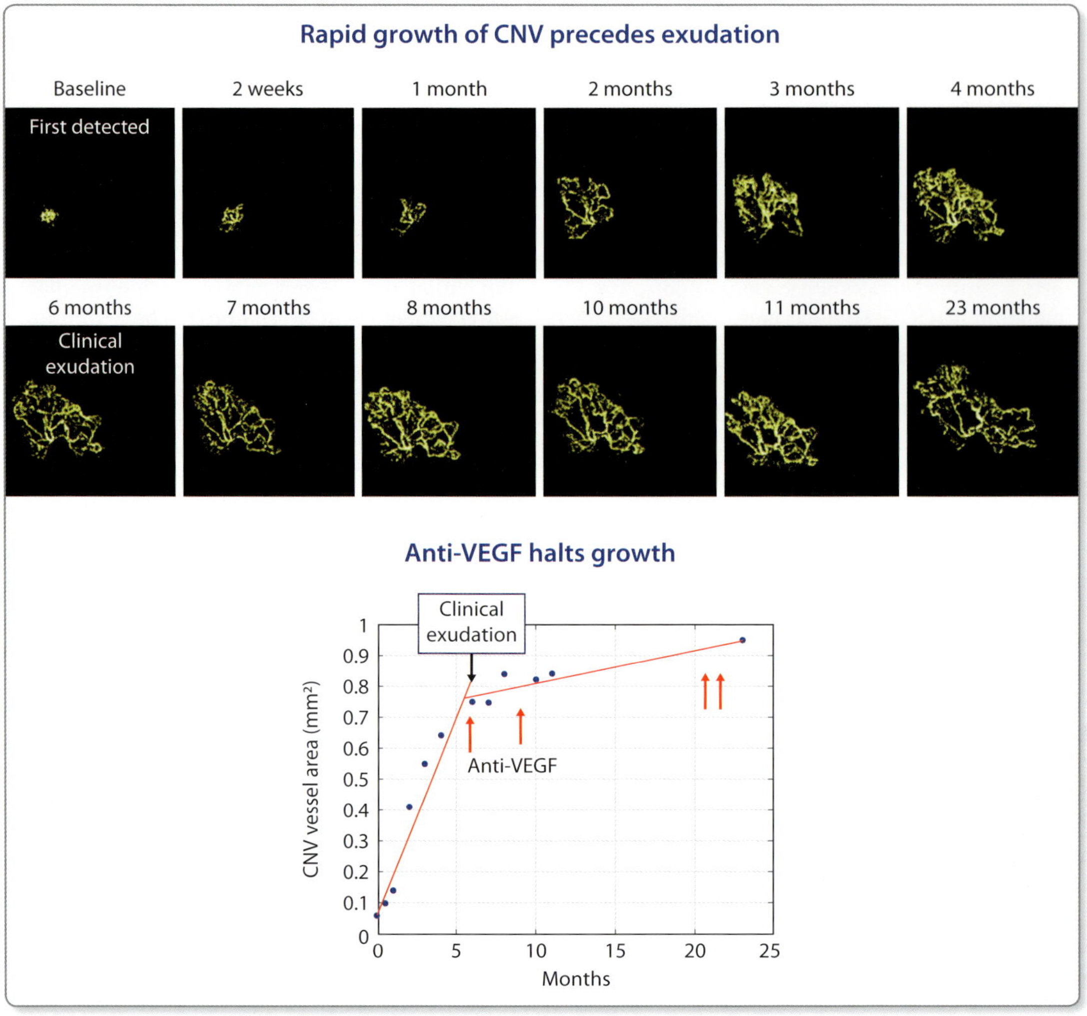

Figure 1 In a typical case of treatment-naïve nonexudative choroidal neovascularization (CNV, type 1), optical coherence tomographic angiography (OCTA) shows rapid growth in vessel area in the 6 months between detection and exudation. After antivascular endothelial growth factor (VEGF) treatment was initiated, the growth rate dramatically slowed down.

References

1 de Oliveira Dias JR, Zhang Q, Garcia JMB, et al. Natural history of subclinical neovascularization in nonexudative age-related macular degeneration Using Swept-source OCT Angiography. Ophthalmology 2018; 125:255–266.

2 Palejwala NV, Jia Y, Gao SS, et al. Detection of nonexudative choroidal neovascularization in age-related macular degeneration with optical coherence tomography angiography. Retina 2015; 35:2204–2211.

3 Yanagi Y, Mohla A, Lee S, et al. Incidence of fellow eye involvement in patients with unilateral exudative age-related macular degeneration. JAMA Ophthalmol 2018; 136:905–911.

4 Carnevali A, Cicinelli MV, Capuano V, et al. Optical Coherence Tomography Angiography: A Useful Tool for Diagnosis of Treatment-Naïve Quiescent Choroidal Neovascularization. Am J Ophthalmol 2016; 169:189–98.

15 Exudative CNV evolution after treatment, CNV activity, CNV quiescence

Bruno Lumbroso, Marco Rispoli

CNV evolution after treatment

Choroidal neovascularization (CNV) treatment should be early, immediately after symptoms appear. Treatment effectiveness is less positive in real life than in clinical trial data. Patient should be treated with accurate loading dose and closely monitored for treatment and retreatment.

Early evolution after treatment

Twenty-four hours after the injection, the vascular network is abruptly reduced and shows capillary fragmentation. The flow is disrupted immediately: secondary branches and most of the loops disappear immediately after the intravitreal injection. This could be due to a slower flow or due to a pulsated flow, which makes circulation invisible, or to a true temporary closure of the capillaries involved. Central efferent branches always remain visible.

The secondary branches and most of the loops continue to decrease slowly until the 10th–15th day. The dark halo dimensions decrease markedly.

About 20–25 days after, few branches reappear.

About 30–50 days after, the main vessels reappear and are wider and thicker compared with the naive vessels. They are less winding, with a faster flow. According to Sarraf, these immature CNVs are formed of many tangled new vessels associated with a form of peripheral 'fringe'. They have significant growth potential.

Later, the increase in flow leads to a histological change and to vessel maturation.

New branches appear and preexisting thin branches reappear whose diameter increased (**Figures 1** to **4**).[1]

Maturation appears after 6 months, permanent after 1 year (Figures 5 and 6)

After 6 months of maturation onset, the main framework vessels are clearly delineated. Small capillaries continue to disappear and reappear following 60-day cycles. Peripheral anastomoses are the first vessels to disappear. After each treatment, the framework vessels reappear with increased flow and decreased branch density. Maturation begins after 6 months: vessels

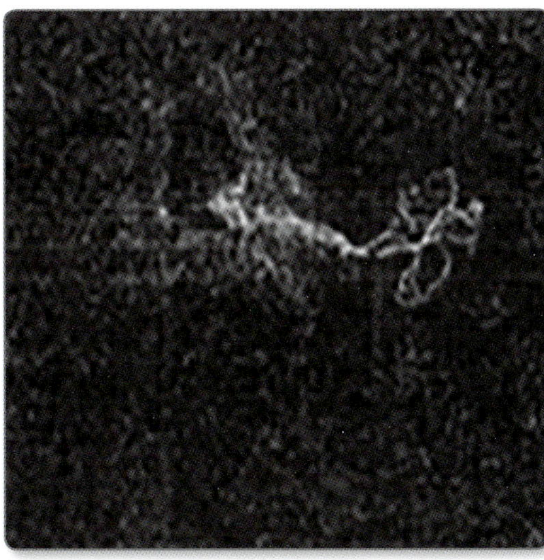

Figure 1 Type 1 choroidal neovascularization (CNV) 1–24 hours after the injection: regression of new vessels. Optical coherence tomography (OCT) angiography, *en face*. The network is smaller in area, precisely reduced, the vascular fringe is smaller and less dense. Vessels are fragmented and disrupted. Thinner branches disappear. Secondary branches are much less visible. Only larger framework vessels coming from the feeder vessel or from the bundle of feeder vessels survive. (Optovue)

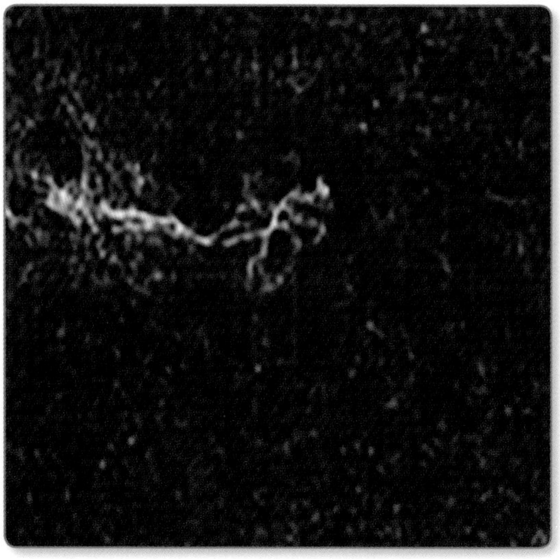

Figure 2 10 days after the injection. The new vessels regression endures and/or progresses lightly. Optical coherence tomography (OCT) angiography, *en face*, the reduction in capillary density progresses up until day 15. Many small capillaries decrease and fade. Larger scaffold vessels coming from the core vessel persist. Finger-like vascular structure is fragmented and partly regressed. (Optovue)

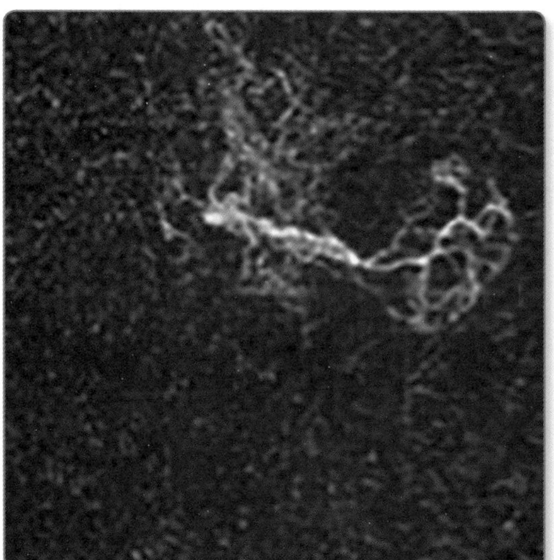

Figure 3 25 days after the injection, progressive reopening of the regressed vessels. Optical coherence tomography (OCT) angiography, *en face*. At 25 days, main framework vessels persist, and some vessels progressively reappear. Branches are thicker and have a higher flow than before treatment. The vessels that re-emerge are straighter and thicker than before the injection. At the finger-like structure, a few fringe capillaries reappear. (Optovue)

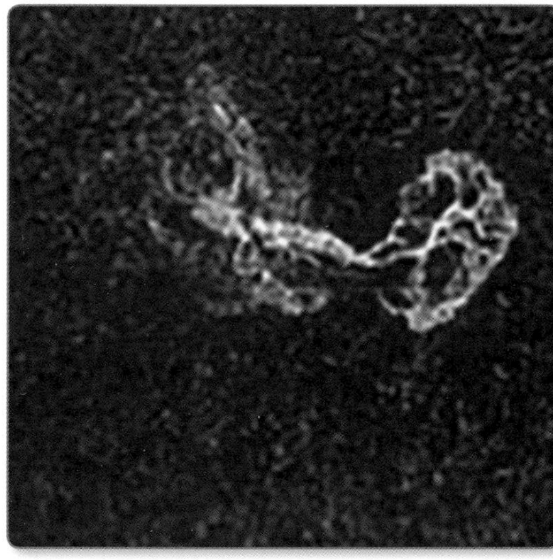

Figure 4 30–35 days after the injection, main scaffold vessels are thicker and small capillaries reappear. Optical coherence tomography (OCT) angiography *en face*. Main scaffold vessels follow the course of the original vessels but are now much thicker and less winding, with a higher flow. The increase in flow and its rapidity act on the walls leading to vessel arterialization. The small capillaries reopen and fringe capillaries recur, very dense again, particularly in the vascular finger. (Optovue)

areless sinuous, thicker, and straighter than the original naïve CNV vessels. Maturation features are permanent 1 year after the first treatment. Scaffold vessels seem to be constant, without variation after new injections. Capillary density decreases permanently.

Sarraf described mature vessels with branches radiating from a central feeder vessel to all directions with dense small capillaries with peripheral arcade and dark halo ring. The sea-fan shape is a variation of the former shape, it displays vessels branching to one side of the main trunk with dense small capillaries with peripheral arcade and dark halo ring.

Later, vessels become hypermature (Sarraf) with the "dead tree" shape, composed by few clipped thick vessels, without small capillaries, without peripheral arcade, and no or small dark halo.

Recurrences (Figure 7)

During evolution, we observe two different kinds of recurrences: the normal, cyclic recurrences that appear after every treatment; and the acute nonperiodic recurrences, occurring independently from treatment.

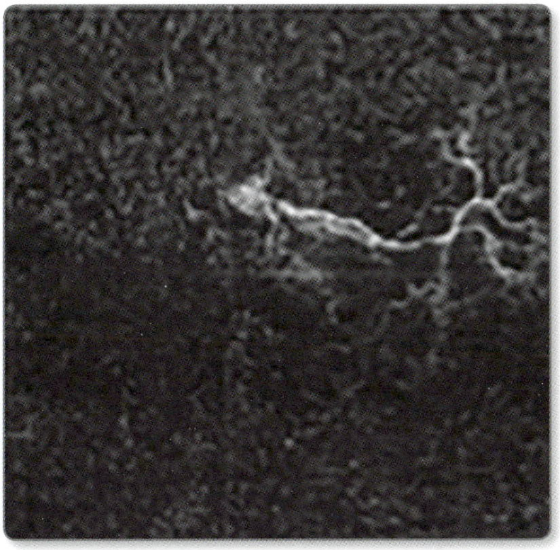

Figure 5 Late evolution, maturation: After many treatments, more than 1 year to 18 months of antivascular endothelial growth factor (VEGF) injections, new vessels show an increased flow, and look mature. Mature vessels are less winding, straighter, and more evident than immature vessels. Altogether their surface is smaller. Residual vessels match with the primary support vessels that had regressed. A very robust vascular framework is able to resist treatment and rematerialize after fading for a few weeks. Few branches are completely new; most are pre-existing thin branches whose diameter increased. Repetitive pruning leads to stalk widening. (Optovue)

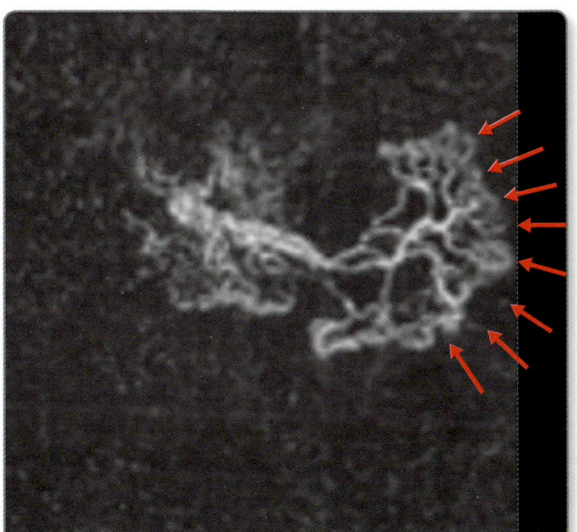

Figure 6 Cyclic recurrence after treatment: Cyclic recurrences are observed regularly after antivascular endothelial growth factor (VEGF) injection treatment. In this case, small capillaries at the end of the finger-like projection replicate and develop again. The cycle duration seems to be quite unvarying: about 60 days. Dense thin capillaries develop at the finger-like vascular stalk (arrows). (Optovue)

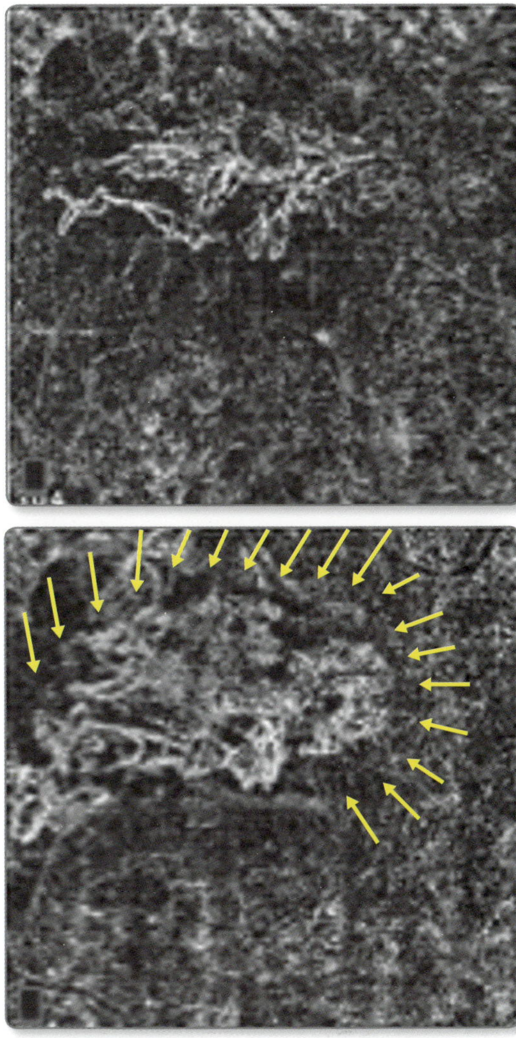

Figure 7 Acute nonperiodic recurrence, optical coherence tomography (OCT) angiography. Upper figure shows quiescent choroidal neovascularization (CNV). Lower figure shows an acute recurrence occurring independently from treatment. All-pervading thin dense vessels sprout from focal hyperdense spots located on CNV loops. In the case shown here, dense thin capillaries develop all over the preexisting CNV. Acute nonperiodic recurrences may occur once or twice a year. (Optovue)

Normal, cyclic recurrences after treatment

The sharp CNV area regression is followed by a slow upwards increase slope till 50–60 days. 30–40 days after injection, a part of lesser vessels reopens. High flow highlights the only large vessels.

The full recurrence is observed 50–60 days after anti-vascular endothelial growth factor (VEGF) injection, after every injection.

After each treatment, the same main vessels seem to reappear with increased flow and decreased branch density. A dark halo area surrounds the CNV. Dark halo dimensions decrease when the vessel density decreases. Before treatment, we observe a complex vascular pattern; after treatment, we see a less complex tangled pattern.

Acute nonperiodic recurrences occurring independently of treatment

Acute nonperiodic recurrences, occurring independently of treatment, show sprout, outgrowth.

They have a specific location: terminal, axillary, lateral, adventitious, localized in different layer. These acute nonperiodic recurrences occur independently of treatment one or twice a year.

Fibrovascular scars (Figures 8 to 12)

After 50 or more injections, the scar develops. Inside the fibrous scar can be seen some large vessels, thick and straight, with an irregular flow, generally nonexudative. The fibrous scar always comprises a residual slow, generally nonexudative, vascular network with dead tree pattern and no thin capillary evident. A dark round halo is present.

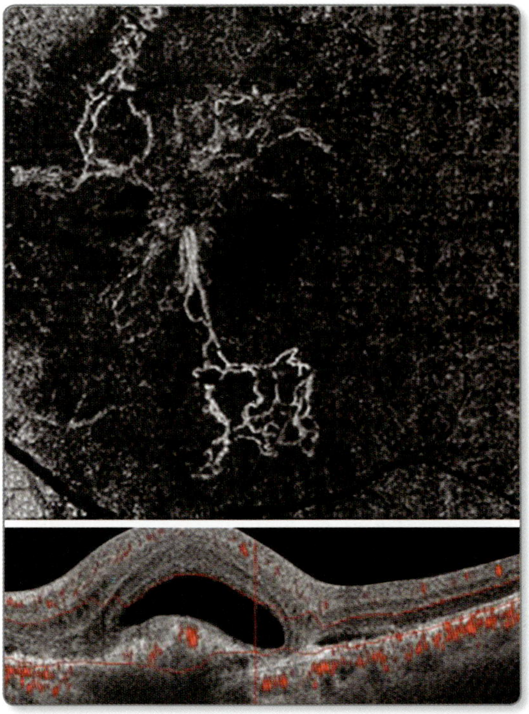

Figure 8 Vascularized fibrous scar. Optical coherence tomography (OCT) angiography. Vascular flow is irregular inside vessels in the fibrous scar. An irregular network includes three apparently separate vascular formations. There are no thin capillaries. A halo (dark round shadow behind and around the neovascular network) is due in this to the fibrous scar shadowing. Angio B-scan shows vascularization inside the scar and retinal serous detachment. (Optovue)

CNV activity features

CNV active or quiescent (Figures 13 to 16)

It is indispensable to detect if a CNV is active or not, in order to decide if treatment is necessary. Sometimes, activity appears evident with structural optical coherence tomography (OCT) imaging. In most cases, OCT angiography shows CNV as an abnormal pattern of vascular flow above Bruch's membrane. OCT angiography (OCTA) is the only imaging technique that can detect nonexudative new vessels. To say if they are active or not is quite another problem. To define 'active' a CNV can be easy during the follow-up of treated new vessels. However, when we see for the first time a naïve nonexudative CNV network, it can be impossible to get to the activity problem solution.[2-7]

Exudative CNV: Active or quiescent?

Histologically, a normal vessel has a well-defined wall structure that does not allow fluids to leak, while the new vessels have an immature and thin wall that may leak fluids. New vessels morphology seems to be very different from the normal vascular tissue. OCTA shows all the CNV features and highlights early vessels and more mature vessels. The wall vessel maturation will create a thicker new vessel with arterial features. These mature new vessels leak less fluids than early new vessels. It is impossible to declare if a CNV is active or quiescent on a single examination.

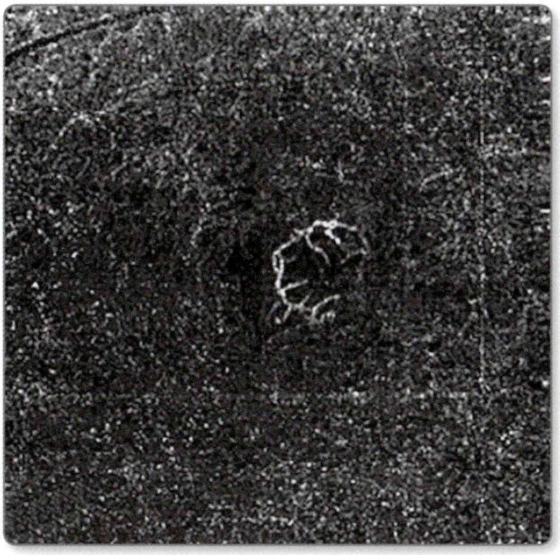

Figure 9 Vascularized fibrous scar. Optical coherence tomography (OCT) angiography. Vascular flow is with rounded shape inside the fibrous scar. (Optovue)

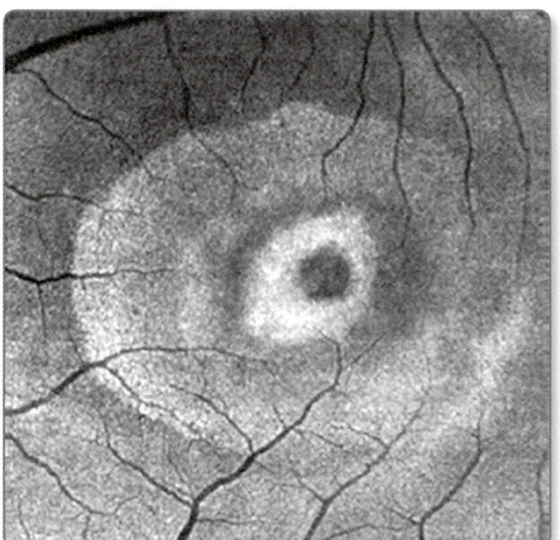

Figure 10 Vascularized fibrous scar. '*En face*' scan. Vascularized fibrous scar seen under a retinal serous detachment. (Optovue)

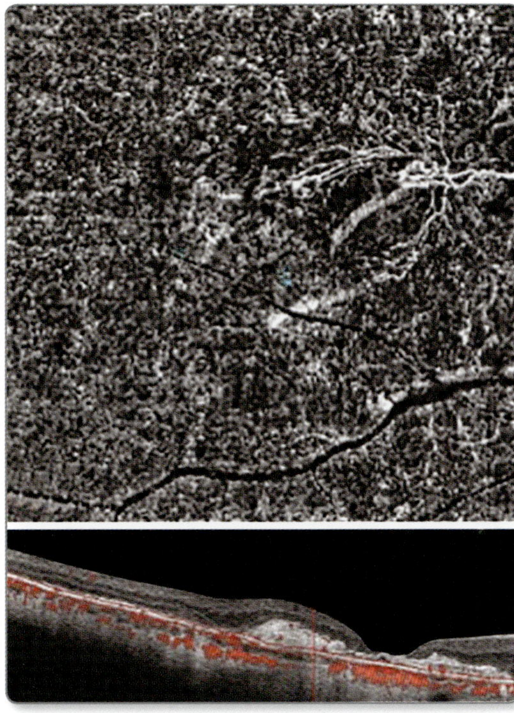

Figure 11 Vascularized fibrous scar. Optical coherence tomography (OCT) angiography and cross-section scan. Irregular vascularized fibrous scar seen inside a fibrous scar. Note retinal atrophy. (Optovue)

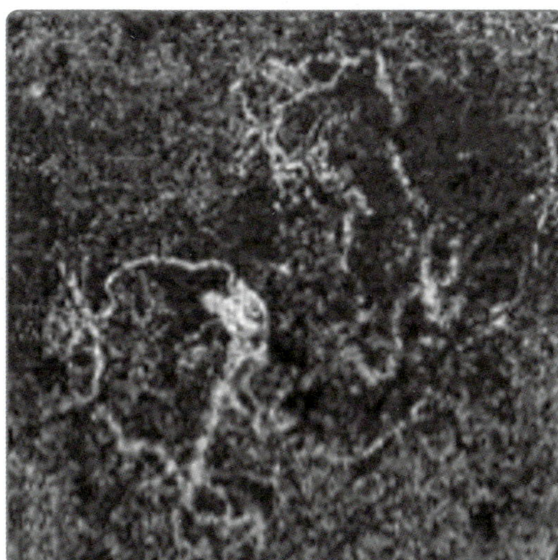

Figure 12 Vascularized fibrous scar. Optical coherence tomography (OCT) angiography. Vascularized fibrous scar seen under a retinal serous detachment. A dense dark halo is caused in this case by the fibrous tissue. (Optovue)

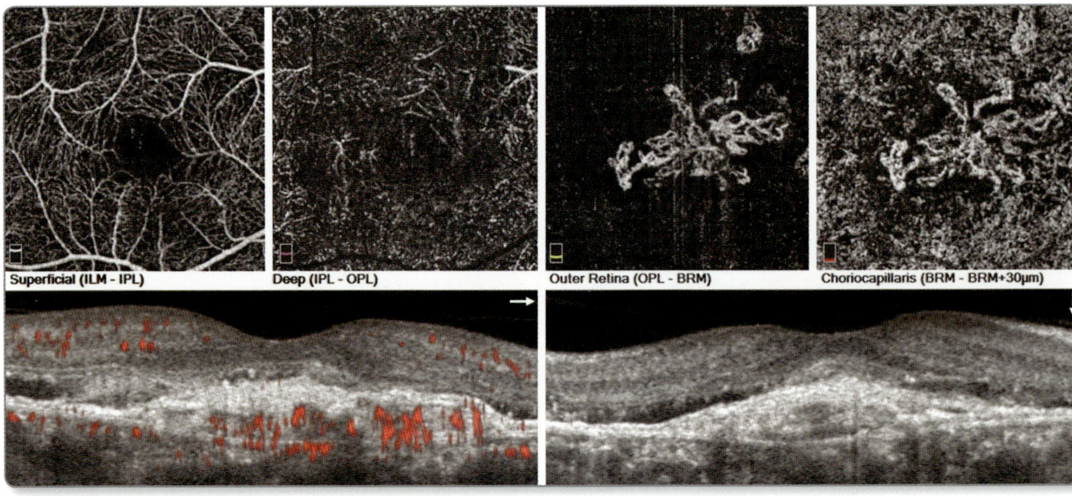

Figure 13 Active choroidal neovascularization (CNV) in optical coherence tomography (OCT) angiography *en face*. Irregularly shaped CNV showing signs of activity: abundant dense, thin capillaries, with anastomoses and full complete vascular arcade. The vessel loops can be seen especially close to the periphery arcade. Vascular density is high, a dark large halo surrounds the lesion. (Optovue)

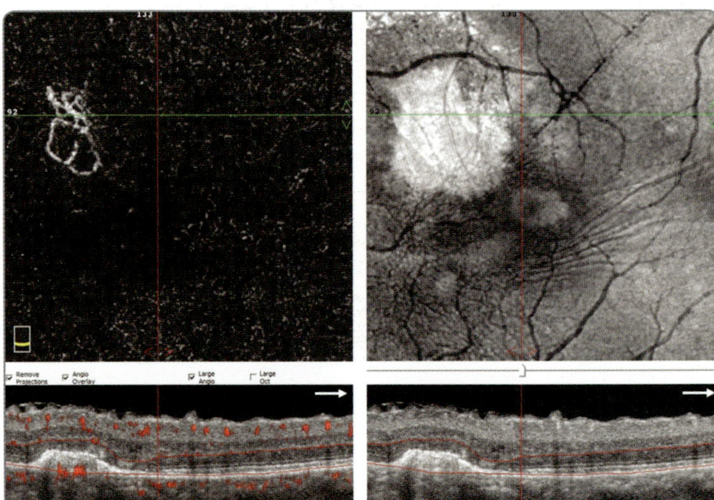

Figure 14 Quiescent choroidal neovascularization (CNV). Optical coherence tomography (OCT) angiography *en face* and angio B-scan. Quiescent new vessels: fragmented, irregular with dead tree features. No fine capillaries, no vessel loops, and no anastomoses. The residual vessels are stiff, and straight tortuous. Greater fractal dimension. (Optovue)

Some parameters are used on OCTA to foresee the activity and progression of the CNV, before and after treatment.

Active CNV features

In the easiest cases, we can rightly think that CNV is active, when the lesion is rounded or globular shaped, (Coral bush, bicycle wheel), when it has a:

- High branching structure
- High capillary density
- Presence of vascular loops at the CNV periphery
- Vascular arcade produced by anastomoses of vessels at the periphery of the lesion
- Dark halo surrounding the lesion

Small fractal dimensions: Sarraf introduced the interesting fact that fractal dimensions are smaller in active CNV and greater in quiescent CNV. Fractals include the idea of a detailed pattern that repeats itself.

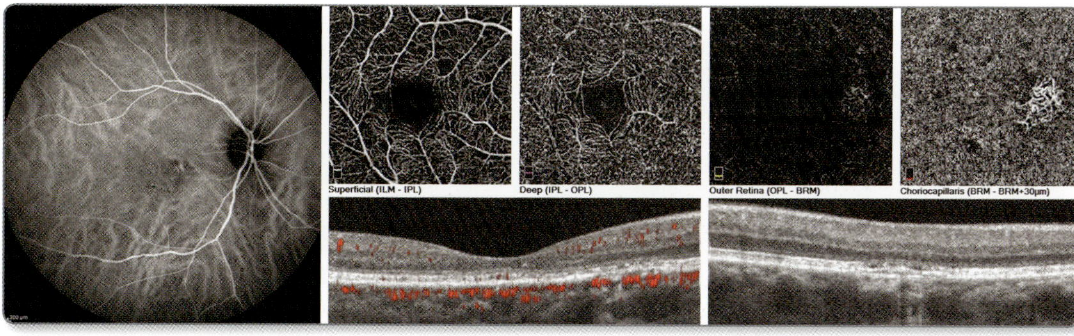

Figure 15 Quiescent choroidal neovascularization (CNV). Indocyanine green (ICG), optical coherence tomography (OCT) angiography *en face* and angio B-scan. New vessels observed during a period of quiescence are fragmented, irregular, and thick. No fine capillaries and vessel loops are seen and there are no anastomoses. (Optovue)

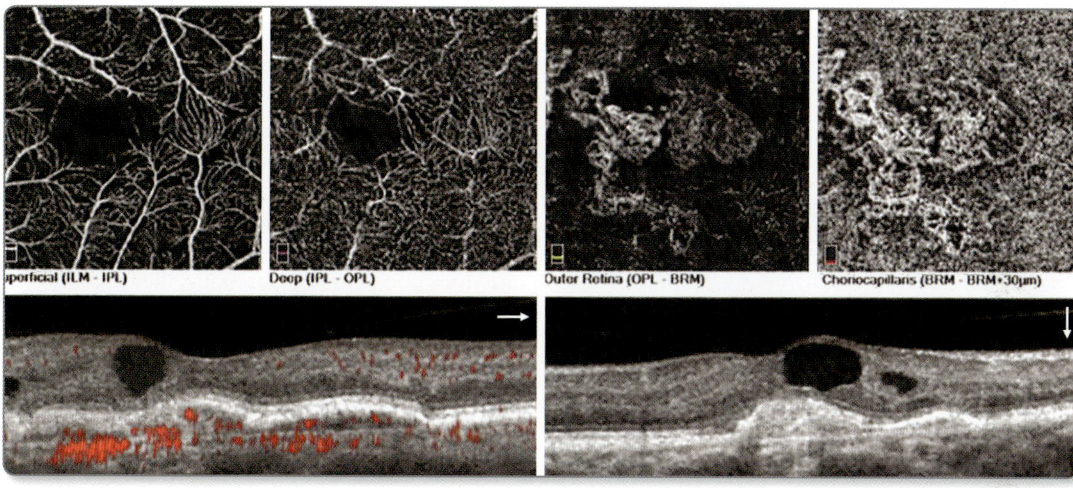

Figure 16 Mixed active and quiescent: optical coherence tomography (OCT) angiography *en face*. Mixed active and quiescent choroidal neovascularization (CNV): mature quiescent vessels are evident with great fractal dimension at left-hand side. They are thick and straight. Active new vessels at right-hand side: there are numerous, very dense showing thin dense capillaries with frequent anastomoses, vessel loops, and small fractal dimension. A dark halo is seen. In this CNV, the left section is nonactive, quiescent, the right-hand section is active. (Optovue)

Quiescent CNV features

We infer a CNV is quiescent when the:

- Lesion shape is irregular, tangled
- Branching structure is sparse and capillary density is low, or
- A total lack of capillaries. There is a greater fractal dimension (Sarraf)
- Vascular loops are missing, there is no vascular arcade and no anastomoses of vessels at the periphery of the lesion. The dark halo surrounding the lesion is small or missing (**Boxes 1** and **2**).

Some authors describe quiescent or nonactive CNV features as a dead tree, as they have no growing loops, and showing only irregular, disaggregated flow. However, this interpretation strategy may be imprecise due the great variety of CNV patterns.

The treatment follow-up highlights some histopathological changes in CNV. After a long intravitreal treatment, we observe the transformation of some capillaries that become mature (arterialized) while other capillaries grow high-flow loops. According to pathological

Box 1: Active choroidal neovascularization (CNV) morphological features

- CNV dimensions, large
- Lesion shape, coral bush, medusa head, cycle wheel
- Dense branching structure
- Dense arborization
- Smaller fractal dimension (Sarraf)
- Capillary density high
- Loops present
- Vascular arcade complete
- Dense anastomoses at lesion periphery
- Dark large halo surrounding the lesion
- Automated quantitative parameters such as vessel density

Box 2: Quiescent choroidal neovascularization (CNV) morphological features

- CNV dimensions, small
- Lesion shape
- Tuft
- Dead tree
- Branching structure low: bare tree
- Greater fractal dimension (Sarraf)
- Capillary density low
- Lacking capillaries
- Loops lacking
- Vascular arcade incomplete or broken
- Anastomoses few
- Dark small halo surrounding the lesion small or lacking
- Automated quantitative parameters such as vessel density

evidence, intravitreal anti-VEGF injection works better on the active growing loops. After treatment, the mature thick trunks show flow decrease, while the active smaller vessels seem to disappear for 3–4 weeks (cyclic recurrence). It is difficult to grade CNV activity with a single OCTA.

Mixed active and quiescent CNV

In mixed active and quiescent CNV, mature quiescent vessels are evident: thick and straight with great fractal dimension. Active new vessels are numerous, very dense showing thin dense capillaries with frequent anastomoses, vessel loops, and small fractal dimension.

Nonexudative CNV: Active or quiescent?

Since OCTA detected nonexudative new vessels, we have the problem to define if they are active or quiescent?

Nonexudative CNV morphology shows generally a sparse capillary density with few branches subdivision and arborization, great fractal dimension. Some loops are present, vessels are thick and sinuous. Generally, they appear as a tangled network or a filament like feature. Arterialized CNV after repeated recurrences and treatments show vessels thicker and straighter, rigid in aspect with lack of the thinner capillaries.

These mature, arterialized vessels can show little or no leakage at fluorescein angiography. Sometimes, nonexudative CNVs are a result of treatment.

We are not sure, if nonexudative CNV describes an atypical quiescent type 1 CNV, or may be sometimes a completely different entity. It is uncertain whether one is the predecessor of the other or if they are two separate clinical entities.

The evolution of nonexudative CNV seems to be very slow, showing some slight morphological changes and enlargement in long follow-up, without vision changes and with no fluid accumulation. According to David Huang, 80% becomes active after less than 1 year (**Boxes 3** and **4**).

The OCTA parameters we have discussed may indicate activity or quiescence in the typical cases. In difficult cases uncertainty endures (**Boxes 5** and **6**).

Management of exudative CNV

Present management of CNV is anti-VEGF treatment; bevacizumab, ranibizumab,[8] and aflibercept have given positive results in reducing CNV activity symptoms and subretinal fluid, reducing PED, and maintaining good vision for years. Unfortunately, we are far from achieving ideal long-term visual results.[9-14]

Intravitreal anti-VEGF therapy does not cure the disease but decreases the rate of progression in many and gives visual improvement in some patients. Our goals in treating neovascular age-related macular degeneration (AMD) are to improve vision, lessen geographic atrophy, and reduce treatment load.

The AMD, OCTA + structural OCT may be sufficient for treatment decision and follow-up in usual care in most cases, but not in all cases.

Treatment should be early, beginning shortly after symptoms appear and before OCT shows structural damage. Patient should be treated with precise loading dose and closely monitored for treatment and retreatment.

Repeated intravitreal injections of bevacizumab, ranibizumab, and aflibercept have become the primary treatment.

Loading phase

All the intravitreal anti-VEGFs approve the need of a loading phase. This approach includes three consecutive injections each 4 weeks as first approach to the treatment.

Monthly injection

Prospective, randomized trials employing current generation anti-VEGF monotherapies show that fixed monthly dosing optimizes visual and anatomic outcomes. Despite the potential value, indefinite fixed monthly dosing poses a substantial burden for subjects and healthcare systems across the globe. Therefore, few physicians report practicing such strict monthly dosing.

Box 3: Nonexudative CNV morphological features

- Dimensions, generally large
- Shape tangled network or filament like
- Capillary density: sparse
- Few branches subdivision and arborization
- Few loops present
- Vessels thick and sinuous
- Arterialized CNV after repeated recurrences shows vessels thicker and straighter, rigid in aspect
- Lack of the thinner capillaries
- Evolution very slow
- Morphological changes slight and small enlargement in long follow-up
- No vision changes
- No fluid accumulation
- Perilesional dark halo small or lacking

Box 4: Nature of nonexudative CNV

- Atypical quiescent type 1 CNV?
- Completely different entity?
- Predecessor of active CNV?
- Two separate clinical entities?

Box 5: David Sarraf optical coherence tomographic angiography (OCTA) biomarkers of activity

- Secondary small vessel branching
- Peripheral arcades with anastomoses
- Greater fractal dimension

Increased areas of geographic atrophy are more seen in subjects treated with monthly ranibizumab than with '*pro re nata*'.

Further, the treatment burden of monthly injections on patients and physicians is significant and the socioeconomic impact on the healthcare system is huge.

Box .6: David Sarraf optical coherence tomography angiography (OCTA) biomarkers of inactivity

- Large dilated straight vessels
- Absent secondary branching
- Absent peripheral arcades
- Lower fractal dimension

Treat and extend

A treat-and-extend (TREX) protocol uses monthly injections until signs of exudation have resolved. Then, the interval between treatments is lengthened, typically sequentially by 1- to 2-week intervals, if there are no signs of recurrent exudation. The interval between treatments is tailored based on exudative disease activity; eyes are treated at each visit, no more frequently than every 4 weeks and no less frequently than every 12 weeks. The time between visits is individualized. Patients are classified as having a dry or wet macula and is treated monthly until a dry macula is achieved.

The results after the 1st year are encouraging compared with the monthly treatment through year 2. TREX dosing achieves similar visual and anatomic outcomes with a significantly reduced treatment burden.

PRN (*pro re nata*)

Lower frequency treatment regimens have been explored in studies in order to assess whether such regimens reproduce visual and anatomical outcomes obtained with monthly ranibizumab treatment regimens as used in the pivotal MARINA and ANCHOR trials. The PIER study employed 3-month loading dose followed by quarterly injections. The PrONTO study used the same 3-month loading dose period, only to be followed by a monthly evaluation and decision to treat based on well-defined criteria including visual acuity (VA) changes and the presence or absence of fluid on OCT: PRN regimen. Currently, there are not scheduled guidelines for the PRN regimen.

Conclusion

Systematic reviews and meta-analyses of randomized clinical trials have shown comparable efficacy between aflibercept and other anti-VEGFs (e.g. ranibizumab) for wet AMD.[15]

Follow-up of CNV treated with anti-VEGF

In a PRN strategy, even if OCTA signs of activity have been described, we prefer with Yves Cohen to treat only when OCT shows exudation. In AMD, OCTA + structural OCT may be sufficient for treatment decision and follow-up in usual care in most cases, but not in all cases. In some difficult cases, fluorescein or/and ICGA may be necessary.

See the Yves Salomon Cohen chart in **Figure 17**.

Alternative delivery methods

Drug delivery systems such as extended-release implants, refillable reservoir-based implants, nanodevices, and cell encapsulation devices vary depending on the technology and design. Currently, there are no FDA approved anti-VEGF extended release systems. Implantable device allowing a large spacing of injections will be very opportune. Patients who are poor responders or who have difficulty in accessing care may

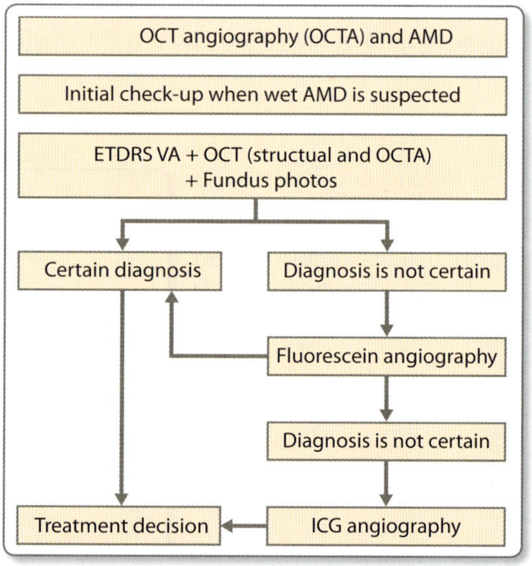

Figure 17 The Yves Salomon Cohen flowchart.
(AMD: age-related macular degeneration; ICG: indocyanine green; OCT: optical coherence tomography)

benefit from this implantable device at pars plana allowing much less frequent injections. Future therapies including modification of cellular transcription via viral infection is a novel approach for therapeutic strategies.

Management of silent subclinical CNV

Close monitoring is advised by most authors, using frequently repeated OCT angiography to follow evolution. These cases should be monitored by structural OCT and OCTA.

Management of subclinical nonexudative NV is discussed. David Huang presented data on a series of eyes with intermediate age-related macular degeneration where 80% subclinical CNV progressed to exudation within 10 months. In most of the eyes, exudation developed within 6 months. Furthermore, the change from nonexudative CNV to exudative CNV was preceded by rapid growth in lesion size as measured by OCTA. Huang study suggests that nonexudative CNV is a precursor to exudation.

A logical next step would be randomized trials to evaluate whether prophylactic treatment of nonexudative CNV could prevent exudation and save vision in the long term at reasonable costs. David Huang thinks that the growth rate of nonexudative lesions as measured by OCTA could be used as the guide for starting and stopping anti-VEGF treatment and should be considered in the design of such trials.

Costs of treatment of neovascular CNV

Parik, Chhablani, et al.[16] examined anti-VEGF medication costs all over the world. They observed that bevacizumab comprises the majority of anti-VEGF medication use in the United States and Singapore, although aflibercept use is growing rapidly.[17] Paradoxically, data demonstrate that there is a significant trend in medication choice towards ranibizumab and aflibercept among practice settings outside of the United States, such as the United Kingdom, China, South Korea, and Australia. The price of anti-VEGF medications ranges from US $30 (ziv-aflibercept) to US $1950 (ranibizumab and aflibercept). Ranibizumab's price ranged from US $240 in India to US $1950 in the United States. Conbercept in China costs approximately US $1150 per dose.

Upcoming treatments in neovascular AMD

Although anti-VEGF therapy has largely replaced other methods of treatment for wet AMD, current treatment algorithms are associated with substantial medical and economic burdens, including the need for repeated treatments with associated cumulative risk of endophthalmitis and other adverse events. In real life, the efficacy results with anti-VGEF therapy are less positive than those published in clinical trial data.

Emerging therapies and delivery methods are presently being investigated to improve patient care and maximize visual outcomes.

The therapeutic action pathways in neovascular AMD pass through endothelial cells and pericytes. The classical track follows the blocking of VEGF. Nevertheless, several pathways under development affect other VEGF (D, B, PIGF), the tyrosine kinase inhibitor, angiopoietin, and integrins.

The main therapeutic target remains the endothelial cell with its different receptors or pericytes.

Conbercept anti-VEGF molecule is a therapy already used in China and some other countries. It is a soluble receptor decoy that blocks all isoforms of VEGF-A, VEGF-B, VEGF-C, and which has a high binding affinity for VEGF and a long half-life in vitreous.

The angiopoietin pathway is promising. The tyrosine kinase pathway is active on endothelial cells and on pericytes.

Ziv-aflibercept, a systemic chemotherapeutic agent approved for the treatment of metastatic colorectal cancer, has potential for intravitreal administration, since it was not associated with signs of toxicity in an experimental study and in human case reports.

Abicipar pegol (Molecular Partners and Allergan) is a second-generation drug with the potential for 12-week treatment intervals. This agent binds to both VEGF and platelet-derived growth factor receptors. In phase 3 results, abicipar administered every 12 weeks was comparable to ranibizumab administered every

4 weeks. However, rates of inflammation were much higher with abicipar.

Brolucizumab: 2-year results from two phase 3 trials (HAWK and HARRIER) of brolucizumab, a new VEGF inhibitor from Novartis, show that intravitreal injections every 12 weeks were sufficient for many patients and that brolucizumab is comparable to bimonthly aflibercept. The gain in visual acuity obtained at 4 months, maintained at 1 year, is also maintained at 2 years. There is less intra- and subretinal edema than under aflibercept and also less detachment of the pigment epithelium. The good anatomical result (with a decrease in central retinal thickness) obtained at 16 weeks is maintained at 48 weeks and at 96 weeks. At this stage, it seems that brolucizumab dries the retina more in OCT. It remains to be seen whether, in the long term, there is no higher risk of progression to atrophy.

Faricimab (Roche) is a bispecific antibody that simultaneously binds to and neutralizes both angiopoietin-2 and VEGF factor A.

A phase 1 study is designed to determine whether a single intravitreal injection of RGX-314, a gene therapy developed by Regenxbio, will induce the production of anti-VEGF antibodies, eliminating the need for more injection.

References

1. Lumbroso B, Rispoli M, Savastano MC. Longitudinal optical coherence tomography-angiography study of type 2 naive choroidal neovascularization early response after treatment. Retina 2015; 35:2242–2251.
2. Palejwala NV, Jia Y, Gao SS, et al. Detection of nonexudative choroidal neovascularization in age-related macular degeneration with optical coherence tomography angiography. Retina 2015; 35:2204–2211.
3. Roisman L, Zhang Q, Wang RK, et al. Optical coherence tomography angiography of asymptomatic neovascularization in intermediate age-related macular degeneration. Ophthalmology 2016; 123:1309–1319.
4. Spaide RF. Optical coherence tomography angiography signs of vascular abnormalization with antiangiogenic therapy for choroidal neovascularization. Am J Ophthalmol. 2015; 160:6–16.
5. Coscas GJ, Lupidi M, Coscas F, Cagini C, Souied EH. Optical coherence tomography angiography versus traditional multimodal imaging in assessing the activity of exudative age-related macular degeneration: A New Diagnostic Challenge. Retina 2015; 35:2219–2228.
6. Cole ED, Ferrara D, Novais EA, Louzada RN, Waheed NK. Clinical trial endpoints for optical coherence tomography angiography in neovascular age-related macular degeneration. Retina 2016; 36.
7. Liang MC, de Carlo TE, Baumal CR, et al. Correlation of Spectral Domain Optical Coherence Tomography Angiography And Clinical Activity In Neovascular Age-Related Macular Degeneration. Retina 2016; 36:2265–2273.
8. Rosenfeld PJ, Brown DM, Heier JS, et al. Ranibizumab for neovascular age-related macular degeneration. N Engl J Med 2006; 355:1419–1431.
9. Sarraf D. Biomarkers of neovascular activity using OCT angiography. Presented at: Angiogenesis, Exudation, and Degeneration 2017.
10. Carnevali A, Cicinelli MV, Capuano V, et al. Optical Coherence Tomography Angiography: A Useful Tool for Diagnosis of Treatment-Naïve Quiescent Choroidal Neovascularization. Am J Ophthalmol 2016; 169:189–198.
11. Jia Y, Bailey ST, Wilson DJ, et al. Quantitative optical coherence tomography angiography of choroidal neovascularization in age-related macular degeneration. Ophthalmology 2014; 121:1435–1444.
12. Rosenfeld PJ, Brown DM, Heier JS, et al. Ranibizumab for neovascular age-related macular degeneration. N Engl J Med 2006; 355:1419–1431.
13. Brown DM, Michels M, Kaiser PK, et al. Ranibizumab versus verteporfin photodynamic therapy for neovascular age-related macular degeneration: two-year results of the ANCHOR study. Ophthalmology 2009; 116:57–65e55–65.
14. Schmidt-Erfurth U, Kaiser PK, Korobelnik JF, et al. Intravitreal aflibercept injection for neovascular age-related macular degeneration: ninety-six-week results of the VIEW studies. Ophthalmology 2014; 121:193–201.
15. Ba J, Peng R-S, Xu D, et al. Intravitreal anti-VEGF injections for treating wet age-related macular degeneration: a systematic review and meta-analysis. Drug Des Dev Ther 2015; 9:5397–5405.
16. Wykoff CC, Croft DE, Brown DM, et al. Prospective trial of treat-and-extend versus monthly dosing for neovascular age-related macular degeneration: trex-amd 1-year results. Ophthalmology 2015; 122:2514–22.
17. Parikh R, Pirakitikulr N, Chhablani J. et al A Multinational Comparison of Anti–Vascular Endothelial Growth Factor Use: The United States, the United Kingdom, and Asia-Pacific. Ophthalmol Retina 2019; 3:16–26.

16 CNV in lesions of Bruch's membrane with normal thickness choroid

Bruno Lumbroso, Marco Rispoli

Introduction

Choroidal neovascularization (CNV) is a procedure of repair response to a lesion of the pigment epithelium and Bruch's membrane. Thus, CNV can be observed in many disorders where lesions, abnormalities, or breaks of Bruch's membrane are observed. Angiogenesis is a normal process in wound healing, the mechanism through which new blood vessels form from pre-existing vessels. The process of CNV formation can be modulated or restrained by treatment. Yet we do not have, so far, the possibility to influence the original cause.

Angioid streaks and CNV

Angioid streaks are breaks or disruptions of the Bruch's membrane due to elastic tissues alteration. After a few years' evolution, type 1 or type 2 CNV almost always appears along the streaks, mainly at the macular area. Optical coherence tomography (OCT) angiography (OCTA) shows commonly a type 2 vascular network above the pigment epithelium. Bruch's membrane ripples seem to precede the Bruch's breaks. These folds are probably produced by high-stretching forces exerted on the Bruch's membrane around the optic nerve head. Type 1 CNV can also be observed, with vascularized pigment epithelium elevations and vascular network between RPE and Bruch's membrane. Type 1 CNVs are seen close to macula, but also farther along the streak. Anti-vascular endothelial growth factor (anti-VEGF) treatment has been reported to give stabilization or improvement in more than 60%, but they do not prevent the affected eyes from progressive visual loss.[1-3]

CNV in inflammatory disorders

CNV in multifocal choroiditis

Multifocal choroiditis (MC) is an inflammatory disorder appearing in young myopic women, after a flu-like episode. A classic type 2 CNV penetrates under the outer retina through a post-inflammatory break of Bruch's membrane and RPE (**Boxes 1** and **2**).

On OCTA, CNVs are similar to type 2 CNV of AMD showing a bicycle wheel, lacy wheel morphology. Thin vessels may grow along with the inflammatory scar margins. OCTA is very useful to differentiate leakage seen in fluorescein angiography imaging, showing if CNVs are present or not. Type 1 CNVs are not seen in multifocal choroiditis. OCTA is also more useful than FA for monitoring anti-VEGF treatment. The feeder vessel may persist and lead to recurrences.

Box 1: Choroidal neovascularization (CNV) in normal thickness choroid with lesions, abnormalities, or breaks in Bruch's membrane

- CNV in choroid traumatic rupture
- CNV in complications of laser photocoagulation
- CNV in angioid streaks
- CNV in inflammatory disorders, choroiditis, and chorioretinitis
- CNV on margin of atrophic areas
- CNV in fibrous scars

Box 2: Choroidal neovascularization (CNV) morphology in choroiditis scars

- Wheel shaped
- Lacy wheel
- Sea-fan–shaped vessels

It will regress when the recovery is complete. The same kind of CNV can be seen in white dot syndromes (**Box 3**).

CNV in choroid traumatic rupture

Choroidal ruptures are breaks in the choroid, Bruch's membrane, and the retinal pigment epithelium that complicate a blunt ocular trauma. They have a crescent shape and are concentric to the optic disc.

Fluorescein angiography may detect CNV at onset, a few weeks after trauma. When CNVs appear, early hyperfluorescence is followed by dye leakage. OCT angiogram shows arcuate choroid break. About 10% develop CNV, mainly when rupture is located close to the macula.

OCT shows subretinal fluid around a disrupted retinal pigment epithelium/Bruch's membrane complex extending into the juxtafoveolar area as an indication of new vessel activity. Older age and location of rupture within the arcades are positively associated with CNV formation.

CNV in laser photocoagulation scars (Box 2)

The CNVs develop mainly when laser spot is close to fovea. New vessels as complication of laser photocoagulation are generally due to errors in applying laser spots too strong and too close to the pigmented macular area. Fluorescein angiography shows in case of CNV, early hyperfluorescence due to intense dye leakage. OCT shows disrupted retinal pigment epithelium/Bruch's membrane complex and fluid as indication of new vessel activity. CNV is generally juxtafoveal, but may also be seen far from macula. On OCTA, CNVs are similar to CNV of choroiditis showing a lacy-wheel morphology. Thin vessels grow along the laser scar margins.[4]

Box 3: White dot syndromes

- Birdshot chorioretinopathy
- Multiple evanescent white dot syndrome
- Acute posterior multifocal placoid pigment epitheliopathy (APMPPE)
- Punctate inner choroidopathy
- Multifocal choroiditis
- Acute retinal pigment epitheliitis or acute retinitis
- Sometimes serpiginous choroiditis is associated in this group of retinal diseases

CNV on margin of atrophic areas

The OCTA may show a vascular network above the pigment epithelium (type 2 CNV), growing along with the atrophic area margin. Shape is very irregular, elongated, and stretched out. Feeder vessels are difficult to identify, and in some cases cannot be seen. Less frequently, the membrane looks rounded with a dense capillary network, and can be large, reaching the same size and aspect of AMD membranes.

CNV in fibrous scars

Subretinal fibrosis is due to repair mechanisms, appearing either during the natural healing process or during anti-vascular endothelial growth factor treatment. It is associated with poor visual outcomes. On structural optical coherence tomography, fibrosis shows a subretinal hyperreflective lesion, involving RPE, limiting membrane and ellipsoid zone.

The OCTA shows a perfused vascular network, as well as structural changes in the outer retina and the choriocapillaris layer. Souied reports that essentially, we see two main phenotypes: dead tree or blossoming tree. While dead tree pattern corresponds to irregular flow in networks formed by major vascular trunks, blossoming tree phenotype (Souied) is correlated with high-flow networks presenting profuse anastomosis with the surrounding vascularization. In fibrous scars, a large, dense *dark halo* represents the masking effect generated by the fibrous scar.[5,6]

References

1. Tilleul J, Mimoun G, Querques G, et al. Intravitreal ranibizumab for choroidal neovascularization in angioid streaks: four-year follow-up. Retina 2016; 36:483–491.
2. Giacomelli G, Finocchio L, Biagini I, et al. Long-term follow-up of choroidal neovascularization due to angioid streaks with pro re nata intravitreal anti-VEGF treatment. Ophthalmologica 2017; 238:44–51.
3. Marchese A, Parravano M, Rabiolo A, et al. Optical coherence tomography analysis of evolution of Bruch's membrane features in angioid streaks. Eye (Lond) 2017; 31:1600–1605.
4. Ament CS, Zacks DN, Lane AM, et al. Predictors of visual outcome and choroidal neovascular membrane formation after traumatic choroidal rupture. Arch Ophthalmol 2006; 124:957–966.
5. Hwang JC, Del Priore LV, Freund KB, et al. Development of subretinal fibrosis after anti-VEGF treatment in neovascular age-related macular degeneration. Ophthalmic Surg Lasers Imaging 2011; 42:6–11.
6. Bloch SB, Lund-Andersen H, Sander B, et al. Subfoveal fibrosis in eyes with neovascular age-related macular degeneration treated with intravitreal ranibizumab. Am J Ophthalmol 2013; 156:116–124.

17 Pachychoroid 1: Polypoidal choroidal vasculopathy

Bruno Lumbroso, Marco Rispoli

Polypoidal choroidal vasculopathy

Presently, there is no unanimously acknowledged definition of polypoidal choroidal vasculopathy (PCV). The PCV was first named posterior uveal bleeding syndrome. It was first discovered and described by Yannuzzi in 1983, in hypertensive middle-aged women of African American ancestry.[1-3] It was thought to be an age-related macular degeneration (AMD) subtype. Many investigators still base the diagnosis of PCV on indocyanine green angiography (ICGA) findings that demonstrate presence of polypoidal dilatations.

Pathophysiology: Pachychoroid and polypoidal choroidal vasculopathy

Polypoidal choroidal vasculopathy has been documented in women and men of all ethnic categories. In Asian populations, polypoidal choroidal vasculopathy is thought to be a common subtype of exudative AMD where it forms 20–50% of the cases, whilst in Caucasian population, it forms less than 5% of the AMD cases.

Freund and his group created the name pachychoroid to describe 'a permanent and abnormal increase in the choroidal thickness', of more than 300 μ, often manifesting dilatation of the large outer Haller layer oval choroidal vessels, compressing the overlying choriocapillaris and Sattler's layer.

Pachychoroid could be an inherited condition, however other factors are present, some of them acquired. This hypothesis suggests that a genetic background may predispose to PCV and that thick choroids could be one of its phenotypic indicators. The similar characteristics shared between PCV and central serous chorioretinopathy (CSC) include choroidal hyperpermeability and increased choroidal thickness as demonstrated with optical coherence tomography (OCT). Histopathology displays dilated thin-walled choroidal vessels in PCV. Recently, the importance of thick choroid in PCV led Bailey Freund to suggest PCV falls within the pachychoroid spectrum of conditions that may have a different cause from AMD (**Boxes 1** and **2**).

Studies into the pathogenesis of PCV, and publications from Bailey Freund and his team suggest that PCV belongs to a spectrum of conditions characterized by pachychoroid. Pachychoroid disease spectrum refers to a group of retinal and choroidal disorders, namely pigment epitheliopathy, central serous chorioretinopathy, neovasculopathy, and polypoid choroidal vasculopathy, all arising from a thickened choroid and hyperpermeable large choroidal vessels. In pachychoroid disorders, disturbance in the choroidal circulation seems to be central to its pathogenesis. Further research is needed to clarify the precise pathogenesis

Box 1: Spectrum of pachychoroid-related disorders (Bailey Freund)

- Central serous chorioretinopathy (CSC)
- Pachychoroid pigment epitheliopathy incomplete, inchoate, 'forme fruste' (incomplete form) of CSC
- Pachychoroid neovasculopathy, which includes type I CNV (PNV)
- Polypoidal choroidal vasculopathy (PCV) probably an eventual progression of PNV
- Focal choroidal excavation, included by some authors

Box 2: Choroid thickness

Increased:

- Hypermetropia (normal)

Pachychoroid disorders:

- Central serous chorioretinopathy, acute and chronic
- Other pachychoroid manifestations are:
  - Pachychoroid pigment epitheliopathy
  - Pachychoroid neovasculopathy, and
  - Polypoidal choroidal vasculopathy

Other disorders:

- Chronic epitheliopathies
- Choroidal inflammations
- Vogt-Koyanagi-Harada disease
- Vascular occlusions
- Sildenafil

Decreased:

- Myopia (normal)
- Age (normal)
- Atrophic macular degeneration
- Hereditary macular dystrophies
- Retinitis pigmentosa
- Tapetoretinal degenerations

of PCV and to clarify the role of angiogenesis, inflammation, complement activation, and lipid metabolism.

Similarities and differences in imaging and natural history between PCV and AMD indicate they share many common pathophysiologic analytic elements, but also point to primary mechanisms leading to the development of dissimilar but comparable disorders.

Clinical features

At the fundus hemorrhages, hemorrhagic retinal detachments are seen in the posterior pole but may be seen outside the vascular arcades, and be associated to nodular, orange, subretinal lesions, red nodular polypoid structure under the retinal pigment epithelium, neuroretinal detachment, lipid exudation. Soft drusen, typical in AMD, may or may not present. Natural evolution is less severe than in CNV associated with other types of AMD, except in case of massive hemorrhage.

Branching network

Polypoidal choroidal vasculopathy presents an intricate pattern of branching vessels. A complex system of splitting vessels is adherent to a flat, undulated fibrovascular pigment epithelium detachment (PED). This elaborate vascular network opens in nodular dilations.

Polypoid dilatations

Vascular saccular dilatations or polyps are located under the retinal pigment epithelium (RPE), close to the fibrovascular PED where polyps are adherent to the elevated RPE. The serous and hemorrhagic detachments are mainly clustered around the optic disc and at the posterior pole but may be also located more peripherally.

Drusen: Pachydrusen

Soft drusen may or may not present. Pachydrusen have been described by Spaide in PCV patients. He highlighted in these eyes, the presence of deposits under the RPE having characteristics different from serous drusen. While the later are rather round, with fuzzy outlines and tend to merge, pachydrusen are often well-defined, isolated, and have a more complex form (oval, or more polylobulated). Cheung et al. found that pachydrusen was significantly associated with choroidal polypoid vasculopathy.

Imaging

The ICGA, OCT, and OCTA show that vascular dilatations or polyps are connected to a complex network of feeder vessels located under the RPE, close to the fibrovascular PED where polyps are adherent to the elevated RPE. A thick choroid is present.

The ICG angiography, SD-OCT, and OCTA are useful for identifying the polyps.

ICG angiography

For many years, ICG angiography was the most important diagnostic tool. Advances in imaging, including enhanced depth imaging, SD-OCT,

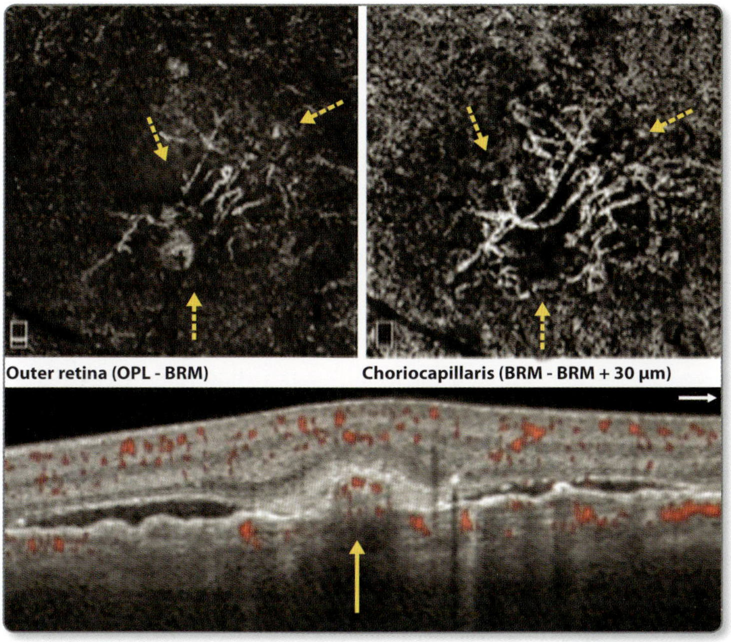

Figure 1 In polypoidal choroidal vasculopathy (PCV), the interconnecting neovascular network is always visible (dotted arrow) under the slightly-elevated retinal pigment epithelium (RPE) detachment. Polypoidal structures (plain arrow) themselves are usually more difficult to be detected due to their perfusion status and their little size.

en face OCT, and OCT angiography (OCTA), have facilitated the diagnosis of PCV. On ICG, one or multiple early hyperfluorescent spots peripheral or above a branching neovascular network represent the essential clues for diagnosis.[4]

Optical coherence tomography

It provides cross-section images showing elevations of the RPE with moderate inner reflectivity due to the polyps, and two highly reflective lines (double-layer sign) corresponding to branching network, dome-shaped serous, or hemorrhagic detachments of the RPE encompass the polypoidal dilatations over the Bruch's membrane. Sometimes, polyps are not detected by OCTA due to their small dimension and to their slow perfusion. Choroid in PCV is much thicker than normally (normal choroid in young persons is 340, at in 60 years old persons 260 microns) (**Figures 1** to 7).

OCT angiography

It shows both polyps and interconnecting neovascular network under the RPE. The polyps are low flow structures.

However, polypoidal dilations are not located on the same plane than the interconnecting neovascular network.

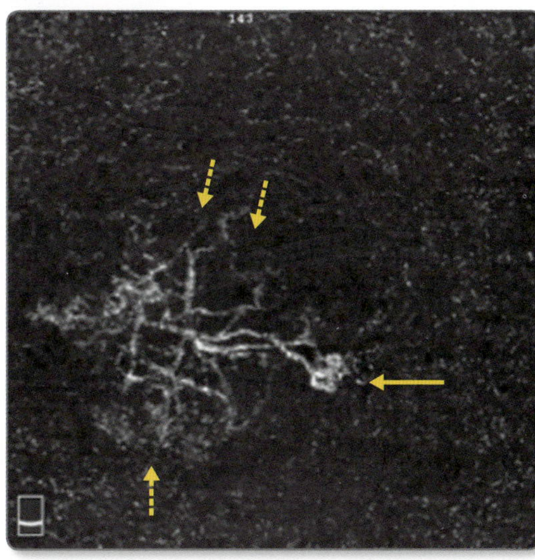

Figure 2 Polypoidal choroidal vasculopathy (PCV), interconnecting neovascular network under the slightly elevated wavy retinal pigment epithelium (RPE) detachment (dotted arrow). Polypoidal structures themselves are usually more difficult to be detected (plain arrow) due to their perfusion status and their little size.

Branching, interconnective networks are high-flow structures. A flat, undulated RPE detachment covers the neovascular branching network.

Polypoidal dilations are usually more difficult to be visualized than the branching vessels because of their location, and difference in level. Sometimes, polyps are not detected by OCTA due to their small dimension and to their slow perfusion. That could mean that there is no flow at the moment OCTA is performed, or that flow is too slow to be detected by the device. Srour, Querques, and Souied suppose the apparent absence of OCTA signal in the polyps could be due to blood turbulence inside the dilatation, or to the fact that blood only circulates at the periphery of the aneurysm.

Recently, OCTA studies conclude that there are two subtypes of PCV: PCV in the strict sense (PCV type 2) and polypoidal CNV (PCV type 1).

In PCV type 2, OCTA shows branching network as a high-flow lesion located above Bruch's membrane and beneath the RPE, and the polypoidal lesion as a low-flow rounded structure, demonstrating that the polyp cavity is devoid of flow signal.[5-18]

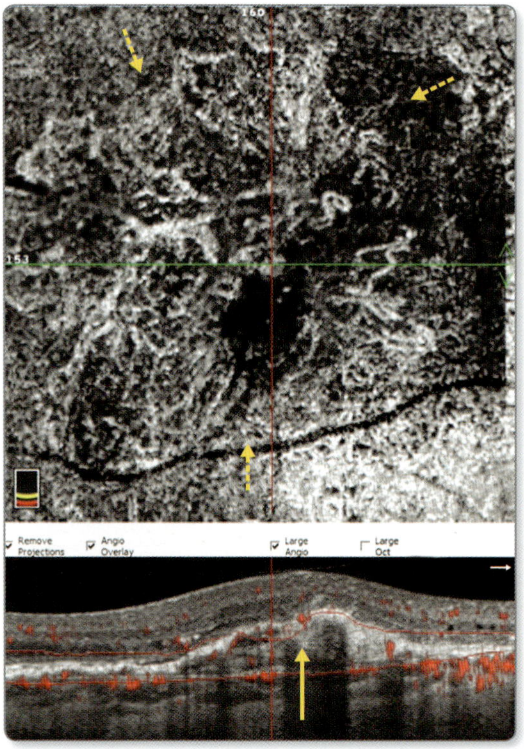

Figure 3 Polypoidal choroidal vasculopathy (PCV): The interconnecting neovascular network is evident (dotted arrow) under the slightly elevated retinal pigment epithelium (RPE) detachment. Polypoidal structures are not seen in the optical coherence tomography (OCT) angiography, as they are located on another level. They may be detected on the angio B-scan (plain arrow).

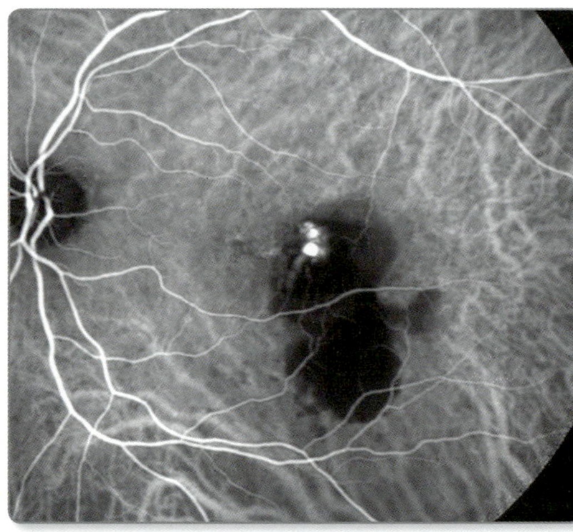

Figure 5 In polypoidal choroidal vasculopathy, indocyanine green (ICG) angiography is still the gold standard imaging technique to visualize polypoidal dilations and guiding photo dynamic therapy (PDT). ICG highlights the pigment epithelial detachment containing the polypoidal dilations. Optical coherence tomographic angiography (OCTA) adds data concerning the perfusion of the polypoidal dilations in PED. In this case, we see two PED and subretinal hemorrhage. (Heidelberg)

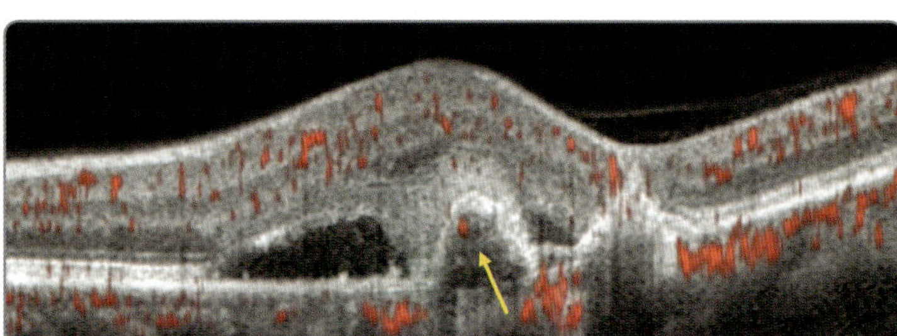

Figure 4 Polypoidal choroidal vasculopathy (PCV): The use of flow data on cross-section scan makes easier the visualization of polyps on the optical coherence tomographic angiography (OCTA) images. One polypoid structure is adherent to the PED inferior face (arrow).

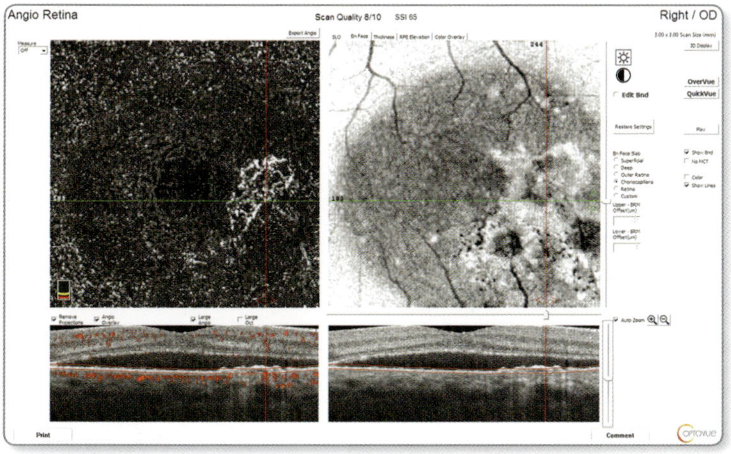

Figure 6 Polypoidal choroidal vasculopathy (PCV), interconnecting neovascular network under the slightly elevated wavy retinal pigment epithelium (RPE) detachment. Polypoidal structures are not detected in this case due to their perfusion status and their little size.

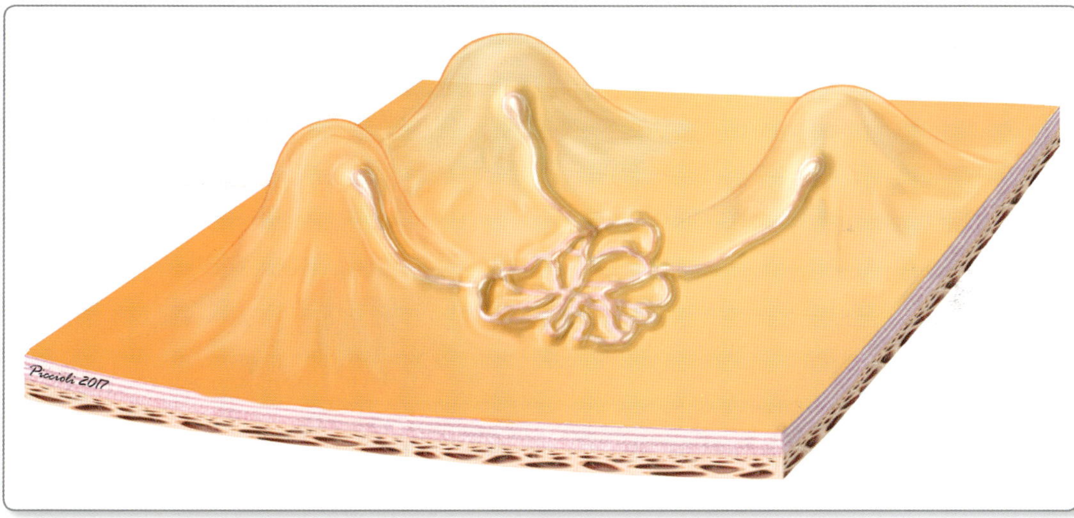

Figure 7 Polypoidal choroidal vasculopathy (PCV), we can see the neovascular network under the retina, and the polypoidal structures in the retinal pigment epithelium (RPE) detachment.

In polypoidal CNV, OCTA reveals a tangled hyperflow network of mature and large caliber type 1 new vessels ending in round, hypo-/ hyperflow polypoidal lesions.

Management

The ICG angiography and OCTA are used for identifying polyps and vascular networks.

Multicentre randomized clinical trials evaluating the safety and efficacy of anti-VEGF monotherapy and combination with photodynamic therapy reported positive outcomes. It results that PCV is less responsive to anti-VEGF therapy than other types of CNV. The best treatment for PCV seems to be photodynamic therapy with verteporfin, associated with anti-VEGF, giving better results than anti-VEGF alone.

References

1. Yannuzzi LA. Idiopathic polypoidal choroidal vasculopathy. Presented at the Macula Society Meeting; 1982.
2. Stern RM, Zakov N, Zegarra H, et al. Multiple recurrent serous sanguineous retinal pigment epithelial detachments in black women. Am J Ophthalmol 1985; 100:560–569.
3. Maruko I, Iida T, Saito M, et al. Clinical characteristics of exudative age-related macular degeneration in Japanese patients. Am J Ophthalmol 2007; 144:15–22.
4. Spaide RF, Yannuzzi LA, Slakter JS, et al. Indocyanine green videoangiography of idiopathic choroidal vasculopathy. Retina 1995; 15:100–110.
5. Ojima Y, Hangai M, Sakamoto A, et al. Improved visualization of polypoidal choroidal vasculopathy lesions using spectral-domain optical coherence tomography. Retina 2009; 29:52–9.
6. Mastropasqua R, Di Antonio L, Di Staso S, et al. Optical coherence tomography angiography in retinal vascular diseases and choroidal neovascularization. J Ophthalmol 2015; 2015:343515.
7. Toto L, Di Antonio L, Mastropasqua R, et al. Multimodal imaging of macular telangiectasia type 2: focus on vascular changes using optical coherence tomography angiography. Invest Ophthalmol Vis Sci 2016; 57:268–276.
8. Toto L, Borrelli E, Di Antonio L, et al. Retinal vascular plexuses' changes in dry age-related macular degeneration, evaluated by means of optical coherence tomography angiography. Retina 2016; 36:1566–1572.
9. Inoue M, Balaratnasingam C, Freund KB. Optical coherence tomography angiography of polypoidal choroidal vasculopathy and polypoidal choroidal neovascularization. Retina 2015; 35:2265–2274.
10. Kawamura A, Yuzawa M, Mori R, et al. Indocyanine green angiographic and optical coherence tomographic findings support classification of polypoidal choroidal vasculopathy into two types. Acta Ophthalmol 2013; 91:e474–481.
11. Coscas G, Lupidi M, Coscas F, et al. Toward a specific classification of polypoidal choroidal vasculopathy: idiopathic disease or subtype of age-related macular degeneration. Invest Ophthalmol Vis Sci 2015; 56:3187–3195.
12. Srour M, Querques G, Semon O, et al. Optical coherence tomography angiography characteristics of polypoidal choroidal vasculopathy. Br J Ophthalmol 2016; 100:1489–1493.
13. Tomiyasu T, Nozaki M, Yoshida M, et al. Characteristics of polypoidal choroidal vasculopathy evaluated by optical coherence tomography angiography. Invest Ophthalmol Vis Sci 2016; 57:324–330.
14. Dansingani KK, Balaratnasigam C, Klufas MA, et al. Optical coherence tomography angiography of shallow irregular pigment epithelial detachments in pachychoroid spectrum disease. Am J Ophthalmol 2015; 160:1243–54.e2.
15. Warrow DJ, Hoang QV, Freund KB. Pachychoroid pigment epitheliopathy. Retina 2013; 33:1659–1672.
16. Pang CE, Freund KB. Pachychoroid pigment epitheliopathy may masquerade as acute retinal pigment epitheliitis. Invest Ophthalmol Vis Sci 2014; 55:5252.
17. Pang CE, Freund KB. Pachychoroid neovasculopathy. Retina 2015; 35:1–9.
18. Dansingani KK, Balaratnasingam C, Naysan J, et al. En Face Imaging of Pachychoroid Spectrum Disorders with Swept-Source OCT. Retina 2016; 36:499–516.

18 Pachychoroid 2: CNV in central serous chorioretinopathy

Bruno Lumbroso, Maria Cristina Savastano, Marco Rispoli

Introduction

Central serous chorioretinopathy (CSC) is a common retinal disease that until a few years ago seemed to be a recognized entity. It was divided in an acute and a chronic retinopathy.

In CSC, a serous detachment of the neurosensory retina occurs over an area of leakage from the choriocapillaris through the retinal pigment epithelium. It affects more men than women (6/1). Serous retinal detachments typically resolve spontaneously in most patients, in 30–60 days, (80%) with vision returning to 20/25. In CSC, choroidal congestion and choroidal hyperpermeability play a role in serous pigment epithelium detachment (PED). There is a 60% risk of recurrence in the same eye and in the contralateral eye. Optical coherence tomography (OCT) angiography shows frequent (20%) nonexudative neovascularization.

About 20% of the cases evolve to a chronic epitheliopathy with recurrent or chronic serous retinal detachments, progressive RPE atrophy. Vision can decrease to 20/200 or worse. These cases of diffuse retinal pigment epitheliopathy evolve toward choroidal neovascularization (CNV) in one-third of cases.

Since 2015, the studies published by Bailey Freund and his group suggested that this entity likely resides within a spectrum of pachychoroid-related macular disorders, thus enlarging the range of disorders connected to CSC.

The term pachychoroid has been coined by Freund to define 'a permanent and abnormal increase in the choroidal thickness', of more than 300 μ, often manifesting dilatation of the large outer oval choroidal vessels (Haller's layer), compressing the overlying choriocapillaris and Sattler's layer. This hypothesis suggests that a genetic background may predispose to central serous chorioretinopathy (CSC) and that thick choroids could be one of its phenotypic indicators, as we will see in the paragraph on risk factors.

Freund et al. included in the spectrum of pachychoroid-related disorders:

- The central serous chorioretinopathy (CSC) in which choroidal congestion and choroidal hyperpermeability play a role in serous pigment epithelium detachment (PED)
- The pachychoroid pigment epitheliopathy (PPE), which likely represents a 'incomplete, inchoate' 'forme fruste' (incomplete form) of CSC
- The pachychoroid neovasculopathy (PNV), which includes type I [subretinal pigment epithelium (RPE)] choroidal neovascularization that usually occurs overlying focal areas of choroidal thickening, and finally
- The polypoidal choroidal vasculopathy (PCV) is probably an eventual progression of PNV. Some authors add—focal choroidal excavation to this spectrum

Central serous chorioretinopathy pathophysiology

Central serous chorioretinopathy has a complex and multifactorial pathogenesis.

The choroid tissue is implicated primarily in the pathophysiology of the pachychoroid disease: The pachychoroid disorders (PPE, CSC, PVN, and PCV) share five main common features (**Box 1**):

1. Choroidal thickness increased to 400 and more micron
2. Choroidal hyperpermeability
3. Vessel dilatation at Haller's layer

Box 1: Pachychoroid disorders

- Central serous chorioretinopathy, acute
- Central serous chorioretinopathy, chronic
- Pachychoroid pigment epitheliopathy
- Pachychoroid neovasculopathy
- Polypoidal choroidal vasculopathy
- Focal choroidal excavation

Box 2: Nonexudative CNV in CSC features

- NV membrane well circumscribed with sharp margins
- NV membrane poorly circumscribed
- NV membrane with long filamentous vessels simple or tangled

(NV: neovascularization; CNV: choroidal neovascularization; CSC: central serous chorioretinopathy)

4. Localized thin choroid in small vessels Sattler's layer
5. Localized alteration and thinning of choriocapillaris. In eyes with a chronic epitheliopathy, focal choriocapillaris atrophy with inward displacement of deep choroidal vessels is noted

Pachychoroid pathophysiology has a few common factors:

- *Genetic factor*: Pachychoroid is probably an inherited condition with dominant transmission mode (Behar Cohen et al.; Lehmann et al., 2015). If confirmed, this hypothesis would suggest that a genetic background may predispose to CSC and that thick choroids could be one of its phenotypic indicators
- Mechanical compression of the choriocapillaris and small vessels Sattler's layer by the pathological enlargement of the already large outer vessels of the Haller's layer
- Choroidal hyperpermeability and congestion[1]

Choroidal neovascularization development could be associated with choroidal flow variations (**Box 2**). Chronic RPE changes and long-standing PED allow the ingrowth of sub-RPE endothelial cells. Presence of shallow irregular PED overlying the area with increased choroidal thickness and dilation of choroidal vein. Because PPE and CSC share similar pathophysiological mechanisms, it could be possible that eyes with long-standing PPE have a predisposition to develop type 1 CNV. Azar, Lumbroso et al. have proposed that the ingrowth of new vessels may represent an effort to reform the choriocapillaris in response to the dilation of the outer choroidal layer.[2] This could, in part, explain optical coherence tomography angiography (OCTA) finding of tangled filamentous vascular networks and, in part, explain why the new vessels are localized adjacent to the border of the dilated choroidal vessels.

However, the exact pathogenesis of this disorder remains discussed. Recently, Francine Behar Cohen and her team have published results from fundamental research studies that inspired the hypothesis that the mineralocorticoid pathway could be involved in CSC. Behar et al. state that in rodents, activation of the mineralocorticoid pathway in ocular cells induced ocular phenotypes carrying many features of acute CSC. Molecular mechanisms include expression of the calcium-dependent potassium channel (KCa2.3) in the endothelium of choroidal vessels, inducing subsequent vasodilation. Inappropriate or overactivation of the mineralocorticoid receptor in ocular cells and other tissues (such as brain, vessels) could link CSC with the known comorbidities observed in CSC patients, including hypertension, coronary disease, and psychological stress.

Central serous chorioretinopathy risk factors

Major risks associated to CSC (Boxes 3 and 4)

- *Genetic predisposition inherited dominant condition*:[3] Probable genetic background may predispose to CSC and thick choroid is phenotypic indicators

Box 3: Central serous chorioretinopathy (CSC) major risk factors

- Genetic predisposition inherited dominant condition
- 'Type-A' personality, stress, and low threshold of frustration
- Endocrine Cushing syndrome
- Corticosteroids
- Stress
- Pregnancy
- Shift work

Box 4: Other CSC risk factors

- Sleep disturbances, sleep apnea
- Cardiovascular diseases and hypertension
- *Gastroesophageal disorders*: High prevalence of *Helicobacter pylori* infection in CSC patients
- *Drug-induced CSC (other than steroids)*:
  - Pseudoephedrine and oxymetazoline
  - MMDA (an illicit amphetamine)
  - Ephedra (contained in body-building dietary products)
  - Sildenafil, tadalafil, and vardenafil
  - MEK-inhibitors (binimetinib) for metastatic cancer
- Allergic respiratory disease
- Autoimmune disorders

- *Psychopathology*: Association between CSC and 'type-A' personality, stress, and low threshold of frustration tolerance

Imaging

Fluorescein angiography imaging

Fluorescein angiography shows one or more leakage dots at the RPE level. At these is associated, after a few years' evolution a diffuse retinal pigment epithelial dysfunction with neurosensory retinal detachment, areas of RPE atrophy, pigment deposits, and large areas of granular hyperfluorescence. Indocyanine green (ICG) angiography shows in late phase choroidal hyperpermeability with staining of the choroidal stroma.

Cross-section OCT

In the central serous retinopathy, a serous retinal detachment is seen in almost all the acute cases. The detached retina forms an angle of 10–15° with the pigment epithelium. The outer nuclear layer, with the photoreceptor nuclei, the outer limiting membrane, and ellipsoid (inner/outer photoreceptor segment junction) are elevated. OCT may reveal a small break in the pigment epithelium at the leakage dot seen on fluorescein angiography. From this break, we may occasionally see fibrin that seems to leak from the choroid toward the inner space of the detachment. At the retinal serous detachment level, the tips of the photoreceptors may be thickened and have increased reflectivity, with granulations or flaking of the internal face of the detachment in the detached area. Choroid is very thick—from 350 μ to 600 μ or more. There is also a further focal increase in choroidal thickness and dilated outer choroidal vessels, and attenuation and thinning of the choriocapillaris and Sattler's layer vessels overlying the dilated vessels.

In the chronic form of serous chorioretinopathy, after detachments waning, there is thinning of the outer nuclear layer associated with changes at the ellipsoid (IS/OS junction) that may be thickened, irregular, or distorted. Areas of retinal atrophy are frequent. Over the course of the natural history, neovascular membranes may appear.

En face OCT

Choroid

En face scans performed deep in choroid shows a dilatation of medium and large vessels. The *en face* OCT choroid images facilitate the visualization of Haller's layer.

Different incidence of choroidal vessel patterns at the posterior pole are observed between healthy and pachychoroid disorders, CSC/DRPE recorded by *en face* OCT (Dansigani, Savastano, and Lumbroso). Five different patterns of Haller's layer are seen in normal choroid. Five different patterns—(1) temporal herringbone, (2) branched from below, (3) laterally diagonal, (4) doubled arcuate, and (5) reticular feature—were observed. Pattern 1 is the most representative in healthy eyes (49.2%) while the pattern 5 (reticular) is characteristic in pachychoroid disorders, CSC (51.22%), and DRPE (46.15%) (**Figures 1** and **5**).

Although the reason of this difference remains unknown, probably the choroid vasculature pattern might play a role in the origin and development of neuroretinal pathologies. Another possible explanation may be changes of morphological pattern during the disease development. It is possible that progressive dilatation of choroid vessels during pachychoroid disorders evolution causes a rearrangement of the previous vascular choroid pattern, probably due to compression of the vessels in choroid tissue. The results of these studies are consistent with the assumption that the angioarchitecture of the choroidal vasculature is not homogeneous throughout the entire choroid and probably are related to the different disease.

Pigment epithelium detachment

In central serous chorioretinopathy, frontal scans show the dimensions of pigment epithelium detachments, and allow precise examination of the photoreceptors. Pigment epithelium detachment shape is predominantly circular and never acquires multilobular or cluster features. Pigment epithelium detachments walls are thin, smooth, and regular. Pigment epithelium detachments shape in chronic diffuse epitheliopathy has different features: circular or irregular ovoid shape and multilobular features on *En face*.

Neovascularization in CSC (Figures 2 to 4)

Clinical features

Exudative or nonexudative new vessels appear under the pigment epithelium flat detachment. These patients with chronic CSC or with vascular age-related macular degeneration (AMD) show frequently no evidence of macular fluid on structural OCT imaging.

Fluorescein angiography features

Most CNVs in CSC are nonexudative. There is no leakage hyperfluorescence. When CNV is exudative, we see the normal dye leakage features. ICG angiography shows in late phase choroidal hyperpermeability with staining of the choroidal stroma.

Structural OCT features

A flat irregular or undulated pigment epithelium elevation can be noted. No fluid is observed. When CNV is exudative, we observe the normal fluid leakage.

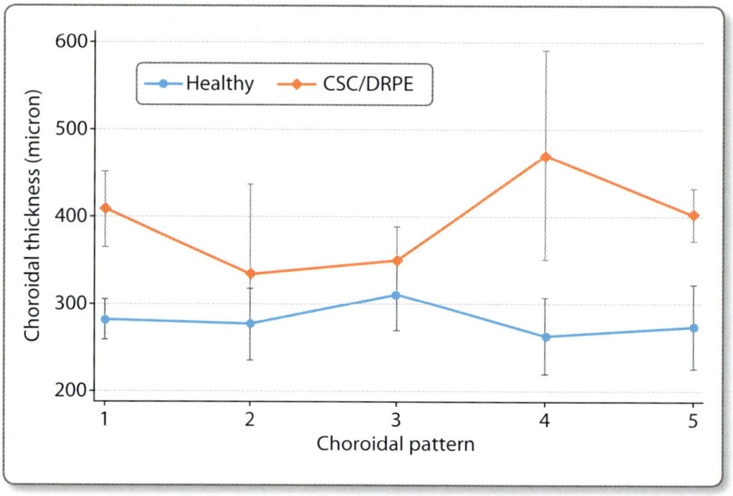

Figure 1 Correlation among the different choroidal patterns (x-axis) and macular thickness (y-axis) between healthy and central serous chorioretinopathy/diffuse retinal pigment epitheliopathy (CSC/DRPE) eyes.

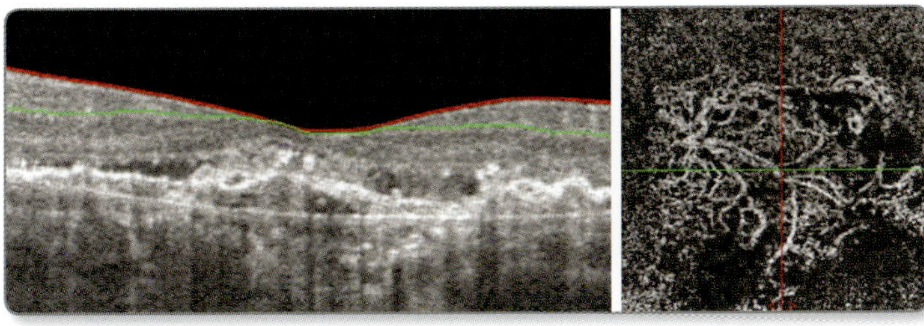

Figure 2 Central serous retinopathy B-scan e angio optical coherence tomography (OCT). Chronic central serous chorioretinopathy (CSC) epitheliopathy: OCT B-scans show a slightly elevated retinal pigment epithelium (RPE) with a wavy profile. OCT angiography shows a wide neovascular membrane with regular new vessels.

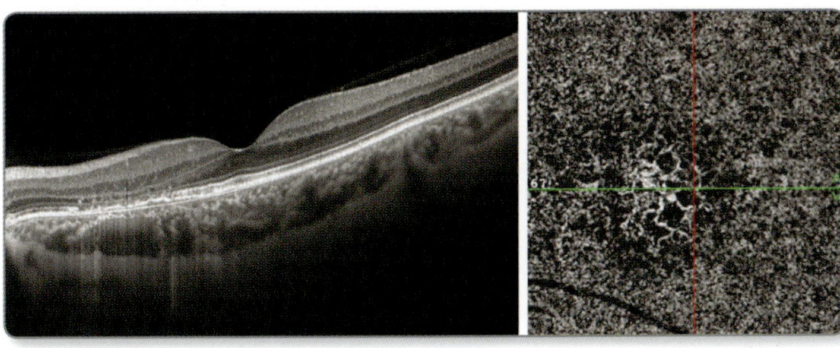

Figure 3 Quiescent (nonexudative) neovascularization complicating this chronic atypical central serous chorioretinopathy (CSC). Slight alteration of the retinal pigment epithelium (RPE) pigmentation. No drusen or other signs of age-related macular degeneration (AMD) are visualized in the macular region. On B-scan optical coherence tomography (OCT), the RPE profile is normal. OCT angiography shows a quiescent (nonexudative) choroidal neovascularization (CNV) complicating this chronic atypical CSC.

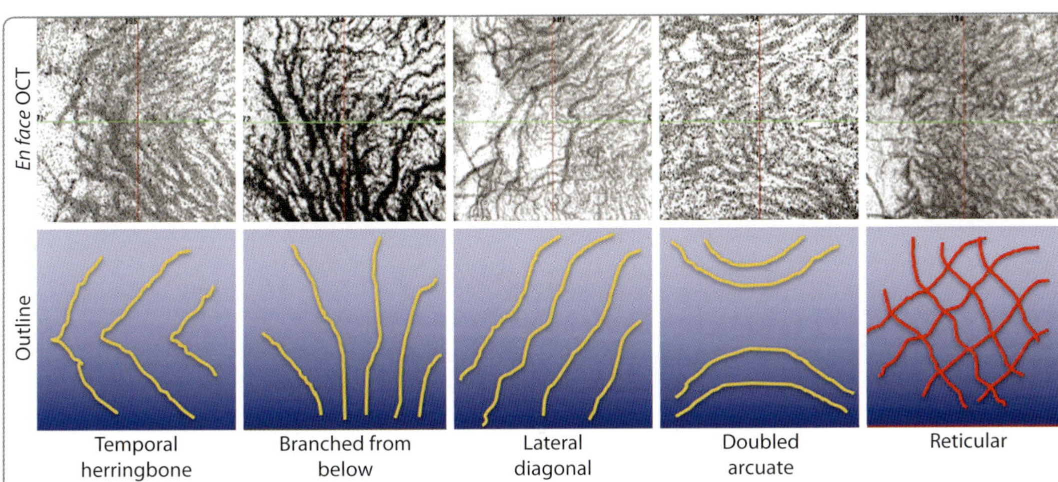

Figure 4 Choroidal patterns in normal eyes. In normal eyes, we observe five different choroidal vessels patterns. In chronic and acute central serous chorioretinopathy (CSC), the most frequently observed pattern is 'reticular'.

OCT angiography features

Choroidal neovascularizations show vessels thick and sinuous and generally filament like. They have a low capillary density with tangled rare branches subdivision and arborization. Some loops are present, nonexudative vessels initially always appear under the pigment epithelium and no flow is observed in the nonvascularized zone. The new vessels may later spread into the avascular area of the external retina and become exudative. Most nonexudative membranes are large vessels with very few or no small capillaries. The neovascular network may be large, but not dense.[3–6]

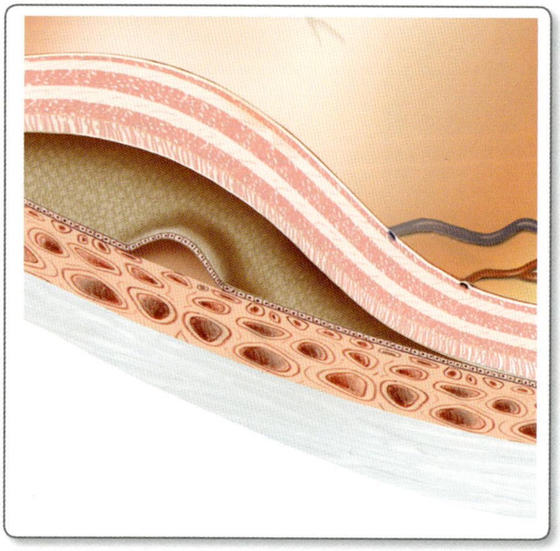

Figure 5 Central serous retinopathy serous retinal detachment in a case of chronic epitheliopathy. Below the retinal elevation, we can observe an optically empty space containing fluid. The detached retina forms an angle of about 15° with the pigmented epithelium. The outer nuclear layer, with the photoreceptor nuclei, the outer limiting membrane and the inner/outer photoreceptor segment junction are elevated.

Morphology

In nonexudative CNV, branching patterns show different shapes. Their margin may be sharp with lacy-wheel shaped or sea-fan shaped vessels. Sometimes, they are poorly circumscribed with long filamentous thick vessels, simple or tangled, long-tangled filaments have rare small sparse capillaries. Their global shape is mostly (80%) irregular, in 20% rounded. No halo is seen around the nonexudative new vessels. This could be due to less choriocapillaris blood flow alterations.

Evolution

The evolution of these nonexudative CNV is very slow. They show some slight morphological changes and sometimes important enlargement in a few years. Normally, there is no vision deterioration and no fluid accumulation. In our cases followed without treatment for 4 years, no vision changes were observed, but they increased in area regularly.

Management

Two-thirds of clinical CSC forms see retinal serous detachment spontaneous regression after 6 months of evolution. Current therapeutic options are based on the traditional retinal laser on the leakage point, dynamic phototherapy, micropulse laser, and oral treatments (antialdosterone).

Dynamic phototherapy

The first thing to do in front of a persistent DSR after photodynamic therapy (PDT) is to repeat complete imaging with fluorescein and ICG angiography for previously untreated diffusion areas and OCT angiography. CSC is one of the few pathologies where FA and ICGA are still necessary. We need to ascertain presence or lack of choroidal neovascularization that could benefit from treatment with antivascular endothelial growth factor (anti-VEGF). In fact, a quarter of patients with chronic CSC have predominantly silent choroidal new vessels (CNV). In the case of associated polyps (66% of NVC complicating CSCs), the occlusion rate of polyps is 50% with PDT and only 25% with anti-VEGF.

Traditional laser

Traditional retinal laser on the leakage area, when it is located more than 400 μ from fovea.

Micropulse laser

A few studies have attempted to compare PDT or traditional laser with micropulse laser. Some studies report complete resolution after the first treatment in 51% of patients treated with PDT versus 13% for micropulsed laser, although 30% required reprocessing in the PDT group (vs. 15%). PDT has the advantage of being widely studied in the literature but its potentially harmful nature on the choroidal circulation, especially in the case of iterative treatments, should be considered. The micropulsed laser has no previously described complication and the procedure can be repeated several times.

References

1. Daruich A, Matet A, Dirani A, et al. Central serous chorioretinopathy: Recent findings and new physiopathology hypothesis. Prog Retin Eye Res 2015; 48:82–118.
2. Azar G, Wolff B, Mauget Faÿsse M, et al. Pachychoroid neovasculopathy: aspect on optical coherence tomography angiography. Acta Ophthalmol 2017; 95:421–427.
3. Lehmann M, Bousquet E, Beydoun T, et al. PACHYCHOROID: an inherited condition? Retina 2015; 35:10–16.
4. Pang CE, Freund KB. Pachychoroid pigment epitheliopathy may masquerade as acute retinal pigment epitheliitis. Invest Ophthalmol Vis Sci 2014; 55:5252.
5. Gallego-Pinazo R, Dolz-Marco R, Gómez-Ulla F, et al. Pachychoroid diseases of the macula. Med Hypothesis Discov Innov Ophthalmol 2014; 3: 111–115.
6. Warrow DJ, Hoang QV, Freund KB. Pachychoroid pigment epitheliopathy. Retina 2013; 33:1659–1672.

19 High myopia, myopic CNV

Bruno Lumbroso

Introduction

In high myopia, or pathologic myopia, individuals present with more than 6 diopters of myopia or an axial length greater than 26–27 mm. It occurs in more than 50% of the world population, mainly in Asia, and is increasing. Choroidal neovascularization (CNV) is frequent, and its evolution is generally negative. It is a significant cause of irreversible vision loss and a common cause of blindness in all continents. It is the leading cause of vision loss in patients younger than 50 years.

Pathophysiology, risk factors: Heredity and environment

Genetic studies have identified more than forty genes that take part in myopic pathophysiological pathways, from retinal phototransduction to scleral remodeling and axial lengthening.

Environmental factors also influence scleral remodeling through visual perception. In the case of near tasks and reading, a physiological feedback leads to axial growth. This problem is particularly apparent in Asia. Population studies suggest that development of myopia is associated with education and the amount time spent doing near work.[1,2]

Myopia is associated with decreased choroidal thickness and thinner choroid is significantly associated with myopic CNV. Mean choroidal thickness less than 200 (µm) for the myopic eye from 3 diopters to 8 diopters in young patients, and 80 (µm) for the high myopia group is associated to neovascular membranes. Choroidal thickness decreases with higher myopia and aging.

Older age and choroidal vascular filling delay are high-risk factors. Highly myopic eyes with lacquer cracks may progress to localized atrophy (40% of eyes) or develop CNV (14%). Eyes with tessellated fundus, lacquer cracks, diffuse or localized atrophy at the initial examination progress to the development of CNV in about 40% of highly myopic eyes, and the progression affects negatively the visual prognosis. Younger patients may retain good vision for a long time. Chorioretinal atrophy always develops around the regressed CNV at 5 and 10 years after the onset of CNV. Some not foveal CNVs may regress spontaneously (**Box 1**).[3-6]

Neovascular membranes in myopia

Myopic CNVs are generally type 2 classical new vessels and frequently small in size. A small proportion may reach greater size. These neovascular membranes develop above the pigment epithelium, generally at level of lacquer cracks or on the edge of a chorioretinal atrophy area. They may penetrate the outer avascular retinal layer. The lesion is roundish and grey, pigmented, without intraretinal fluid nor subretinal fluid pooling without pigment epithelium detachment, nor edema. At times, dot or flame hemorrhages can be seen.[7-9] A roundish or spindle-shaped dark area can be noticed around CNV margin (**Box 2**).

Fluorescein angiography features

Hyperfluorescence is initially dot like in the first frames and enlarges with dye leakage.

Box 1: Choroid thickness

Decreased:

- Myopia (normal)
- Age (normal)
- Atrophic macular degeneration
- Hereditary macular dystrophies
- Retinitis pigmentosa
- Tapetoretinal degenerations

Structural optical coherence tomography features

Choroidal neovascularization appears as a small hyper-reflective formation with sharp limits, above retinal pigment epithelium (RPE). There is hardly ever any cystoid edema nor diffuse edema. A hyper-reflective ring is frequently noticed along the CNV margin.

> **Box 2: Morphology of myopic choroidal neovascularization (CNV)**
>
> *Generally:*
> - Rounded
> - Tuft shaped
> - Clump shaped
> - Glomerular shaped
> - Globular
> - Irregular, elongated at atrophic area margin
>
> *Rarely:*
> - Medusa head
> - Coral bush shaped

Optical coherence tomographic angiography features

In high myopia, segmentation is difficult and artifacts are frequent, due decrease in thickness and irregularity of its layers that causes difficulty in automated but also in manual segmentation. It is technically awkward to obtain a very good optical coherence tomographic angiography (OCTA) scan due to ocular length and eventually staphyloma.

The myopic neovascular membrane is frequently a glomerular, globular, or tuft shaped. The membrane forms an irregular sphere with sharp margins. Less frequently, the membrane is bigger, elongated, growing on the margins of an atrophic area, with a dense capillary network, reaching the size and features of AMD membranes (**Figures 1** to **3; Box 2**).[7–9]

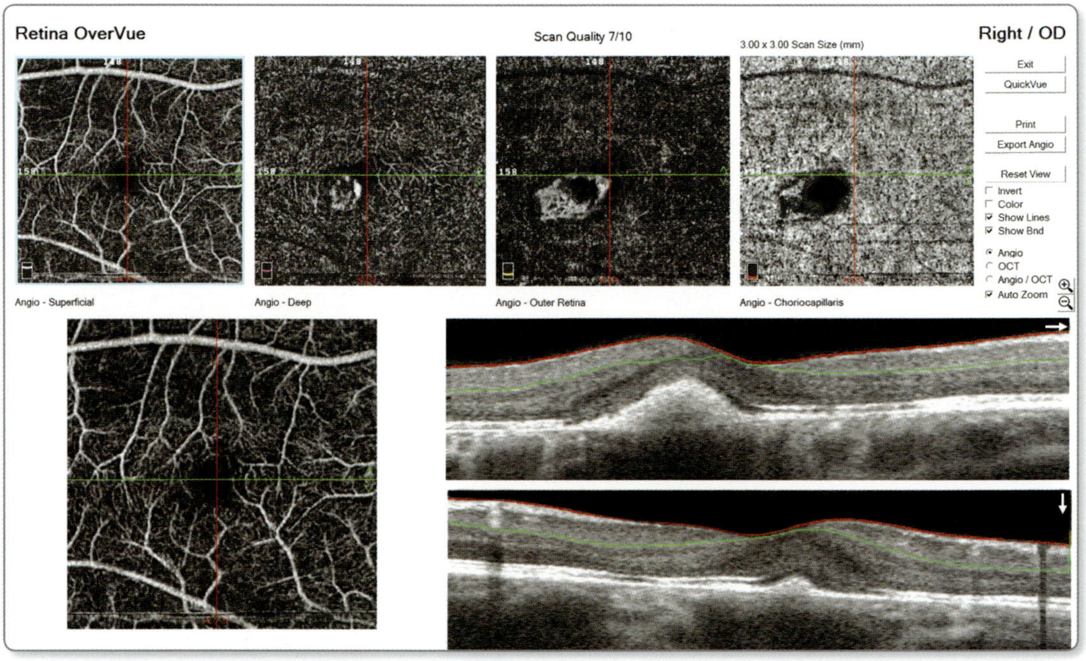

Figure 1 Glomerular myopic type 2 new vessels. New vessels in myopia are generally small, tuft like, or glomerular. This myopic choroidal neovascularization (CNV) is tuft like with ring new vessels. There is no exudation. (Optovue)

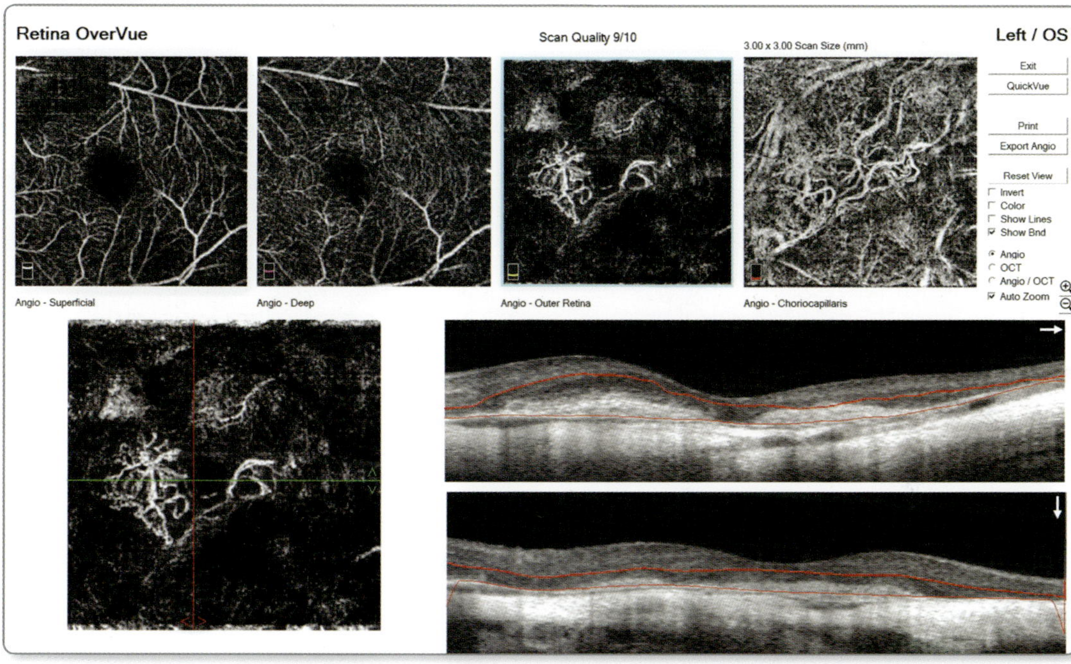

Figure 2 Myopic type 2 new vessels. In this case, the myopic membrane is larger than in glomerular cases. The neovascular membrane is located at an atrophic area margin. No exudation is seen. Limits are sharp. (Optovue)

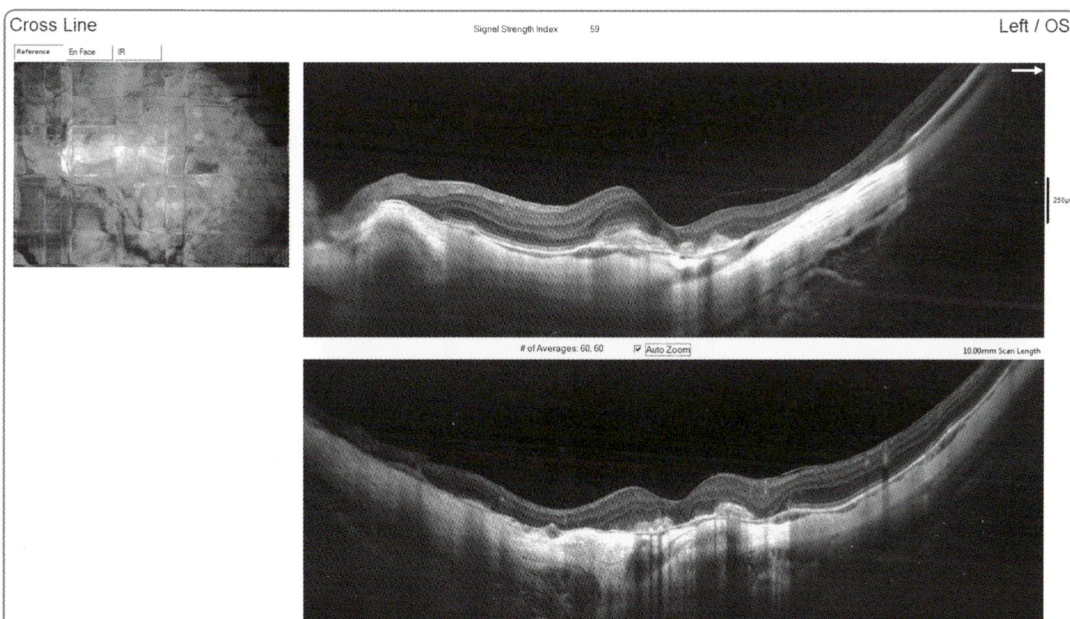

Figure 3 Myopic type 2 new vessels, cross-section scan. The myopic membrane is large, located at an atrophic area margin. No exudation is seen. Limits are sharp. (Optovue)

References

1. Cassagne M, Malecaze F, Soler V. Pathophysiology of myopia: nature versus nurture. J Fr Ophtalmol 2014; 37:407–414.
2. Cooper J, Tkatchenko AV. A Review of Current Concepts of the etiology and treatment of Myopia. Eye Contact Lens 2018; 44:231–247.
3. Miller DG, Singerman LJ. Natural history of choroidal neovascularization in high myopia. Curr Opin Ophthalmol 2001; 12:222–224.
4. Bottoni F, Tilanus M. The natural history of juxtafoveal and subfoveal choroidal neovascularization in high myopia. Int Ophthalmol 2001; 24:249–255.
5. Hayashi K, Ohno-Matsui K, Shimada N, et al. Long-term pattern of progression of myopic maculopathy: a natural history study. Ophthalmology. 2010; 117:1595–1611.
6. Kumaran N, Sim DA, Tufail A. Long-term remission of myopic choroidal neovascular membrane after treatment with ranibizumab: a case report. J Med Case Rep 2009; 3:84.
7. Avila MP, Weiter JJ, Jalkh AE, et al. Natural history of choroidal neovascularization in degenerative myopia. Ophthalmology 1984; 91:1573–1581.
8. Silva R. Myopic maculopathy: a review. Ophthalmologica 2012; 228:197–213.
9. Secrétan M, Kuhn D, Soubrane G, et al. Long-term visual outcome of choroidal neovascularization in pathologic myopia: natural history and laser treatment. Eur J Ophthalmol 1997; 7:307–316.

20 Pathophysiology of diabetic retinopathy

Maria Cristina Savastano

According to global estimates of the prevalence of diabetes, diabetes mellitus (DM) is expected to affect around 550 million people all over the world.[1]

Although the exact pathophysiological mechanism is not perfectly understood, DM is characterized by constant hyperglycemia that damages various organs and manifests in macrovascular complications. Premature atherosclerosis resulting in strokes, peripheral vascular disease, myocardial infarctions, nephropathy, neuropathy, and retinopathy are the most common complications secondary to diabetic disease.[2]

Hyperglycaemia and in particular glycemic variations caused aberrant regulation of a number of biochemical pathways, ultimately leading to superoxide production and the burden of oxidative stress in retinal tissues. Multiple factors are implicated in diabetic retinopathy (DR) pathophysiology that generates mitochondrial dysfunction, inflammation, and hypoxia with secondary vascular endothelial growth factor (VEGF) secretion, give rise to vascular and neuronal apoptosis, neovascularization, and elevated vasopermeability.

In DR, inner blood-retinal barrier (BRB) dysfunction is characteristic. The leakage of blood constituents into the retinal tissue occurs in conjunction with the degradation of the inner BRB, and this often leads to diabetic macular oedema (DMO).

In the pathophysiology of DR, it is possible to recognise four different steps that cause the microscopic alterations to macroscopic clinical observations (**Figure 1**).

Hyperglycemia induces an obliteration of small vessels through the glycosylation of the basal membrane of endothelial cells. Further, hyperglycemic states favor the activation of alternative pathways leading to reactive oxygen species (ROS) formation and augmented concentrations locally and in the rest of the body.

Central to the degenerative capillary pathophysiology seen in DR is the loss of pericyte function. Pericytes play a crucial role in normal retinal function, facilitating the differentiation, migration, and proliferation

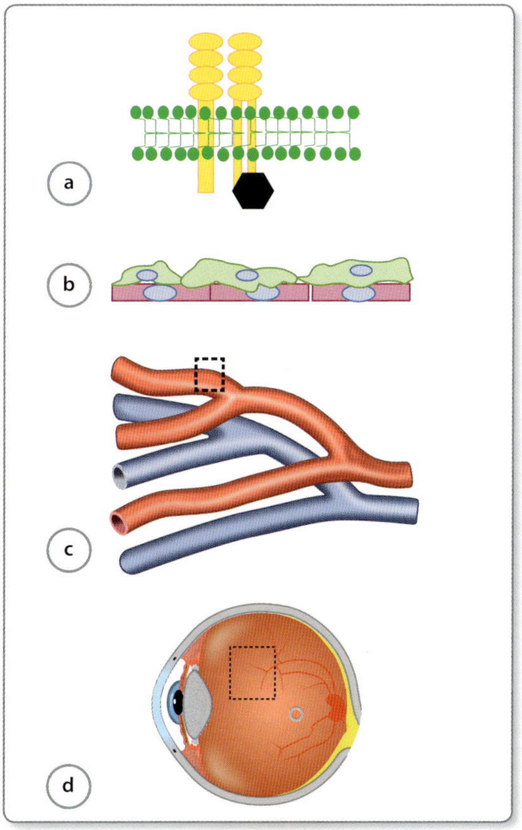

Figure 1 Pathophysiology of diabetic retinopathy. Early damages of diabetic retinopathy are reported in outline. (a) Microscopic events involve pericyte with their apoptosis secondary to dephosphorylation of platelet-derived growth factor (PDGF) receptors (black hexagon). (b) Vessel instability is directly attributed to apoptotic cell death of pericytes and uncoordinated proliferation of endothelial cells. (c) Retinal tissue damages show the microvasculature changes with microhemorrhages and macular edema. (d) Macroscopic event observed by standard ophthalmoscopy with severe retinal diabetic signs.

of angiogenic endothelial cells. The loss of pericytes and the presence of 'pericyte ghosts' are therefore considered a key histopathological hallmark of DR. VEGF is strongly implicated in the leakage of blood vessels and acts as a potent vasopermeability agent. Thickening of the vascular basement membrane is also common in DR and is thought to arise from the upregulation of fibronectin, collagen, and laminin, which in turn lead to changes in the microenvironmental factors mediating the growth, survival, and function of pericytes and endothelial cells (**Figures 2** and **3**).

Mitochondrial aberrations may induce apoptosis and inflammatory factors may elevate hypoxia-mediated VEGF secretion. Neurovascular dysfunction, vascular hyperpermeability, and/or neovascularization may follow and give rise to the pathological hallmarks of PDR and DMO.

Recently, particular interest is turned to Muller cells and the cells of the pigment epithelium that seem to be directly susceptible to hyperglycemia.

This new evidence has induced researchers to consider new hypotheses for the early histopathological changes occurring in DR linked in particular to paracrine secretions and consequently to the increase in the glial fibrillary proteins in Müller cells and in the retinal pigment epithelium.

Hyperglycaemia associated with poor DR management drives the aberrant regulation of five biochemical pathways in DR patients, resulting in excess glucose being metabolised via the polyol pathway through an aldose reductase (AR)-mediated pathway, which leads to the deposition of advanced glycation end products (AGEs). AGEs can induce prooxidant and proinflammatory events, thus exacerbating oxidative stress and leukocyte adhesion.

In the nonproliferative stage of DR, the following lesions can be seen in the fundus of the eye:

- Microaneurysms
- Microhemorrhages and intraretinal hemorrhages
- Hard exudates
- Cotton-wool
- Exudates
- Intraretinal microvascular abnormalities (IRMA)
- Irregular size of the veins
- Retinal edema

Proliferative retinopathy is characterized by development of new vessels to overcome

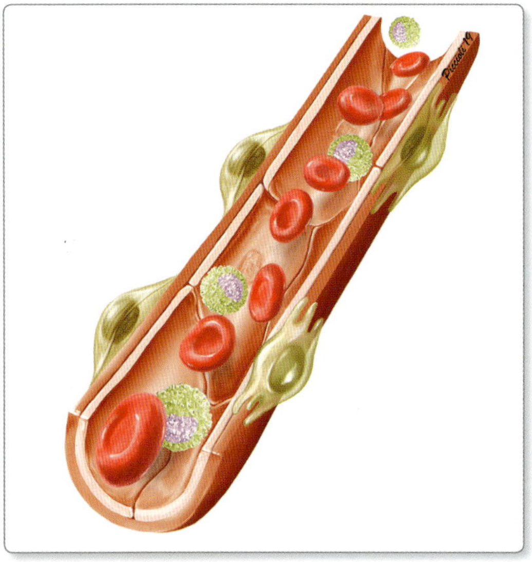

Figure 2 Normal retinal capillary with red blood cells and white blood cells. On the walls pericytes are drawn in light green.

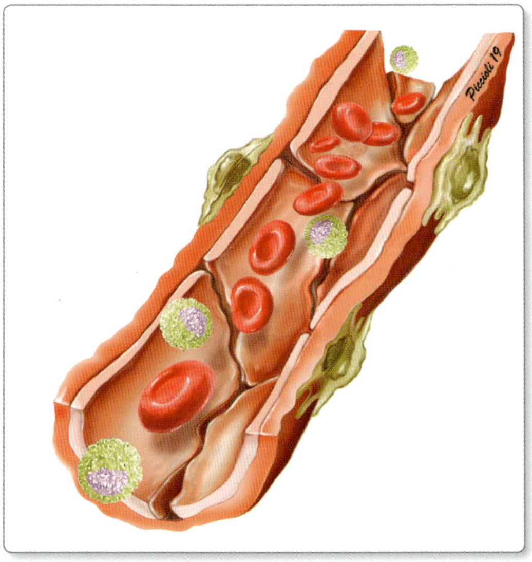

Figure 3 Retinal capillary in diabetic retinopathy showing wall alterations, leaking cell junctions. On the walls pericytes are damaged.

the hypoxic stimulus and guarantee retinal perfusion. However, new vessels formed have a wall that consists only of the endothelium and makes them sensitive to bleeding causing preretinal and endovitreal hemorrhages. New vessels may generate on the retina and/or optic disk and are accompanied by a fibrous structure that arises from the retinal level and from inside the vitreous cavity. The contraction of this tissue may be the cause for secondary retinal detachment.

A fearful consequence is reduced perfusion of retinal tissue and the development of new vessels in the anterior segment with the ensuing neovascular glaucoma.

Both early retinopathy and its proliferative advanced form may be complicated by the presence of macular damage that may be of the edematous and/or ischemic form with ensuing impairment of vision.

As reported, the most important inflammatory factor linked to hypoxia and released in the early stages of DR is VEGF. Many retinal structures have VEGF receptors: Muller cells, endothelial cells, astrocytes, retinal pigment epithelium, and ganglion cells. This occurrence determines the participation of the entire retinal stroma in triggering of DR. Further, VEGF, inducing increase in vascular permeability with extravasal leakage, is precursor of neovascularization and of macular edema (**Figure 4**).

Besides VEGF, in DR, many other molecules are produced having the ability to transmit and amplify the signal of hypoxic distress. Among these, mention can be made of the metabolites of arachidonic acid, tumor necrosis factor-α (TNF-α), and various interleukins (IL) among which IL-1b and IL-6.

Underlying the greater predisposition to the more aggressive forms of DR that do not respond to possible treatments, one must always consider genetic predisposition. Indeed, there are factors that cannot be influenced like the genetic factors that determine the aggressiveness of the disease. Knowledge about genetics of this disease will be useful to identify the genome variants that are associated with the higher possibility of complications among individuals with DM.

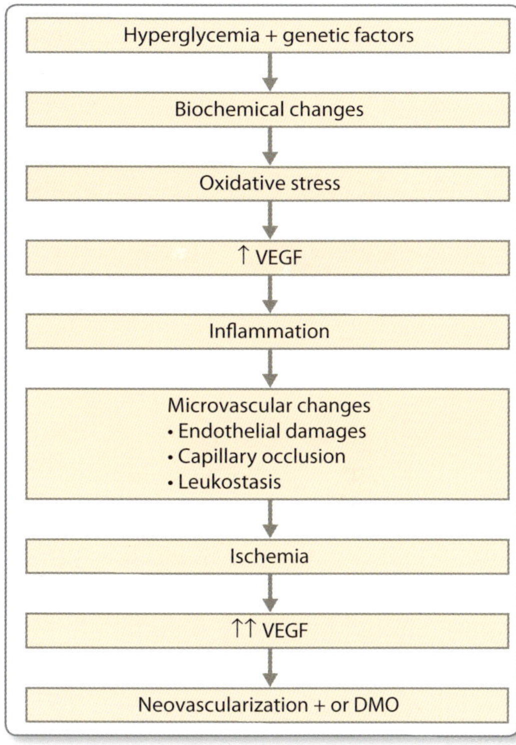

Figure 4 Flowchart of pathophysiology of diabetic retinopathy.
(DMO: diabetic macular oedema; VEGF: vascular endothelial growth factor)

Treatment

Optimizing glycemic and lipid controls is the first-line therapy in diabetes control, which also reduces the DR progression.

A number of large clinical trials have demonstrated that the onset and severity of DR can be prevented by a good blood hyperglycemia control that often implies the use of insulin injections.

In case of proliferative DR, the use of laser photocoagulation is still to be considered the election therapy. DMO management is currently controversial although the use of intravitreal anti-VEGF is considered the most effective to reduce the risk of visual acuity loss. The use of intravitreal glucocorticoid showed visual acuity preservation in a large number of cases (**Figures 5** to **7**).

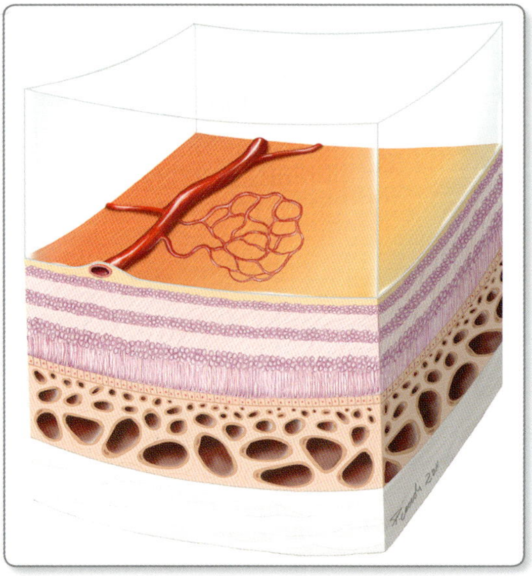

Figure 5 Proliferative diabetic retinopathy. A vascular proliferative membrane is creeping on the retinal surface.

Although a number of therapeutic strategies are available to clinicians for the treatment of DR, no treatment is yet to fully attenuate clinical progression to reverse damage to the retina. Further, a large number of patients do not respond to certain treatments at all, and patient outcomes are often limited in many cases.

Future prospective treatments

Future prospective treatment probably will be the gene therapy. The anatomy of the eye is highly favorable and the small size enables the use of low doses of vector for gene delivery. Further, the possibility of fundus examination allows to easily evaluate the results of treatment efficacy.

One of the most relevant aspects of the research interest is aimed at artificial intelligence.

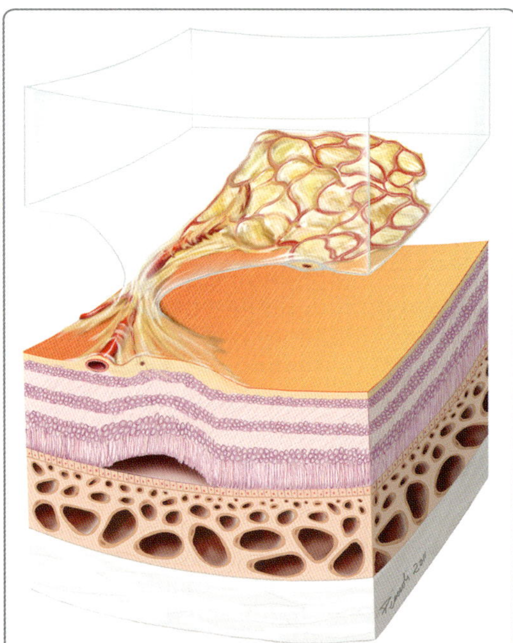

Figure 6 Proliferative diabetic retinopathy. The proliferative membrane is now fibrovascular. Vitreous traction lifts slightly the retinal surface.

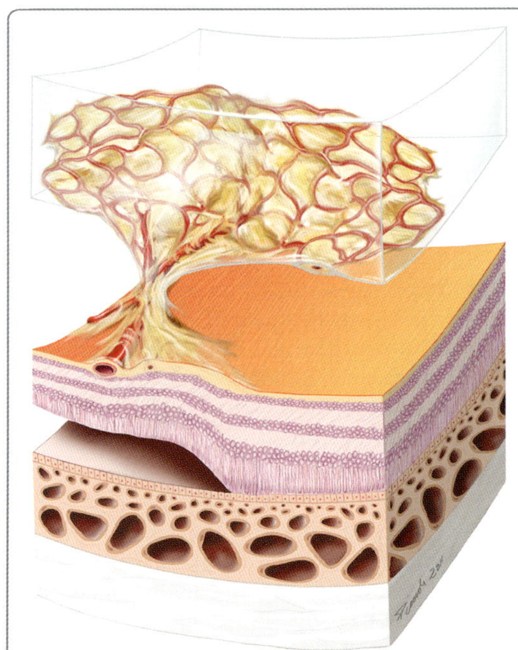

Figure 7 Proliferative diabetic retinopathy. The fibrovascular proliferative membrane lifts strongly the retinal surface, resulting in retinal traction detachment.

The early phase or predicting DR signs and their identification might help to reduce the risk of complicated DR. New machine learning algorithms able to identify and interpret biomedical features, and can help the clinician in everyday clinical practice.[3]

References

1 Shaw JE, Sicree RA, Zimmet PZ. Global estimates of the prevalence of diabetes for 2010 and 2030. Diabetes Res Clin Pract 2010; 87:4–14.
2 Cecilia OM, José Alberto CG, José NP, et al. Oxidative Stress as the Main Target in Diabetic Retinopathy Pathophysiology. J Diabetes Res 2019; 2019:8562408.
3 Tsao HY, Chan PY, Su EC. Predicting diabetic retinopathy and identifying interpretable biomedical features using machine learning algorithms. BMC Bioinformatics 2018; 19:283.

21 Diabetic retinopathy

Bruno Lumbroso, Maria Cristina Savastano

Introduction

Fluorescein angiography (FA) was, until a few years ago, gold standard for studying diabetes. Currently, structural optical coherence tomography (OCT), '*en face*' OCT, and OCT angiography are necessary for the evaluation and quantification of vascular alterations, for deciding treatment and for post-treatment monitoring. OCT angiography is replacing FA in everyday clinical routine to study diabetic retinopathy. It is essential to get a detailed imaging of the normal and pathologic vascularization. Quantitative optical coherence tomographic angiography (OCTA) vascular evaluation has become an integral part of diabetic retinopathy assessment and follow-up. As clinicians get more familiar with the technology, the images appear more meaningful and useful than dye angiography images. OCTA visualizes better retinal flow, allows quantifying vascular lesions, and permits a close clinical monitoring. Diabetic retinopathy is subdivided into proliferative and non-proliferative retinopathy and is seen in patients with diabetes evolution for more than 8 years. We use the American Academy of Ophthalmology classification (**Box 1**).

Box 1: 2003 American Academy of Ophthalmology classification

This classification is used all over the world and includes five levels:

1. No diabetic retinopathy
2. Mild nonproliferative diabetic retinopathy (NPDR)
3. Moderate nonproliferative diabetic retinopathy (NPDR)
4. Severe nonproliferative diabetic retinopathy (NPDR)
5. Proliferative diabetic retinopathy (PDR)

Nonproliferative diabetic retinopathy

The first retinal manifestations of diabetic retinopathy are caused by a microangiopathy. Microaneurysms, intraretinal hemorrhages, cotton-wool spots, microvascular abnormalities, vascular dropout areas are seen in mild and severe nonproliferative diabetic retinopathy (NPDR). Diabetic macular edema (DMO) can occur at any stage. OCT angiography highlights the following alterations: dilated and irregular capillaries, coarser capillary network, widening of the avascular area with interruptions in the capillary arcade, capillary micro-occlusions, and microaneurysms. It allows already to highlight nonperfused areas even before the clinical retinopathy onset (**Boxes 2** to **6**).

Box 2: Optical coherence tomographic angiography (OCTA) in nonproliferative diabetic retinopathy

Superficial network:

- FAZ widening
- Enlarged perifoveal intercapillary areas
- Capillary dropout
- Disappearance of small capillaries
- Areas of capillary nonperfusion
- Capillary tortuosity
- Neovascularization of the retina

Deep network:

- FAZ widening
- Microaneurysm
- Vessel congestion
- Capillary tortuosity
- Capillary dropout

(FAZ: foveal avascular zone)

Box 3: Diabetic maculopathy

- Maculopathy with diffuse edema
- Maculopathy with cystoid edema
- Macular serous elevation of the retina
- Ischemic maculopathy
- Traction maculopathy

Box 4: Microaneurysms on optical coherence tomography (OCT) angiography

Visualization of microaneurysms is possible when:

- Intravessel flow
- Thrombosed microaneurysms silent
- Microaneurysms with very slow flow silent
- FA shows more microaneurysms than OCTA.

(FA: fluorescein angiography)

Box 5: Causes of microaneurysms

- Diabetic retinopathy
- Venous occlusions
- Sickle cell disease
- Hypertensive retinopathy
- Peripheral telangiectasia
- Coats' disease
- Eales' disease

Some microaneurysms seen in retinal periphery in normal persons

Structural OCT and '*en face*' OCT show macular edema as leading cause of visual impairment in NPDR. The irregular microcavities merge, giving rise to the initial pseudocysts of cystoid edema. When cystoid edema evolves over a long period, the pseudocysts merge forming large confluent irregular and angular cavities.

Box 6: Causes of proliferative retinopathy other than diabetic retinopathy: extensive retinal ischemia

Frequent causes:

- Occlusions of the central retinal vein
- Occlusions of the venous branches
- Eales' disease
- Other vasculitis
- Pars planitis
- Sicklecell anemia
- Thalassemia

Rare causes:

- Leukemia
- Cryoglobulinemia
- Waldenstrom's disease
- Multiple myeloma
- Unknown causes

In the mild NPDR, nonperfused zones are seen close to the foveal avascular zone and partly merge with it. Avascular foveal zone is enlarged, with first small then wide breaks of the vascular arcade. Later, temporal dropout areas will merge with the avascular foveal zone. Dilated capillaries and irregularly enlarged vessels and few microaneurysms can be observed. Vascular density map is very useful to assess retinopathy severity, highlighting the dropout areas.[1-5]

A potential level of ischemic retinal injury is superficial capillary plexus with its disorganization of retinal inner layers (DRIL). DRIL, if occupying the macular center, represents a negative prognostic factor for the visual acuity. Cross-sectional images within the disorganization of retinal inner layers area show a loss of inner retinal layers from the ganglionar complex to the inner nuclear layer while NFL and outer retina remain unaffected. These structural changes correspond to the distribution of retinal hypoperfusion on OCT angiography. The maximum of flow signal void lies within superficial capillary plexus, but intermediate and deep plexus also demonstrate hypoperfusion. Disorganization of retinal inner layers may be identified as a component of severe and complex retinal pathology in diabetic retinopathy.

In later evolution, superficial plexus shows more advanced dropout lesions, large ischemic areas, and numerous microaneurysms. Large nonperfused zones merge with the foveal avascular zone. Vascular dilatations and loops at the ischemic areas' margins are the first symptoms of proliferative retinopathy. Diabetic retinopathy evolution is more severe and network disruption is more marked at deep vascular plexus level. The possibility given by OCTA of separately examining the superficial and deep retinal vascular plexus makes it possible to differentiate the retinal involvement in various diabetic lesions.

Widening of the foveal avascular zone (FAZ) and vascular dropout areas are best seen in the superficial capillary plexus, nonperfused zones are most important in superficial network. Dilatations of the microaneurysms are best seen in the deep capillary plexus. In OCT angiography, thrombosed microaneurysms are silent. Microaneurysms with very slow flow are also silent.

Diabetic macular edema occurs at every stage of diabetic retinopathy evolution in 30% of the cases. It is the most frequent cause of low vision and blindness in diabetic eye disease, OCT and OCTA help in confirming diagnosis, deciding treatment, and monitoring the evolution with or without treatment.

The quantitative assessment of OCT scans in DMO is important in predicting outcome. Vascular congestion is highest at the border of ischemic areas with normal retina.

Traction edema is seen when the traction applied by the epiretinal membrane leads to retraction of the internal limiting membrane.

Quantitative changes are important in following the structural changes progression and the response to therapy. AngioAnalytic software consents to see enlargement of the foveal avascular zone and the capillary dropout areas. We can study capillaries in real time and get precise measurement and study perfusion density maps to grade progressive vascular changes. A new algorithm makes it possible to objectively estimate flow density in any retinal layer (**Figures 1** to **8**).

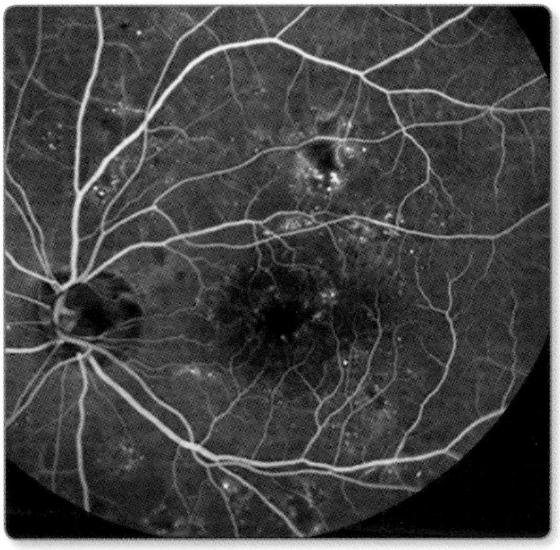

Figure 1a Early nonproliferative diabetic retinopathy: Fluorescein angiography (FA) highlights irregular diameter on retinal vessels, numerous microaneurysms clusters, non-perfused zones, rare hemorrhages, areas of dye leakage. However, in FA, superficial and deep networks are overlaid and cannot be observed separately.

Proliferative diabetic retinopathy

Diabetic new vessels proliferation appears initially inside retina. Slowly, it reaches retinal surface and later develops at preretinal, pre-papillary, and intravitreal level. New vessels can be seen at the optic disk or the edges of ischemic retinal areas in severe ischemic retinopathies. Later, new vessels appear in the iris angle inducing iris rubeosis and neovascular glaucoma. These new formed capillaries are very fragile, due to thin single cell walls and may cause vitreous hemorrhages with ensuing glial proliferation and retinal detachment. Proliferative retinopathy is most frequent among younger people: it may be a developmental stage of nonproliferative retinopathy or it may appear early. Fluorescein angiography produces an intense dye leakage that masks the vessels in the late frames.

OCT and OCT angiography features

Proliferative diabetic retinopathy shows loops of blood vessels protruding from the retina or the optic disk into the vitreous. Intraretinal

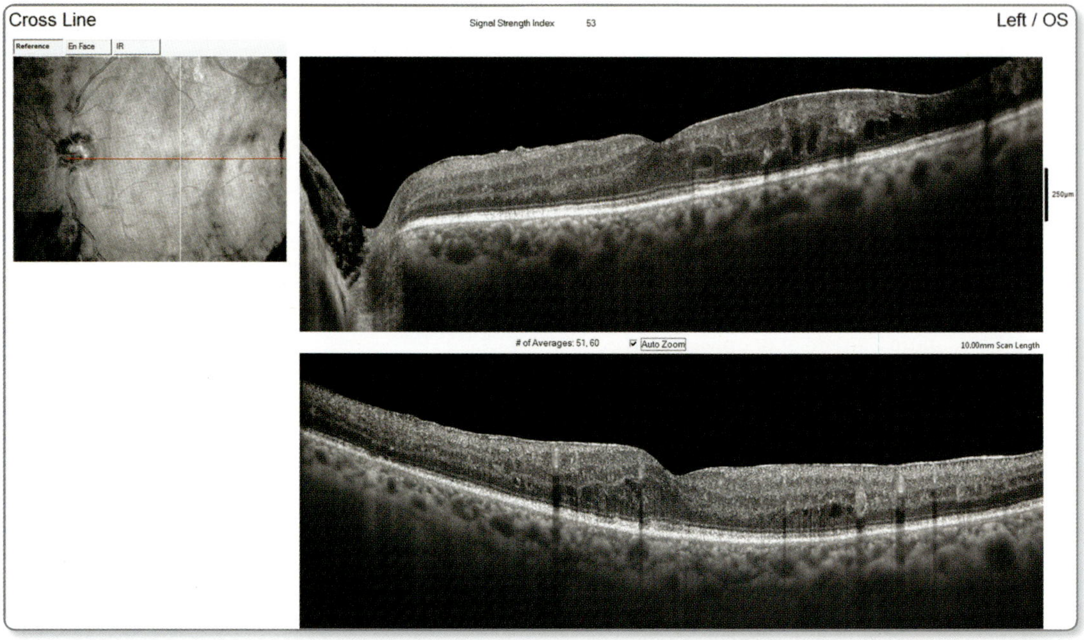

Figure 1b Nonproliferative diabetic retinopathy. Structural optical coherence tomography (OCT). There are few microaneurysms and rare small cystoid cavities. A thin epiretinal membrane can be seen. (Optovue)

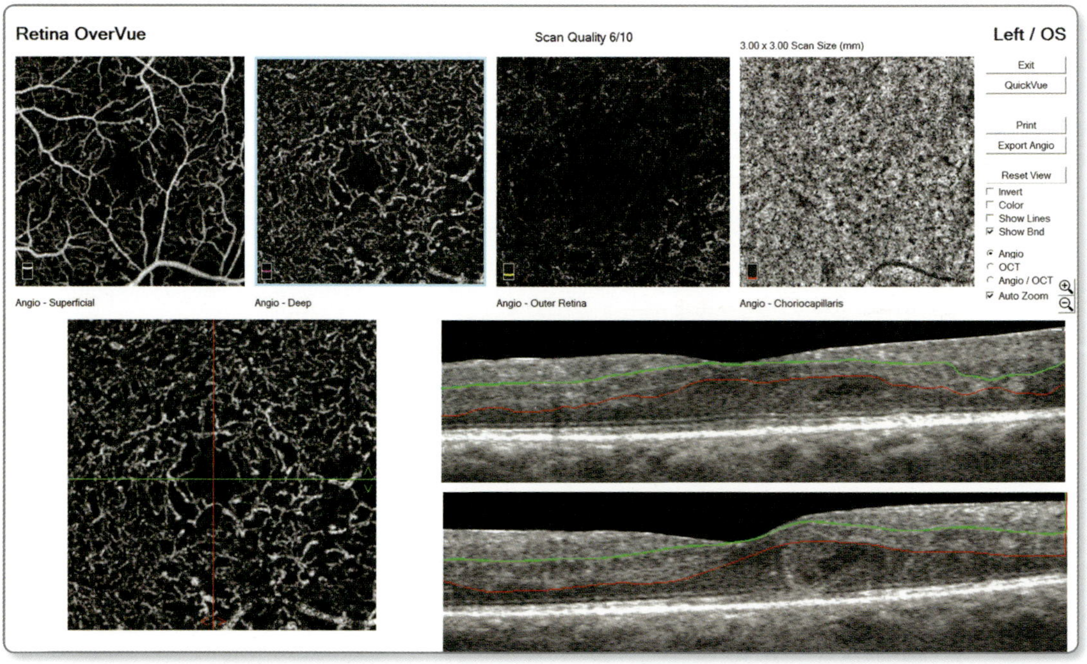

Figure 1c Early nonproliferative diabetic retinopathy. Optical coherence tomography (OCT) angiography. The superficial network shows few microaneurysms, an enlarged avascular foveal zone, with irregular breaks of the vascular arcade, dropout areas around the foveal avascular zone and rare microaneurysms. The deep network shows irregularities of the net, with few irregular microaneurysms. B-scans highlight diffuse edema and some cavities. (Optovue)

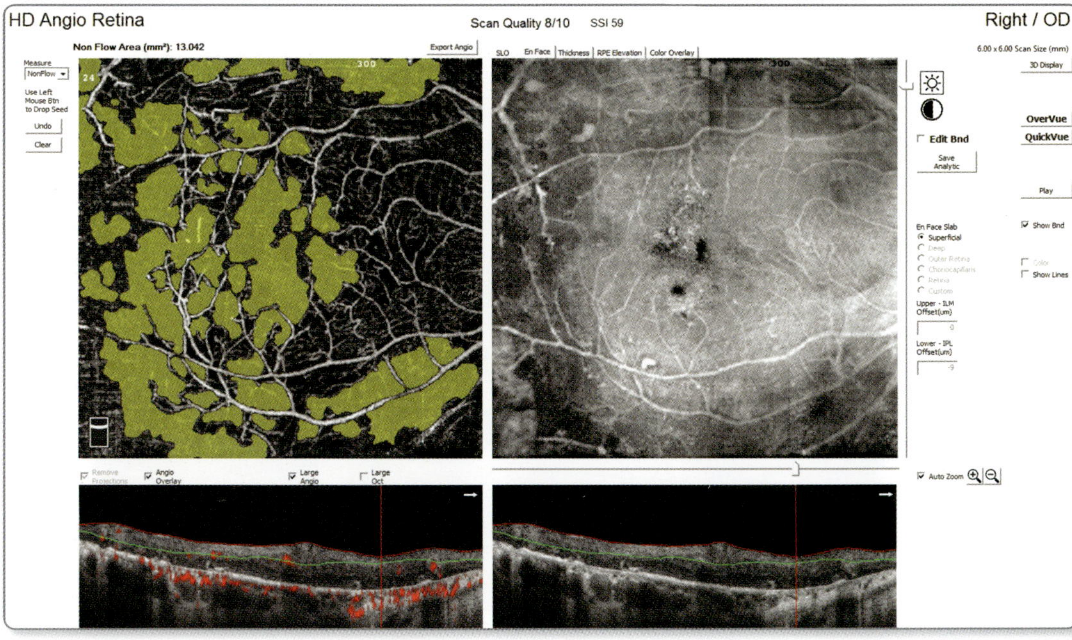

Figure 2a Nonproliferative diabetic retinopathy. Optical coherence tomography angiographic (OCTA) angio analytic superficial network. Vessels at superficial network level are irregular and there are some vasodilatations and microaneurysms. Nonperfused area in nonproliferative diabetic retinopathy case is present. Dropout areas are highlighted in yellow. At bottom, a B-scan OCT angiography showing intraretinal flows. (Optovue)

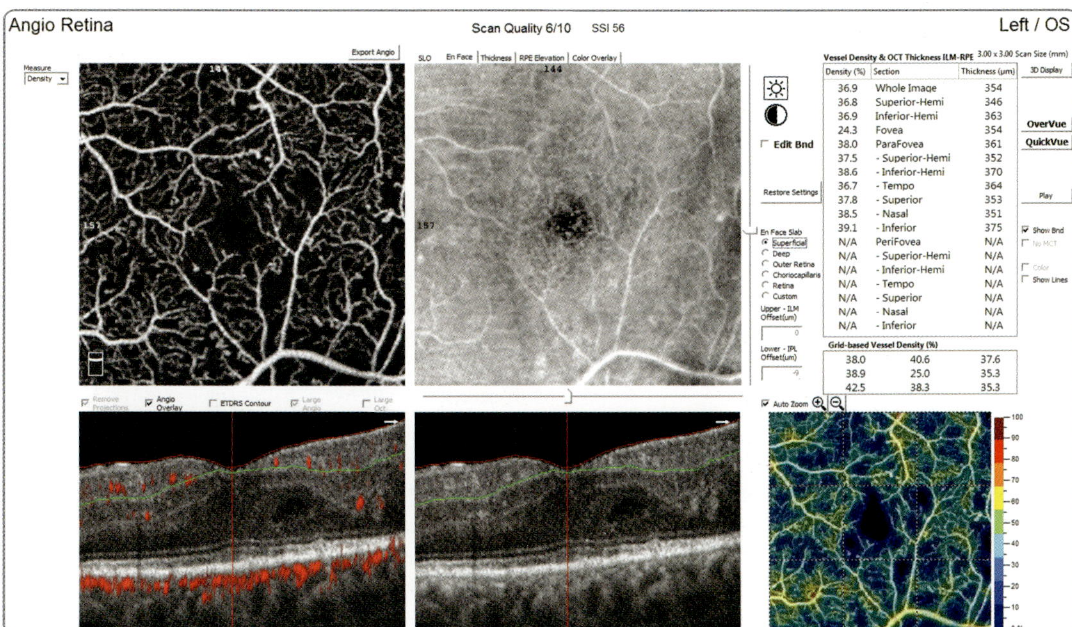

Figure 2b Nonproliferative diabetic retinopathy. Optical coherence tomography angiography (OCTA) angio analytic superficial network. Vessels are irregular and there are some vasodilatations and microaneurysms. Nonperfused area case is present. At bottom, a vessel density scan showing intraretinal flows. (Optovue)

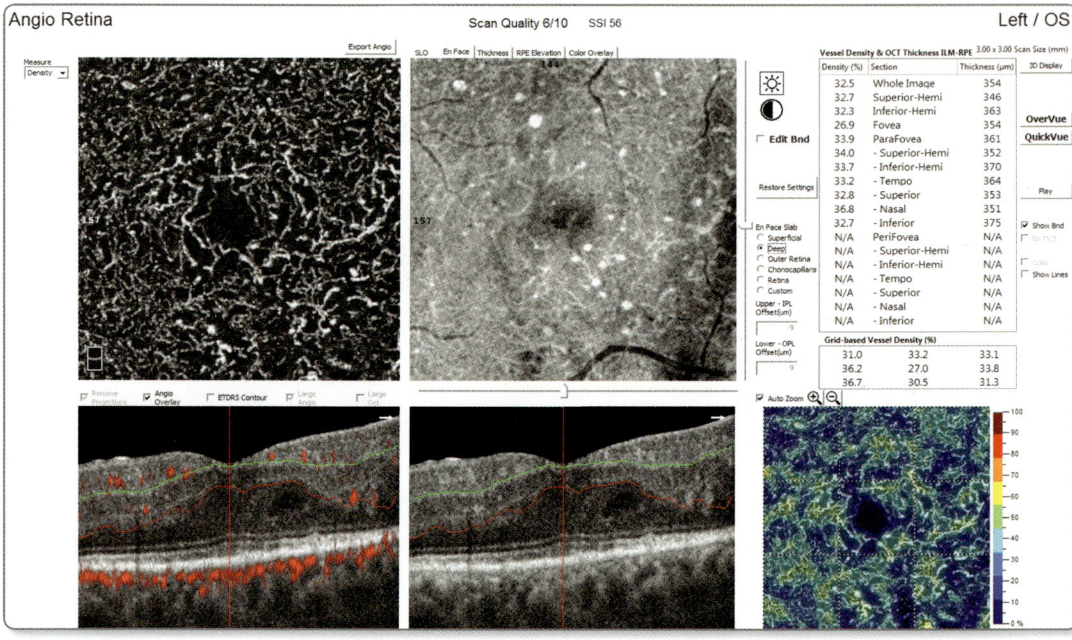

Figure 2c Nonproliferative diabetic retinopathy (same case). Optical coherence tomographic angiography (OCTA) angio analytic deep network. Vessels at deep network level are irregular with frequent vasodilatations and microaneurysms. Nonperfused area is present. These dropout areas are more important in superficial than in deep network. At bottom, a B-scan OCT angiography showing intraretinal flows. Right-hand side figure shows '*en face*' vascular density map with dropout areas. (Optovue)

microvascular abnormalities (IRMAs) are seen as hyper-reflective lesions of the inner retinal vascular nets. Ischemic areas are well delineated on the OCT angiography and allow precise quantification and evolution monitoring.

The OCT angiography shows loops, branching, and irregularity of the neovascular network. It allows to see the circulating blood flow in the vessels. Preretinal new vessels proliferation appears creeping on retinal surface. Later, they penetrate vitreous. Prepapillary new vessels infiltrate deeply in the vitreous cavity surrounded by fibrovascular tissue (**Figures 9a** and **9b**).

Management of diabetic retinopathy

Management of early (background) nonproliferative diabetic retinopathy

Glycemic, blood lipid levels control, and monitoring hypertension are the basis of management of NPDR. No effective treatment of ischemic maculopathy is known at present.

Management of diabetic macular edema in nonproliferative diabetic retinopathy

Treatment should be started early. Currently, antivascular endothelial growth factor (VEGF) therapy and dexamethasone implant have been the new standard of care in center-involved DMO. Retinal periphery should be monitored and treated by laser in case of large ischemic areas.

Two VEGF-bindings drugs are approved for treatment of DMO: ranibizumab (Lucentis; Novartis) and aflibercept (Eylea; Bayer).

Intravitreal steroid therapy has been available for some years to treat DMO. DMO treatment by dexamethasone low release implant (Ozurdex; Allergan) reducing the number of treatments compared to anti-VEGF drugs. However, dexamethasone implants may induce ocular hypertension and cataract development.

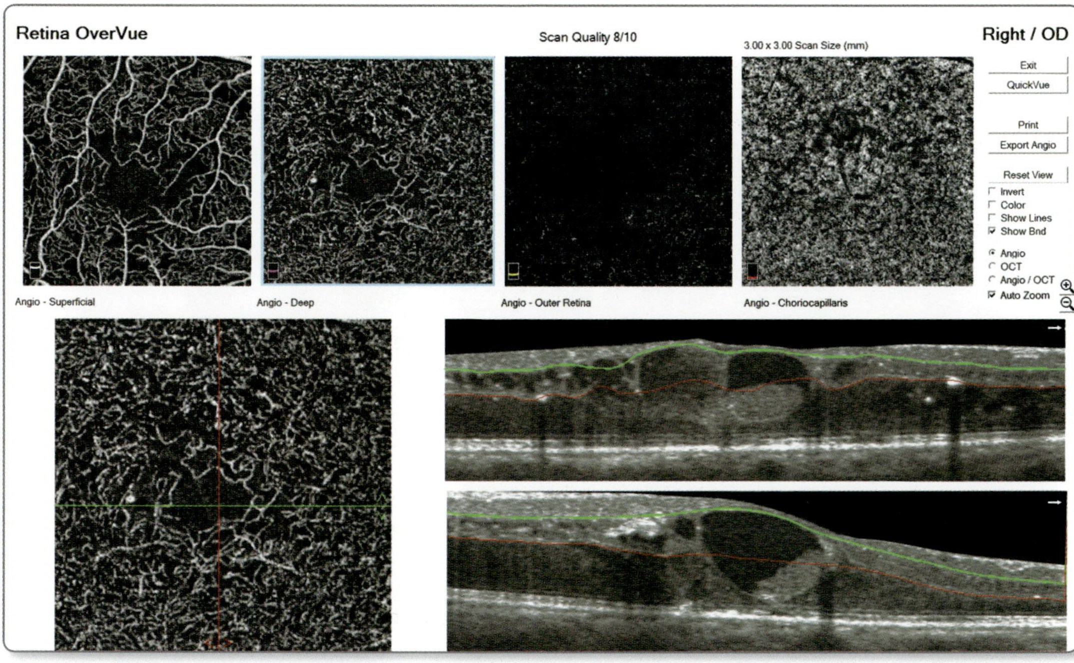

Figure 2d More advanced nonproliferative diabetic retinopathy. Optical coherence tomography (OCT) angiography. The superficial network shows few microaneurysms, an enlarged avascular foveal zone, with breaks of the vascular arcade, dropout areas all around the foveal avascular zone. The deep network shows irregularities of the net, with one microaneurysm. B-scans highlight cystoid edema cavities that can show dense contents. Some hard exudates with shadow below them. Vascular density map shows irregular dropout zones. (Optovue)

Laser photocoagulation treatment for DMO has a decreased role in current management. Safer subthreshold micropulse laser has shown edema reduction.

American Academy of Ophthalmology (AAO) states: 'However, in applying these findings to clinical practice, factors such as frequency of follow-up, treatment cost, and patient preference must be considered in addition to these safety and efficacy outcomes.'

Suggested guidelines (Figure 10)

Two main circumstances may be present:

1. Macular edema involving the fovea center with good vision
2. Macular edema involving the fovea center with decreased vision
   a. The first situation in a standoff as the patient may be reluctant to accept any type of treatment when vision is not impaired. In this case, we consider observation if vision is good (20/20) and the central macular edema is inferior to 400 μm and subfoveal retinal detachment is absent. Good metabolic control is mandatory in this phase and a new control is recommended after 3 months or before in case of visual acuity worsening
   b. Anti-VEGF therapy or slow release dexamethasone implant is required in center-involving DMO with moderate to severe vision loss. Due to possibilities of increased IOP and early cataract formation associated with dexamethasone implant, anti-VEGF injection is our suggestion as the first-line treatment

In case of macular edema not involving mainly the center, subthreshold micropulse laser therapy could be considered hoping that it will decrease the number of injections, however. However, this is not evidence based.

In case of recent (less than 3 months) cerebrovascular or cardiovascular accident, we

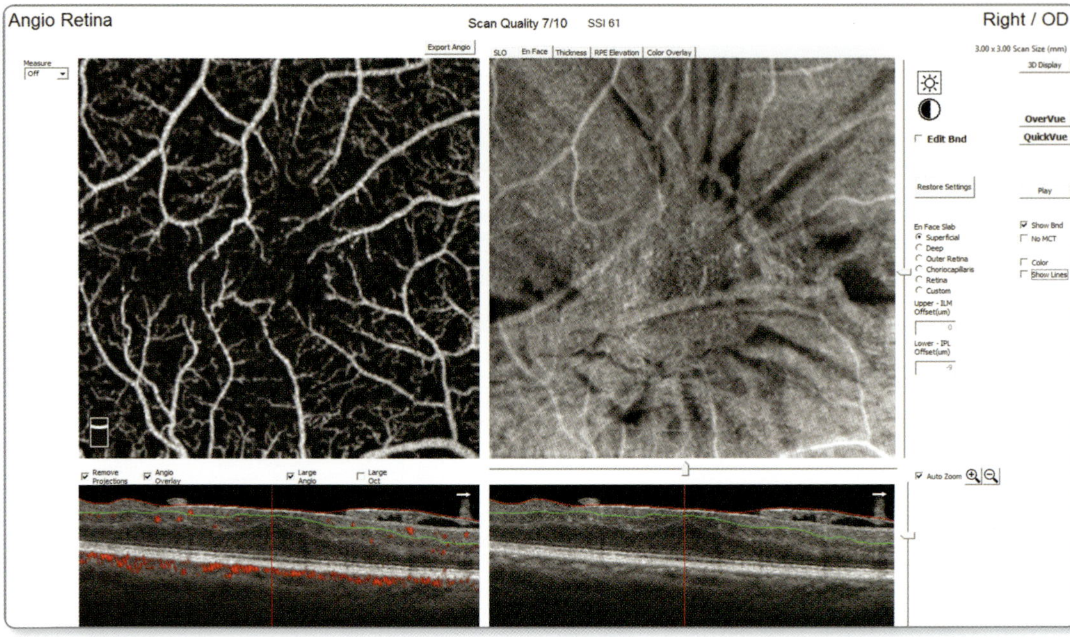

Figure 3a Nonproliferative diabetic retinopathy, superficial network, retinal folds, epiretinal membranes. In the superficial network, the avascular foveal zone is swollen, with large breaks of the vascular arcade. There are few microaneurysms. Nonperfused zones are close to the foveal avascular zone. The '*en face*' scan shows stellar retinal folds shaped by epiretinal membranes traction, seen on B-scans. (Optovue)

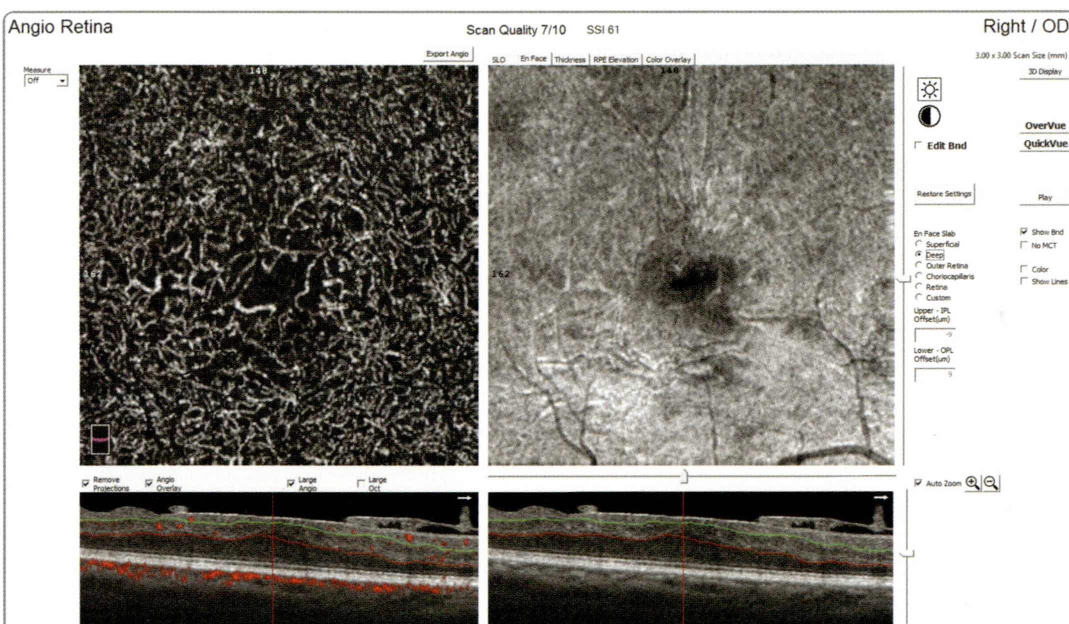

Figure 3b Same case, nonproliferative diabetic retinopathy, deep network, retinal folds, epiretinal membranes. In the deep network, we see a small avascular foveal zone, with irregular dilated vessels and few microaneurysms. Nonperfused zones are less important in deep than in superficial network. The '*en face*' scan shows the same, but less evident stellar retinal folds due to traction by epiretinal membranes, seen on B-scans. (Optovue)

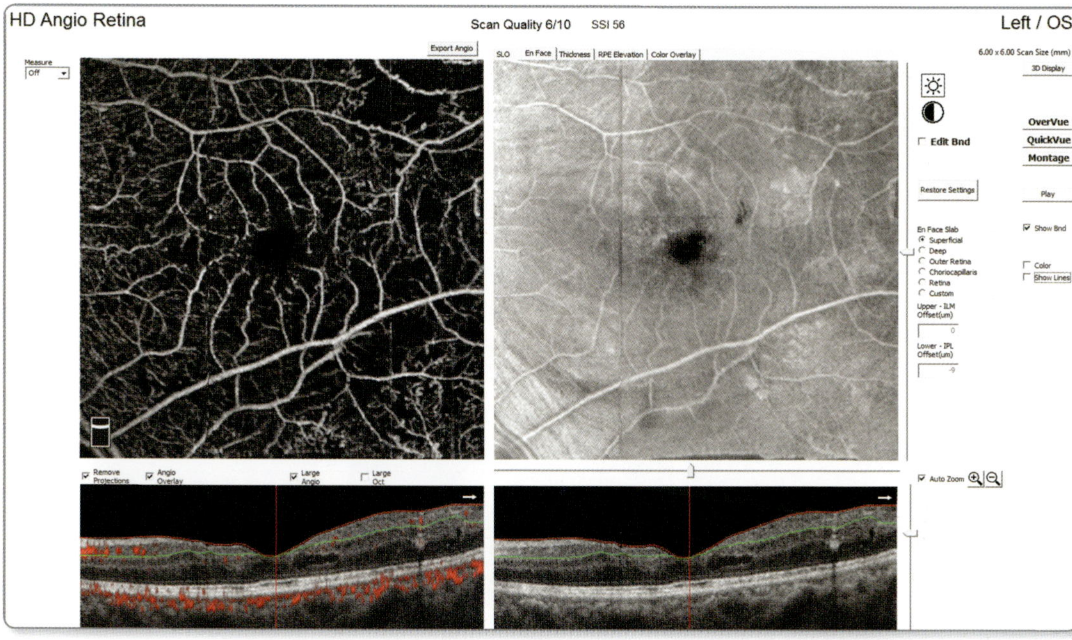

Figure 4a Advanced nonproliferative diabetic retinopathy. Fluorescein angiography. Nonperfused zones are seen close to the foveal avascular zone and partly merge with it on the temporal side. (Heidelberg)

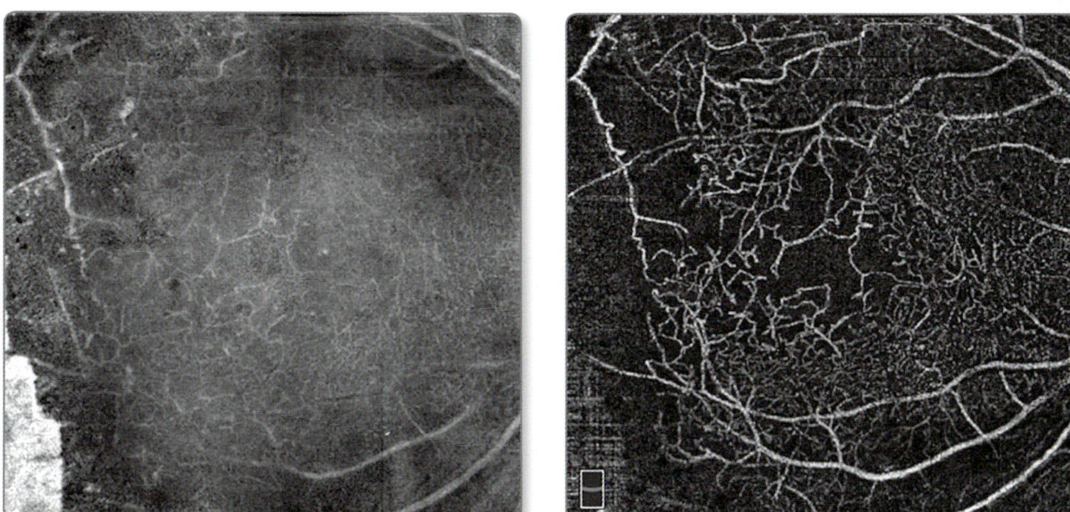

Figure 4b Advanced nonproliferative diabetic retinopathy. Fluorescein Angiography and Optical coherence tomography (OCT) angiography of the same case. Large nonperfused zones are seen on the temporal side, close to the foveal avascular zone, and partly merging with it. Enlarged avascular foveal zone, with disruption of the vascular arcade, dilated capillaries, and rare microaneurysms. (Optovue)

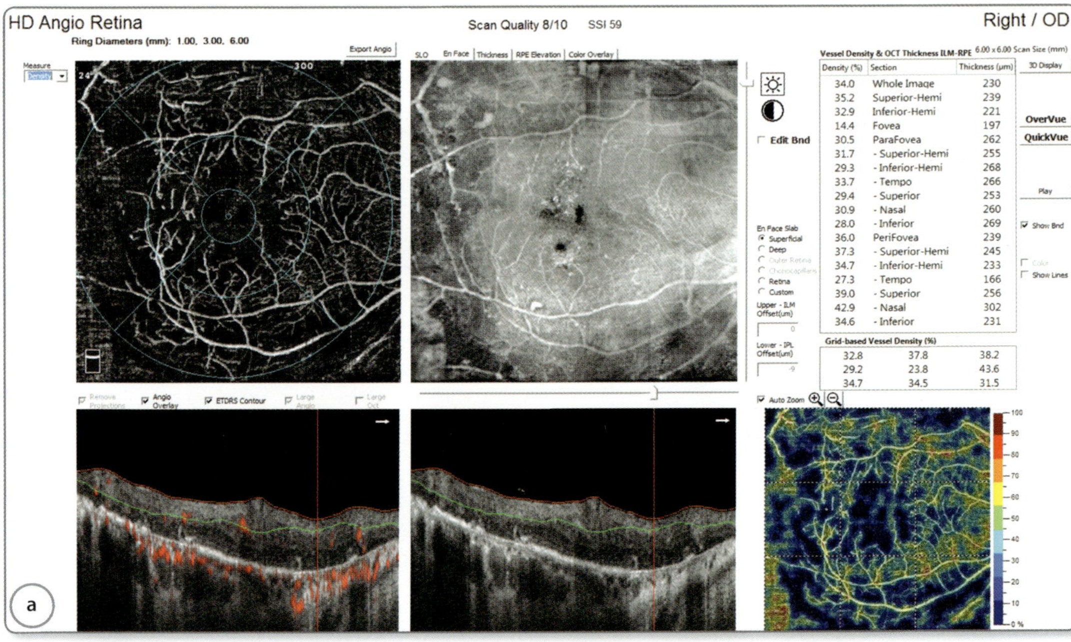

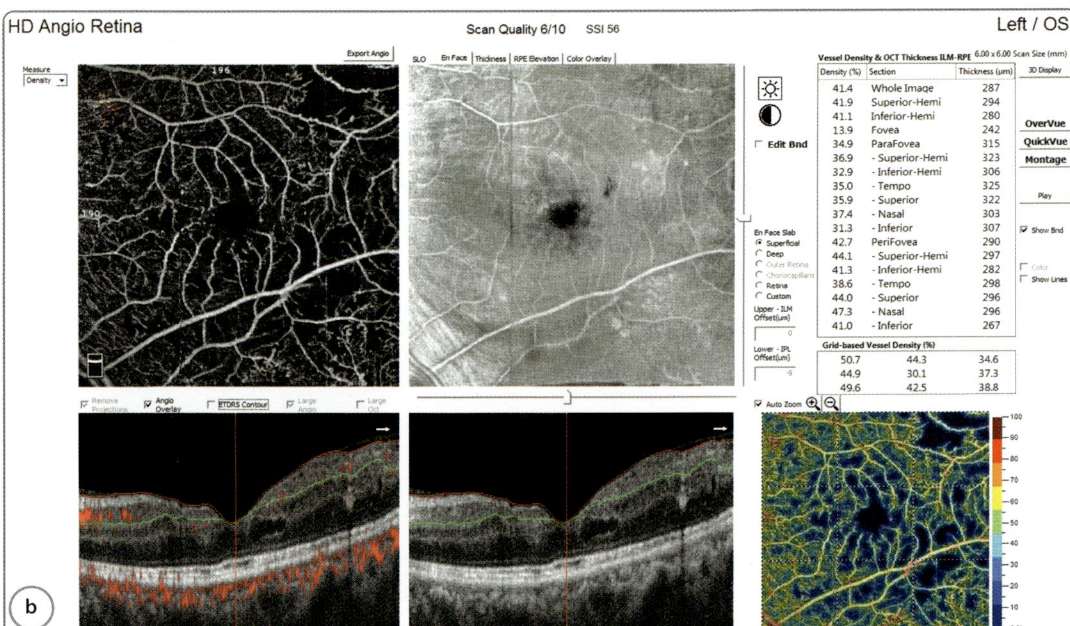

Figure 5a and b Advanced nonproliferative diabetic retinopathy quantitative assessment. Superficial vascular network, vascular density map. Vascular density map is very useful to assess retinopathy severity and for follow-up, highlighting the dropout areas. It shows irregular vessels, few microaneurysms. The nonperfused zones are close to the foveal avascular zone that is enlarged with some interruptions of the vascular arcade. B-scans show retinal thickening with some edema cavities. (Optovue)

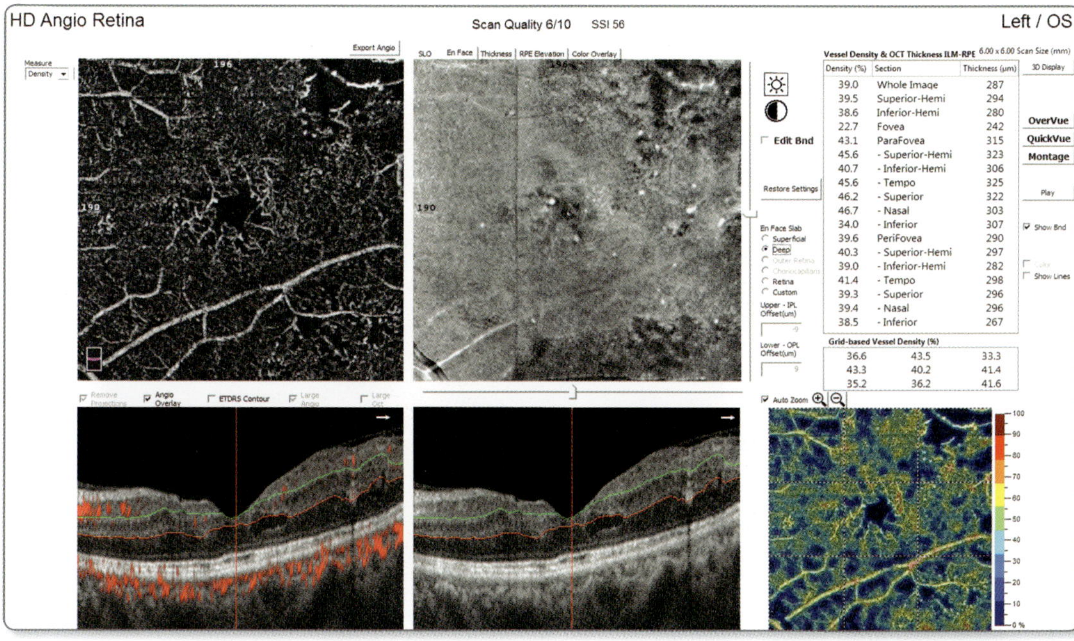

Figure 6 Same case, advanced nonproliferative diabetic retinopathy. Deep vascular network density map. Nonperfused zones show a wide interruption of the vascular arcade. Vascular density map shows the retinopathy severity. B-scans show retinal thickening with some edema cavities. (Optovue)

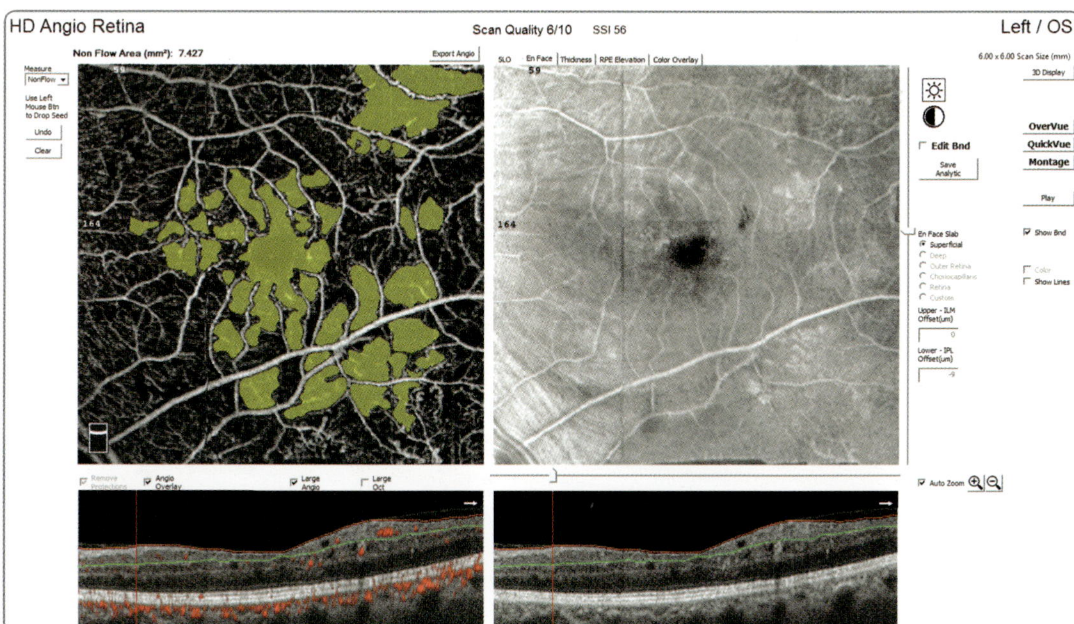

Figure 7 Mild nonproliferative diabetic retinopathy. Angio analysis: quantitative analysis of no flow area. AngioAnalytics software gets precise measurement of dropout areas and allows to quantify enlargement of the foveal avascular zone and the capillary no-flow areas, highlighted in yellow. (Optovue)

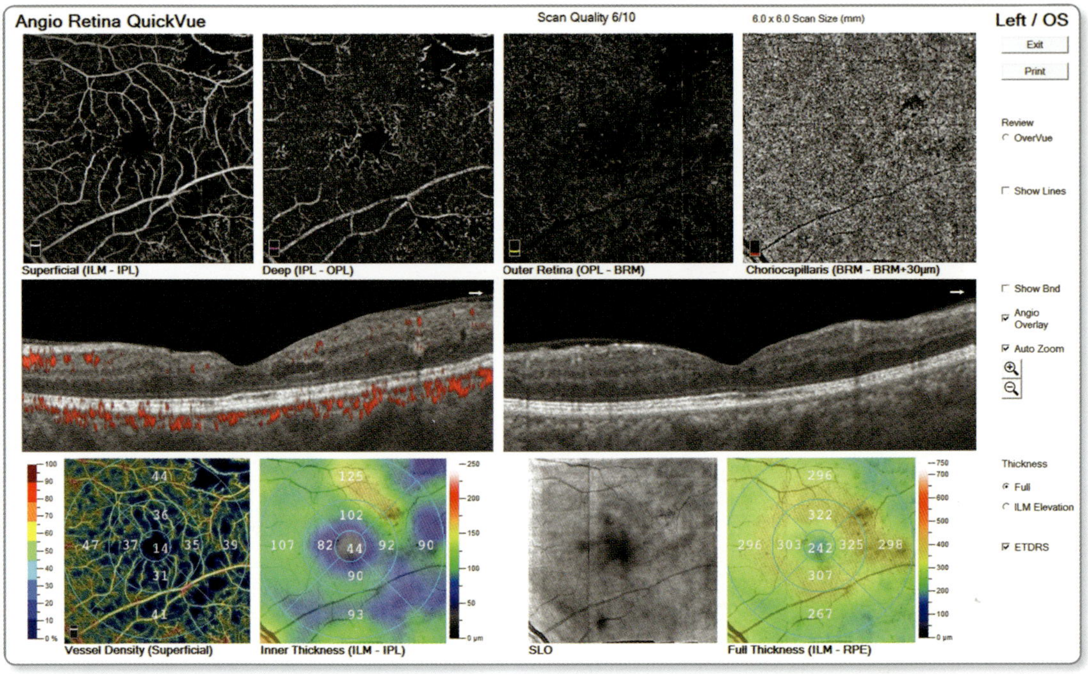

Figure 8 Mild nonproliferative diabetic retinopathy quantitative analysis with flow density map of superficial network. Perfusion density maps allow grading progressive vascular changes. In both plexuses, we can see vessel congestion that is highest at the margin of ischemic areas with normal retina. Diabetic retinopathy evolution is more severe and network disruption is more marked at deep vascular plexus level. (Optovue)

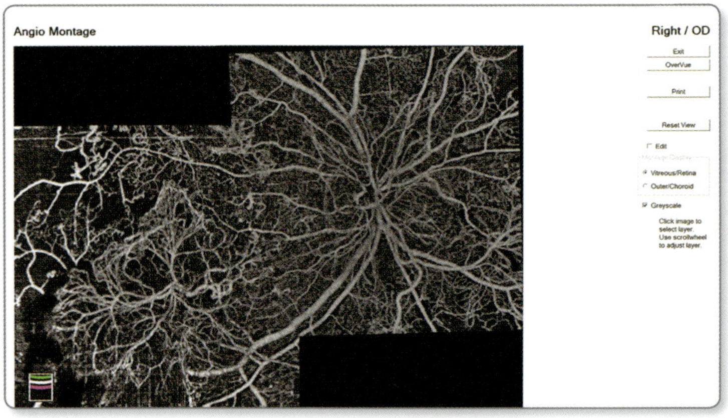

Figure 9a Severe proliferative diabetic retinopathy. Optical coherence tomography (OCT) angiography, composite. OCT angiography allows to assess vessel proliferation even when it is impossible to perform fluorescein angiography for the general conditions of the diabetic patient. At posterior pole, vascular proliferation is located close to wide ischemic lesions of the macula and of the temporal retina. We can see truncated vessels and of microaneurysms clusters. New vessels form tangled loops penetrating in the vitreal cavity. (Optovue)

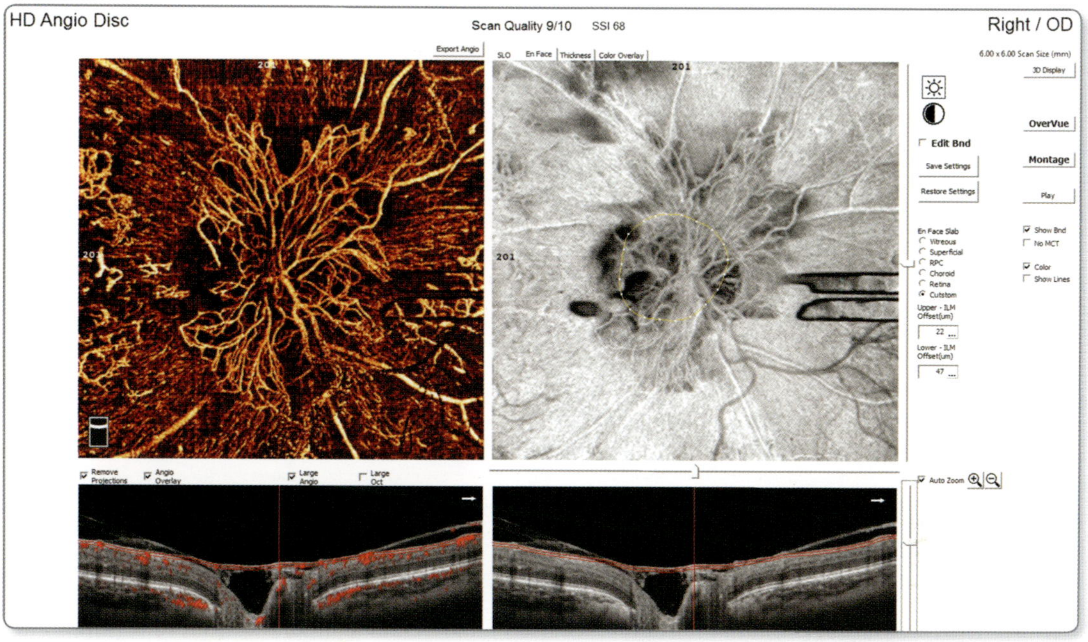

Figure 9b Severe proliferative diabetic retinopathy in pregnant patient. Proliferative retinopathy with new vessels growing on the optic disk in a pregnant young woman. Fluorescein angiography was not possible. Vascular proliferation is located close to wide ischemic lesions of the nasal and temporal retina. Prepapillary new vessels form tangled loops penetrating deeply in the vitreal cavity. From the retina and the optic disk, they enter the vitreous. Angio B-scans show the fibrovascular vessel filling the optic disk cavity. (Optovue)

prefer to suggest slow release dexamethasone implant.

Therapy shifting is indicated in nonresponders. The options are either shift to another anti-VEGF or use slow release dexamethasone implant.

Vitrectomy is necessary in eyes with vitreoretinal traction.

Treatment of neovascularization in proliferative diabetic retinopathy

Laser pan photocoagulation is still one of the main treatments of proliferative retinopathy. As high levels of VEGF induce neovascularization, anti-VEGF therapy is being used as an adjunct to the treatment, or instead of laser. However, anti-VEGF injections may induce regression of proliferative diabetic retinopathy but they can increase fibrosis of the regressing neovascularization. Vitrectomy is necessary when it is not possible or it is dangerous to perform panretinal laser photocoagulation.

Future treatments

Future treatment probably will be the gene therapy. The anatomy of the eye is highly favorable and the small size enables the use of low doses of vector for gene delivery and fundus examination allows to easily assess the results of treatment efficacy.

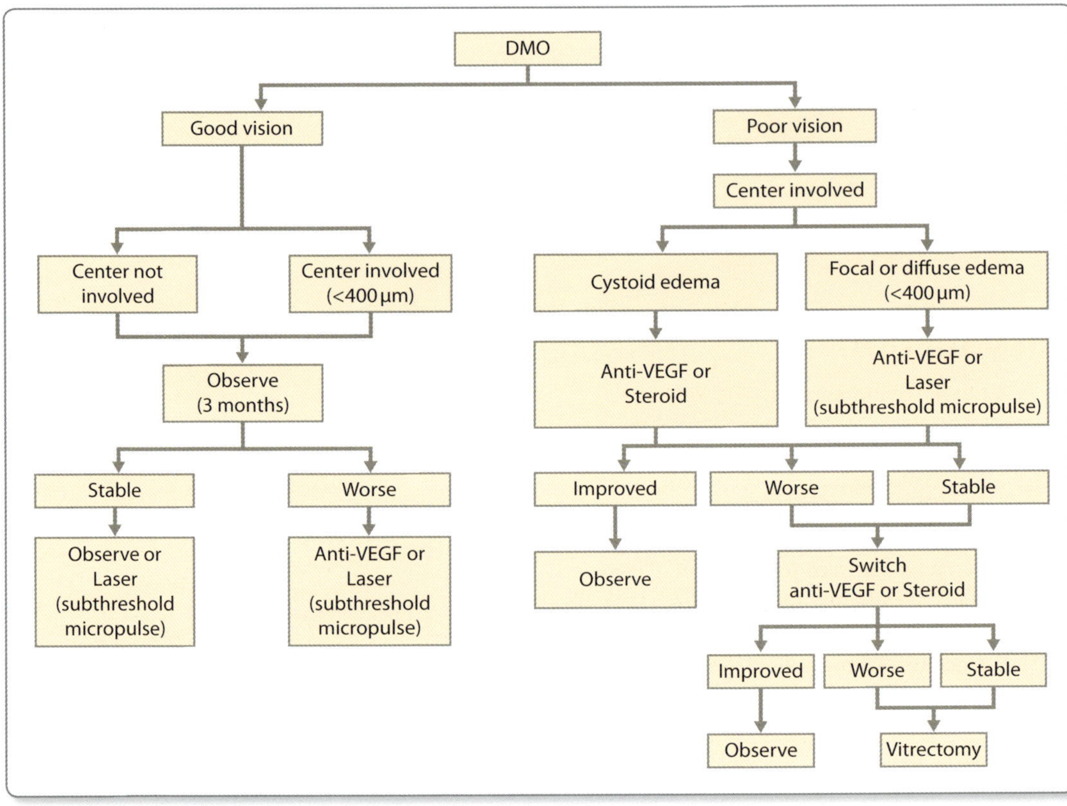

Figure 10 Suggested guidelines for treatment of Diabetic Macular Edema.
(DMO: diabetic macular edema; VEGF: vascular endothelial growth factor)

References

1. Agemy SA, Scripsema NK, Shah CM, et al. Retinal Vascular Perfusion Density Mapping Using Optical Coherence Tomography Angiography in Normal and Diabetic Retinopathy Patients. Retina 2015; 35:2353–2563.
2. Early Treatment Diabetic Retinopathy Study Report Number 2. Early Treatment Diabetic Retinopathy Study Research Group. Treatment techniques and clinical guidelines for photocoagulation of diabetic macular edema. Ophthalmology 1987; 94:761–774.
3. Hwang TS, Jia Y, Gao SS, et al. Optical coherence tomography angiography features of diabetic retinopathy. Retina 2015; 35:2371–2376.
4. Ishibazawa A, Nagaoka T, Takahashi A, et al. Optical Coherence Tomography Angiography in Diabetic Retinopathy: A Prospective Pilot Study. Am J Ophthalmol 2015; 160:35–44.
5. Soares M, Neves C, Marques IP, et al. Comparison of diabetic retinopathy classification using fluorescein angiography and optical coherence tomography angiography. Br J Ophthalmol 2017; 101:62–68.

22 Central retinal vein occlusion, branch retinal vein occlusion, retinal artery occlusion

Marco Rispoli, Bruno Lumbroso

Introduction

Optical coherence tomography (OCT) angiography provides a detailed imaging of the vascular networks and allows to include a quantitative assessment in the study of branch retinal vein occlusion (BRVO) and central retinal vein occlusion (CRVO); however, it does not detect leakage and staining seen on dye angiography. OCT angiography visualizes retinal circulation better than fluorescein angiography.

Venous occlusions may affect the central retinal vein, one of its main branches or a smaller subdivision. Venous occlusions give origin to two fundamental pathologic responses: increase of vascular permeability or/and retinal ischemia. For clinical reason study, we classify them in:

- Edematous occlusions
- Ischemic occlusions
- Mixed edematous and ischemic occlusions type
- Occlusive phlebitis may happen in patients less than 40 years old. These generally regress spontaneously or after treatment

Central retinal vein occlusion pathophysiology

Retinal vein occlusion happens when in all or part of the venous retinal vascular flow is obstructed by a thrombus at lamina cribrosa level: pressure builds up in the capillaries, leading to hemorrhage and leakage of fluid and blood. This high pressure in turn causes macular edema.

When capillaries supplying oxygen to the retina are obstructed, retina downstream is nonperfused and ischemia occurs. Ischemia later results in neovascularization that will cause vascular glaucoma, vitreous hemorrhage, fibrosis, retinal traction and retinal detachment, and painful blindness. In both ischemic and edematous CRVO, obstruction of the central retinal vein occurs, but the edematous, non-ischemic type allows a better blood flow through collaterals.

Intravascular thrombus formation in RVO is associated with Virchow's triad: venous stasis, endothelial lesion, and hypercoagulability. The vein is occluded by fibrin and platelets at level of the lamina cribrosa leading to turbulent flow and venous stasis. The central retinal vein and artery share a common adventitial sheath at arteriovenous crossings posterior to the lamina cribrosa, so that sclerotic lesions of the artery constrict and squeeze the vein and induce flow sharp decrease. Damage to the retinal artery wall from atherosclerosis and compression modifies blood flow in the adjacent central vein, contributing to stasis, thrombosis, and thus occlusion.

There is frequently compression of the adjacent vein by atherosclerotic retinal arteries at the site of AV crossing, leading to turbulent flow and venous stasis (**Figures 1** and **2**). This predisposes to thrombus formation in the

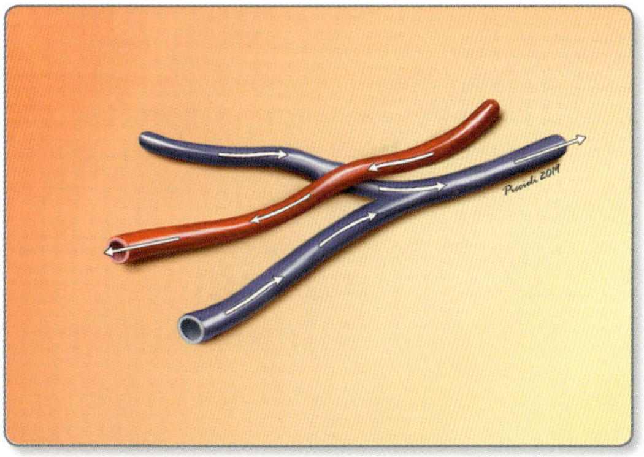

Figure 1 Normal retinal artery crossing vein.

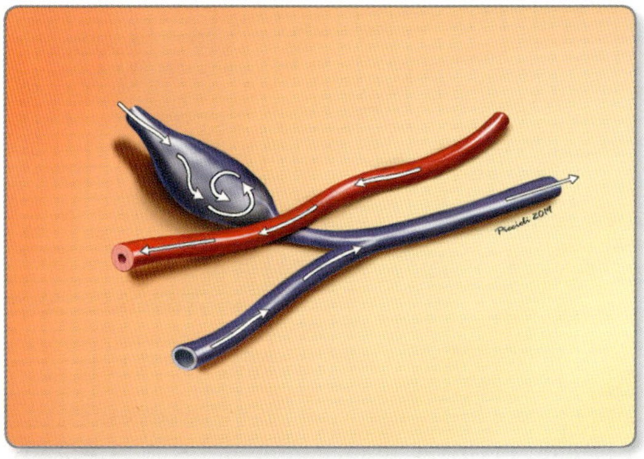

Figure 2 Compression of the vein by the artery at crossings is the main cause of BRVO causing blood flow turbulence.

central retinal vein by slowing of the blood flow, alteration in vessel wall, endothelial changes and causing hemodynamic disturbances. Stagnation of the blood brings ischemic damage to the retina. It increases production of vascular endothelial growth factor (VEGF) in the vitreous cavity that stimulates neovascularization and causes capillary leakage leading to macular edema. In RVO, there is a combination of increased hydrostatic pressure behind the occlusion, causing the deterioration of the endothelial cell integrity, instigating a secondary inflammation with an increase of VEGF production.

The edematous CRVO is less damaging than the ischemic type and occurs in 80% of cases (**Figures 3** and **4**). Untreated macular edema will lead to legal blindness. Ischemic CRVO evolution leads to vascular glaucoma, retinal traction detachment, massive, hemorrhages, and painful blindness.

Risk factors include mainly age, smoking and hypertension, and glaucoma. In younger patient's risk factors include hyperlipidemia, diabetes, blood diseases, vasculitis, and oral contraceptive use.

Central retinal vein occlusion clinical features

In the acute phase, we observe in the retina edema, hemorrhages, veins congested and irregularly dilated associated with optic disc

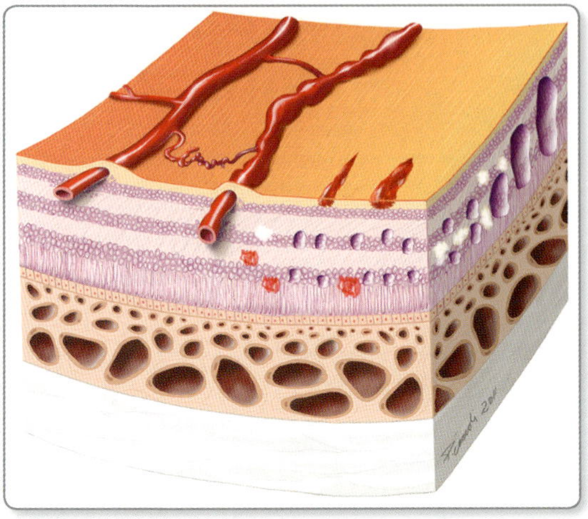

Figure 3 Retinal vein congested and dilated, some hemorrhages.

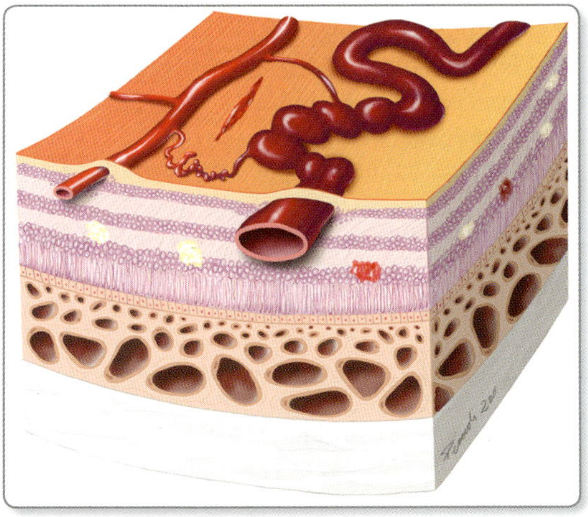

Figure 4 Occluded dilated vein.

papilledema. Large no-flow areas affect most retina in ischemic occlusions (**Figures 5** and **6**). The central retinal vein is obstructed at the lamina cribrosa level.

Ischemic occlusion immediately causes very bad vision (less than 20/200–1/100) confluent hemorrhages and cotton-wool spots. Edematous (nonischemic) occlusion usually gives better visual acuity (80/200–3/10) and less hemorrhages. Nonischemic occlusions may evolve to ischemic type in a few months, in about a third of cases.

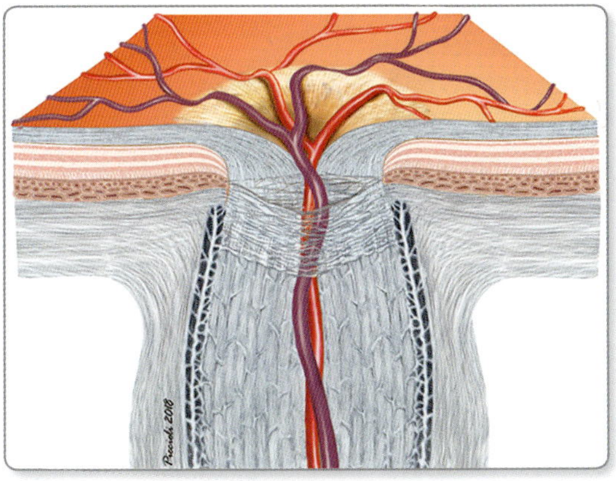

Figure 5 Normal optic disc.

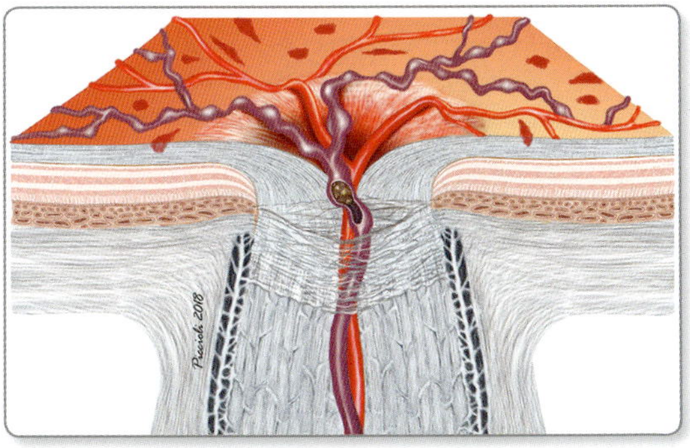

Figure 6 Optic disc in central venous occlusion: edema, hemorrhages, veins congested and irregularly dilated associated with optic disc papilledema. The central retinal vein is obstructed at the lamina cribrosa level.

Central retinal vein occlusion in young people frequently is inflammatory, occlusive periphlebitis.

Fluorescein angiography features: Delayed arteriovenous phase, blocked fluorescence from hemorrhages, nonperfused areas, and dye leakage.

Cross-section OCT signs of central vein occlusion

Retina is thickened with diffuse edema cystoid spaces and subretinal serous elevation. Retinal profile is irregular with swollen retina and dilated and misshapen blood vessels; hemorrhages are located in the fibers layer and the external plexiform layer. Cystoid cavities are located mainly in the outer layers. The outer limiting membrane and the ellipsoid are disrupted. Central edema cells will soon expand to the full retina thickness.

OCT angiography

Hemorrhages and massive edema increase retina thickness and distort retinal architecture. It is difficult or impossible to obtain correct automated segmentation in case of central vein occlusion. It is even difficult to obtain good segmentation by hand. Vascular congestion affects both vascular networks but is more important in the deep one. Capillaries are widened and swollen. When it is possible to acquire a relatively good segmentation, the vascular network shows large dropout areas at both superficial and deep plexus. Vessel course presents deviations; the wall thickness is irregular with focal segmentation and lumen narrowing. Vessels show terminal dilatations.

In ischemic CRVO, the avascular foveal zone is enlarged and irregular with breaks in the vascular arcade; peripheral dropout areas merge with the enlarged avascular zone. The main superficial vessels lose most of their collateral branches. In recent ischemia, capillary dropout concerns mainly the superficial vascular plexus, with some conservation of the morphology, caliber, and flow of the deep plexus capillaries. Neovascularization appears a few months after the occlusive event. New vessels grow first at the borders of the ischemic areas, then from the optic disc. In long-standing ischemia, shunts develop, linking superficial and deep plexus. The deep network shows changes in caliber, flow, and morphology.

Preretinal and retinal neovascularization appear around the no-flow zones 6 or more months after the occlusive event. The circulating blood flow is manifested in the new vessels. These abnormal capillaries at first creep on retinal surface and then penetrate vitreous. Prepapillary new vessels appear later and intrude the vitreal cavity. OCT angiography shows clearly loops, branching irregularity of the neovascular network and fibrous tissue (**Box 1**).

Box 1: Central retinal vein occlusion (CRVO) risk factors

- *Age:* over 55 years
- *Hypertension*: High blood pressure is observed in 70% of CRVO patients over 50 years and in 25% of younger patients. Adequate control of hypertension is necessary to prevent recurrence of CRVO in the same or fellow eye
- Hyperlipidemia
- Diabetes
- Glaucoma
- High intraocular pressure
- Smoking
- Contraceptive medication

Other uncommon predispositions:

- Myeloproliferative disorders
- Polycythemia
- Abnormal plasma proteins (e.g. myeloma, Waldenström's macroglobulinemia)
- Acquired hypercoagulable states
- Hyperhomocysteinemia
- Lupus anticoagulant and antiphospholipid antibodies
- Dysfibrinogenemia
- Inherited hypercoagulable states
- Activated protein C resistance (factor V Leiden mutation)
- Protein C deficiency
- Protein S deficiency
- Antithrombin deficiency
- Prothrombin gene mutation
- Factor XII deficiency

Inflammatory disease associated with occlusive periphlebitis:

- Behçet syndrome
- Sarcoidosis
- Wegener's granulomatosis

Miscellaneous:

- Chronic renal failure
- Causes of secondary hypertension (e.g. Cushing syndrome) or hyperlipidemia (e.g. hypothyroidism)
- Orbital disease
- Dehydration in young patients in hot countries

(CRVO: central retinal vein occlusion)

Branch retinal vein occlusion

Pathophysiology

In most of the eyes, there is an anatomical predisposition to intravascular thrombus formation at arteriovenous crossings. When the artery is anterior to the vein, it may crush the venous walls. Compression of the vein by the artery at crossings is the main cause of BRVO causing blood flow turbulence. The localized endothelial vascular damage leads to thrombus formation and vessel occlusion. Other factors are hypertensive, atherosclerotic, inflammatory, or thrombophilic conditions that may lead to retinal endothelial vascular damage. BRVO causes an impaired recruitment of lymphocytes and macrophages to the injured area, cell death, and deterioration of blood-retinal barrier with increased edema. Pathophysiologic processes from venous occlusions comprise macular edema, serous retinal detachment, and intraocular neovascularization.

Risk factors comprise age, smoking, hypertension, and glaucoma. In younger patient's hyperlipidemia, diabetes, blood diseases, vasculitis and oral contraceptive use.

Retinal branch vein occlusion clinical features

Occlusions of branch vein present localized edema in the area of the affected branch. Some hard exudates are visible. Veins are enlarged, irregular, swollen, and distorted, with flame and dot hemorrhages. Cotton-wool exudates appear around the dropout areas. Most BRVOs occur in the supratemporal quadrant due to the specific anatomy of this zone and to frequency of arteriovenous crossings in this area. Nasal BRVOs go frequently ignored by patients. Decrease in visual acuity for ischemic BRVO and for edematous BRVO is generally about 20/60 (4/10).

Fluorescein angiography

It shows vessel abnormalities associated with dropout areas, dye staining of vessel walls but in the late frames lesions are masked by dye leakage.

Structural OCT features

Optical coherence tomography shows retinal thickening and edema in the occluded area and at macula level. Hard exudates are seen as hyper-reflective intraretinal deposits in the outer retina at limit between normal and edematous tissue. There are diffuse retinal edema and/or cystoid cavities in the outer retina with cystoid edema cells. Cystoid edema small cells occupy the inner nuclear layer while the outer plexiform layer is involved with larger and more irregular cystic cavities. Later large edematous cystoid cavities invade the entire thickness of the retina. The outer limiting membrane and ellipsoid are fragmented. A limited serous central retinal elevation is frequent.

OCT angiography

It allows to study separately the lesions at the superficial and deep vascular network level. Vascular modification, congestion, and dropout areas are mainly localized at the border between occluded zone and normal retina. The no-flow areas margins are sharper at superficial network level and the capillaries are sparse in the ischemic zones. Arterial-venous anastomoses and vascular loops are easy to see. Retinal edema induces wider and distorted meshes. Deep vascular plexus shows more changes than the superficial plexus, mainly in the ischemic areas. The capillary distribution is irregular and tortuous in the no-flow area. There are irregularities in vessel size, localized dilatations, macro- and microaneurysms. Dilated capillaries alternate with closed or with thinner capillaries. Vascular congestion is increased in the deep plexus, at the border with normal retina. The foveal avascular zone is wider and more irregular than normal. The perifoveal arcade is locally fragmented. The dropout temporal areas frequently merge with the avascular zone thus widening the macular no-flow areas on the temporal side.

AngioAnalytics software allows to assess quantitatively OCT angiography data: flow area, vascular drop out area, flow density map: warm colors show high-density vascular areas and the cold colors the low flow or no-flow zones, measuring the percentage of vascular areas on *en face* angiograms **(Figures 7 to 12).**

Management of retinal vein occlusions: Suggested guidelines

We differentiate three groups **(Figure 13)**:

1. Branch retinal vein occlusion (BRVO):
   - Macular edema not involving the fovea center with a good functional vision
   - Macular edema involving the fovea center with compromising of functional vision

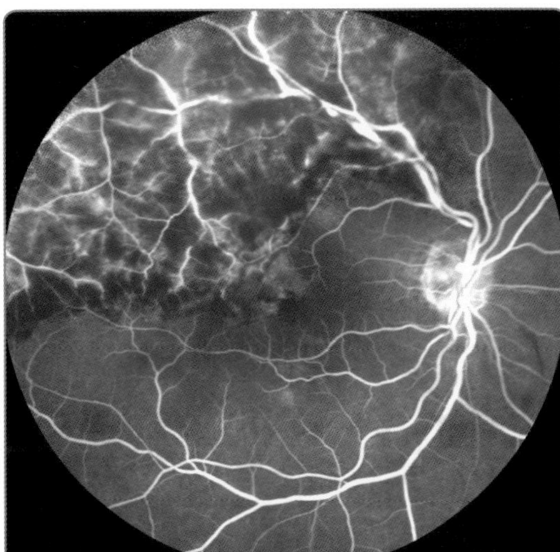

Figure 7 Fluorescein angiography. Superior temporal branch vein occlusion: the occluded vessels are intensely stained, dilated, and irregular, with tortuosity of the smaller branches, rare microaneurysms. Some hemorrhages are seen in the superior retina. Diffuse hyperfluorescence at macular area highlights retinal edema with blurring and leakage. The optic disc is slightly hyperfluorescent. (Heidelberg)

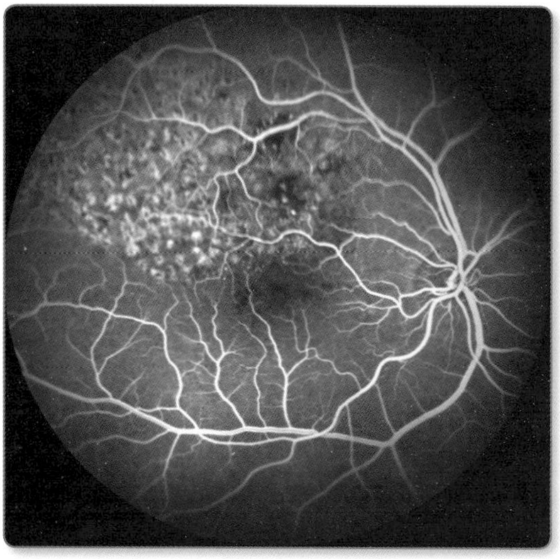

Figure 8 Fluorescein angiography: mixed edematous ischemic branch vein occlusion treated by laser. Hyperfluorescent dye staining of the major veins close to the optic disc. Hypofluorescence for lack of perfusion in the occluded area. Truncated vessels and early shunts can be seen. The occluded zone has been intensely treated by laser spots. (Heidelberg)

2. Central retinal vein occlusion (CRVO)
3. Occlusive periphlebitis may happen in young patients. These generally regress spontaneously or after corticosteroid treatment.

When macular edema involves the fovea and compromises vision or in case of CRVO, treatment should be initiated immediately.

In the BRVO and edema not involving the centre of fovea with a good functional vision, we prefer to observe or treat with laser. Monitoring is scheduled after 3 months or before in case of visual acuity decrease.

We prefer the use of anti-VEGF agents (ranibizumab or aflibercept indifferently) as first-line therapy and typically reserve corticosteroids for pseudophakia patients unresponsive to anti-VEGF agents.

The increased risk of cataract formation and transitory increased IOP with steroids should be extensively discussed with the patients before proceeding.

After the induction treatment, the anti-VEGF administration timing is PRN, according to

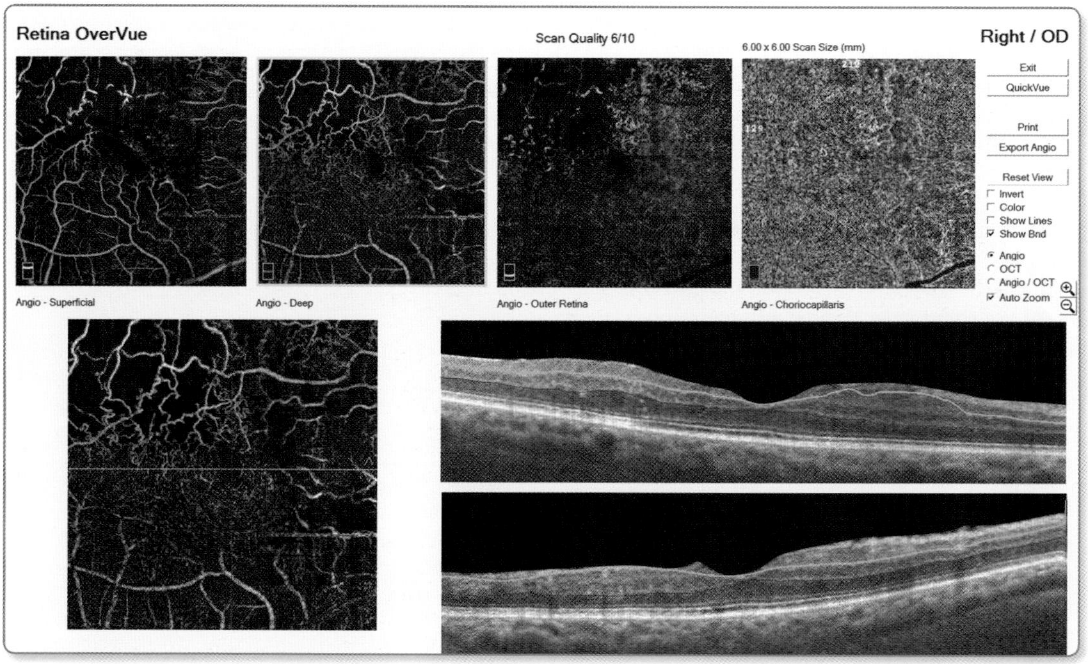

Figure 9 Optical coherence tomography (OCT) angiography of ischemic area in a branch vein occlusion. In both superior and deep networks, we see tortuosity of the smaller vessels, irregular vascular diameter, and dilated capillaries. The foveal avascular zone is enlarged. (Optovue)

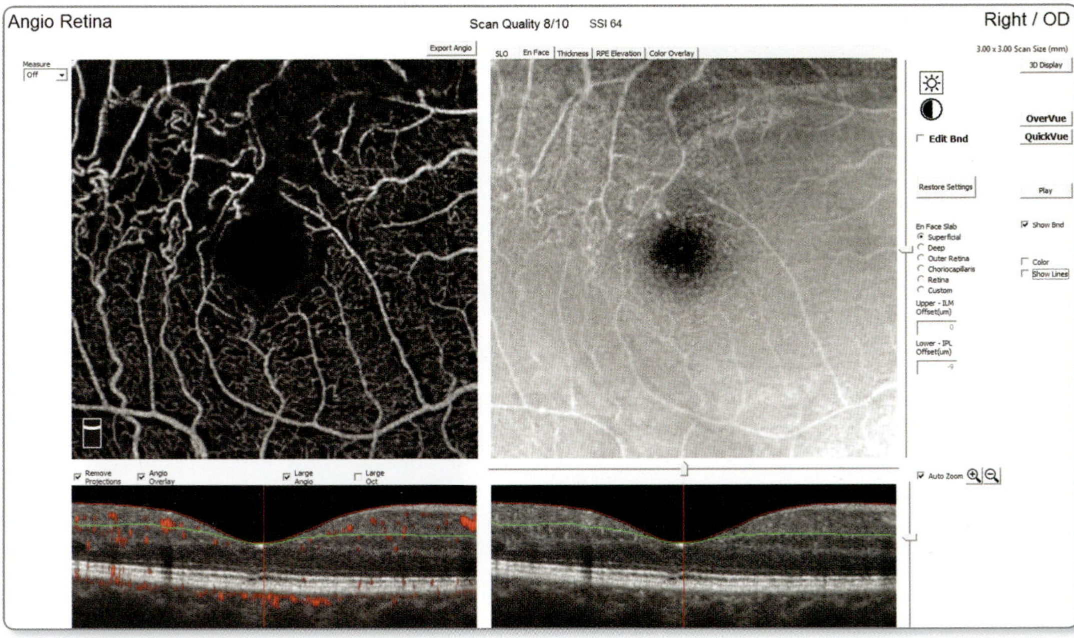

Figure 10a Optical coherence tomography (OCT) angiography of ischemic area in a branch vein occlusion. Superficial network. Truncated vessels with sharp disruptions in the areas of nonperfusion. Tortuosity of the smaller vessels. Irregular vascular diameter. No collateral branches are seen in the occluded area. Some vessels are thick and irregular. Enlarged foveal avascular zone with interruptions in the vascular arcade. (Optovue)

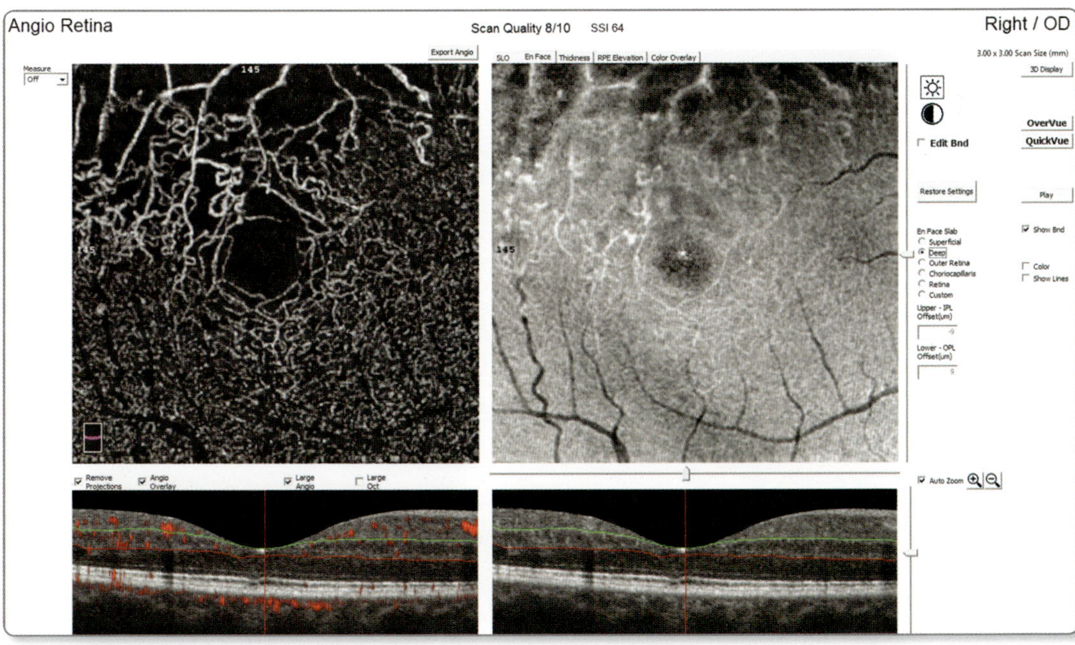

Figure 10b Same case. Deep vascular network in branch retinal vein occlusion. Enlarged foveal avascular zone with interrupted vascular arcade. Some vessels are thick. Vein dilatations and irregularities, mainly at the border between occluded and normal retina. Vessels are irregular in diameter, frequently segmented and dilated, with areas of nonperfusion. Some vascular loops in the occluded area. Enlarged foveal avascular zone merging with more peripheral nonperfused areas. (Optovue)

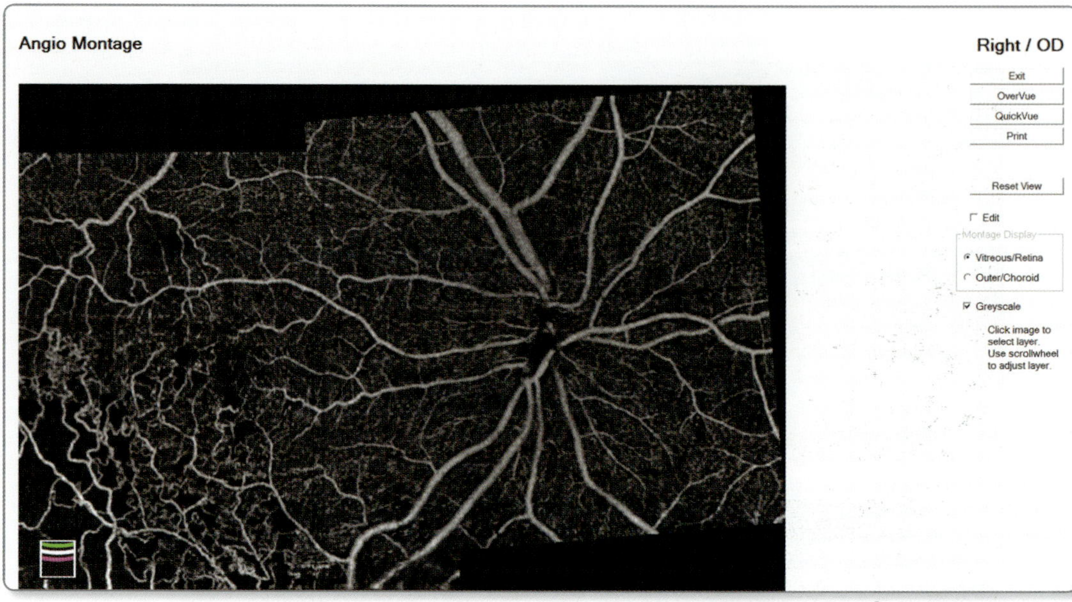

Figure 11A Optical coherence tomographic angiography (OCTA) composite of a branch retinal vein occlusion (BRVO) case, superficial network. Ischemic areas are clearly seen. The foveal avascular zone is increased in size with interruption of the normal vascular arcade. Vessels in dropout area are thick. Vein are dilated and irregular mainly at the border between occluded and normal retina. Vessels are segmented and dilated, with areas of nonperfusion. (Optovue)

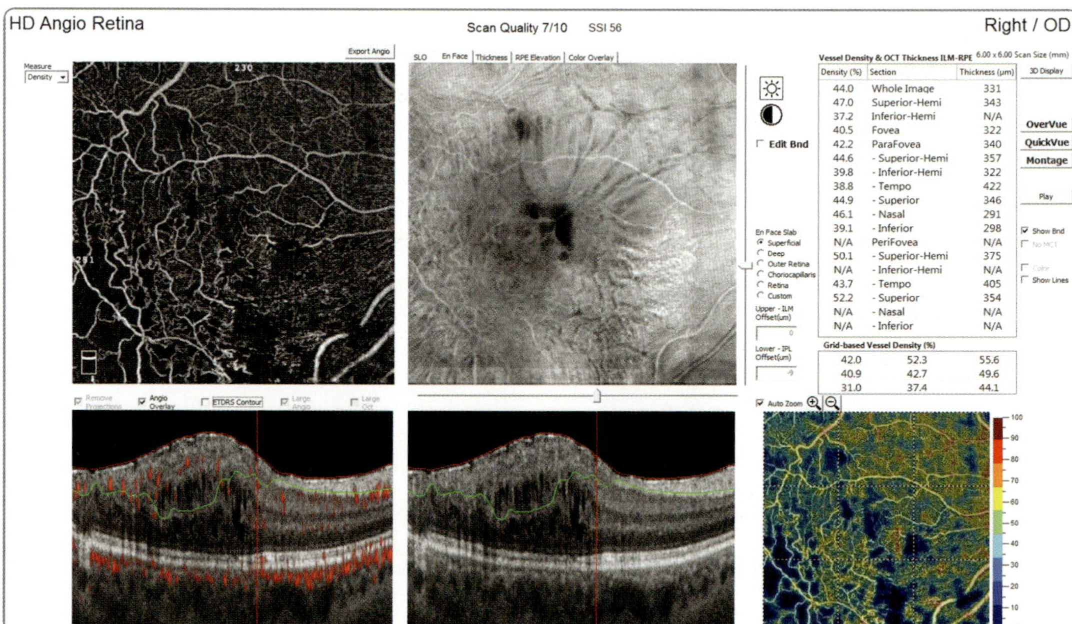

Figure 11B AngioAnalytic, Perfusion Density map, AngioFlow of the superficial vascular plexus. Dropout areas show in some zones a complete ischemia with no flow. '*En face*' scan highlights stellar retinal folds above an area of cystoid edema. Cross-section scans show retina thickening with cystoid edema cavities. Traction by epiretinal membranes induces retinal folds. (Optovue)

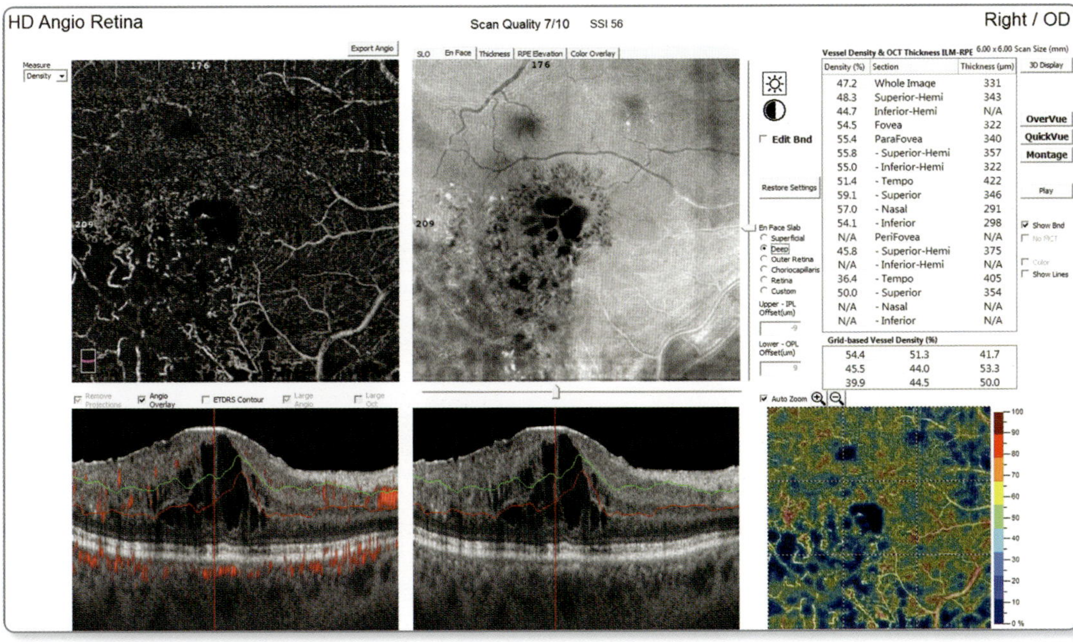

Figure 11C Same case, AngioAnalytic, Perfusion Density map. AngioFlow of the deep vascular plexus, Cystoid edema cells. Dark areas combine no-flow zones and cystic cavities. The inferior part of the angio scan shows dilated and segmented deep capillaries and cystoid edema cavities. The superior part of the figure shows normal deep vascular plexus capillaries.

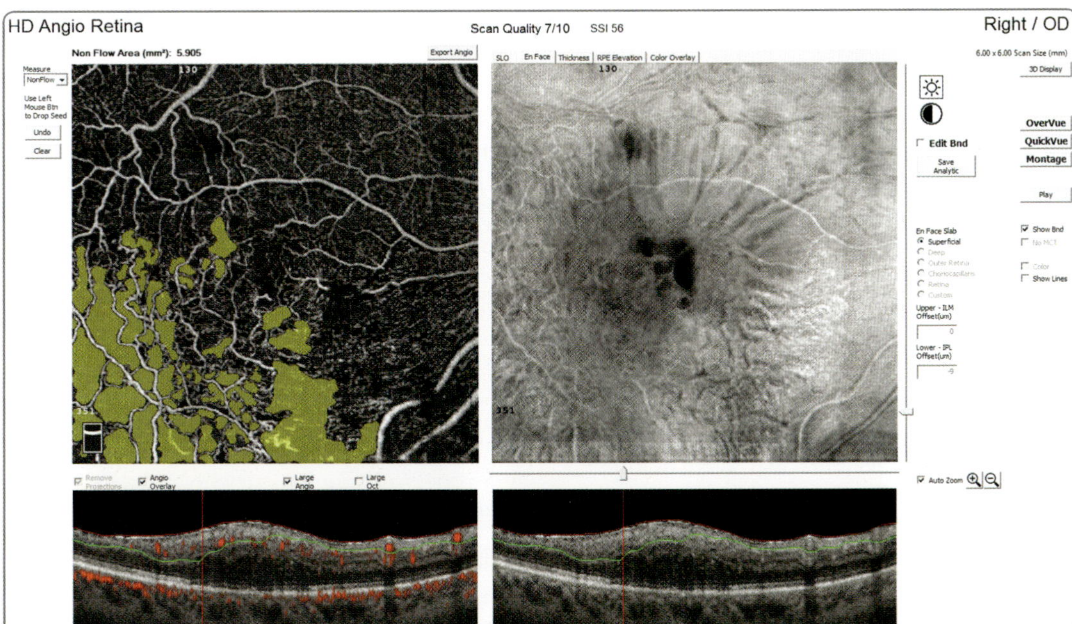

Figure 12 AngioAnalytic. No-flow area branch retinal vein occlusion (BRVO), superficial vascular plexus. No-flow area shows relative or total ischemia and vascular 'dropout'. Dropout areas are highlighted in yellow and show in some zones a complete ischemia with no flow. The measurements can be compared with later examinations during the follow-up. '*En face*' scan highlights stellar retinal folds above macular cystoid edema. Cross-section scans show retina thickening with cystoid edema cells. Traction by epiretinal membranes induces retinal folds. (Optovue)

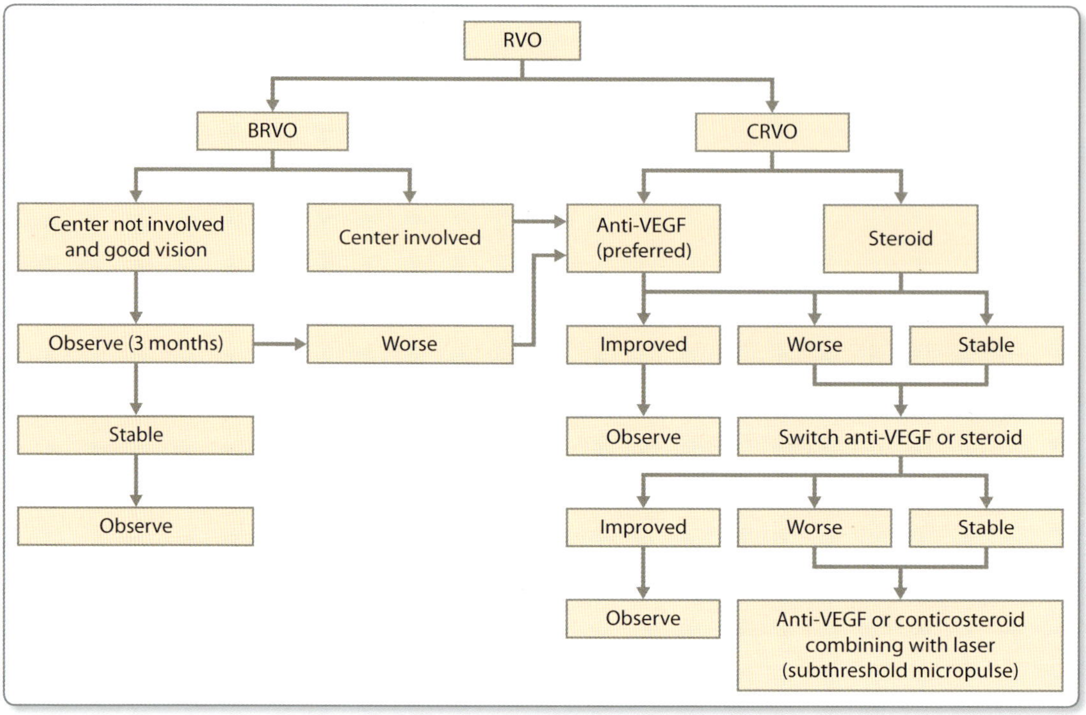

Figure 13 Suggested macular edema postretinal vein occlusion (RVO) management guideline.
(BRVO: branch retinal vein occlusion; CRVO: central retinal vein occlusion; RVO: retinal vein occlusion; VEGF: vascular endothelial growth factor)

edema observation on OCT and to visual acuity reduction.

The laser subthreshold micropulse is suggested to complete intravitreal therapy of recurrent edema, although no evidence-based results for this treatment are reported.

In case of recent cerebrovascular or cardiovascular accident, we prefer to use the dexamethasone sustained delivery implant.

Therapy shifting is suggested in non-responders or refractory cases. The options are either shift to another anti-VEGF agent or implant sustained release dexamethasone.

Retinal artery occlusions

Main causes of arterial occlusions are hypertension, atheroma, carotid disorders, and emboli. Giant cell arteritis causes 2% of central retinal artery occlusions.

In central and arterial branch occlusions, the superficial vascular network shows a capillary dropout with loss of collateral vessels. The deep vascular network is totally disrupted with capillary loss and total closure in a considerable number of others. The deep capillary network presents larger than normal meshes. When occlusion is recent, OCTA shows a dense edema that interests the inner retina. There is opacity of the inner layers, large dropout areas at deep network level. Capillary density is decreased in occluded areas. In structural OCT, the edematous inner retinal layers appear to be quite reflective. Atrophy of the inner retinal layers initiates after a few weeks **(Box 2; Figures 14** to **17)**.

Box 2: Causes of arterial occlusions

Emboli:
- Cardiac lesions
- Mitral valve lesions
- Artificial cardiac valves
- Endocarditis
- Aortic aneurysms
- Cardiac catheterization
- Arteriography and other diagnostic procedures
- Talcum in self-injected drugs
- Fat emboli in open bone fracture
- Purtscher syndrome

Vascular occlusion

Temporal arteritis:
- Hypertension
- Atheroma of the carotid artery
- Other internal carotid diseases
- Giant cell arteritis
- Polyarteritis nodosa
- Oral contraceptives
- Migraine
- Scleroderma
- Orbital cellulitis
- Wegener granulomatosis
- Dermatomyositis
- Takayasu syndrome

Ocular high pressure:
- Angle closure glaucoma
- Ocular trauma
- Accidental ocular high pressure during surgical procedure

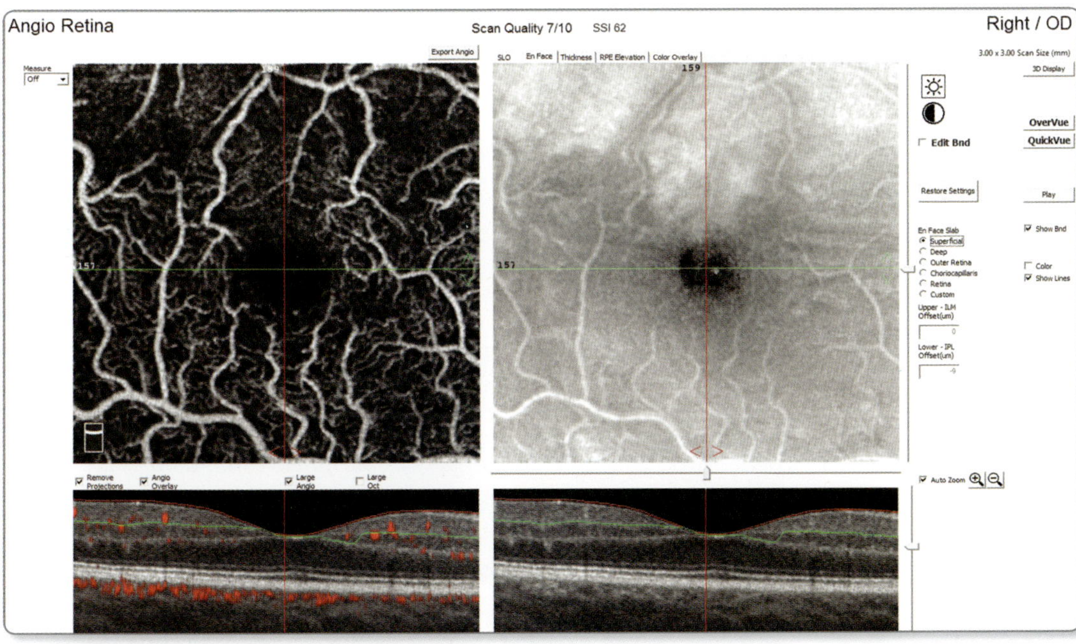

Figure 14 Branch artery occlusion, superficial network. Angio-optical coherence tomography (OCT) highlights the main superficial retinal vessels in the arterial occluded area. Part of the collateral branches is not perfused after the ischemic event. This feature concerns mainly the superficial vascular plexus. The '*en face*' scan shows white retinal edema with sharp margins that appears immediately in the occluded area. (Optovue)

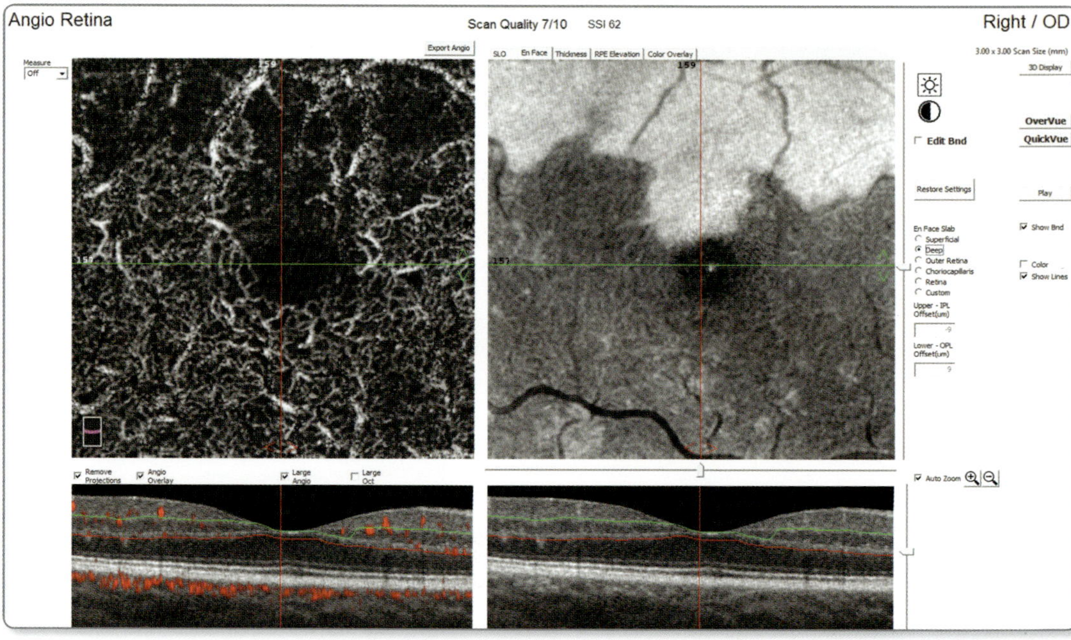

Figure 15 Branch artery occlusion, same case, deep network. The capillaries of the deep plexus are intensely interested by arterial occlusion. In the occluded area, most capillaries are closed, a few are dilated. The '*en face*' scan shows white retinal edema in the occluded area. (Optovue)

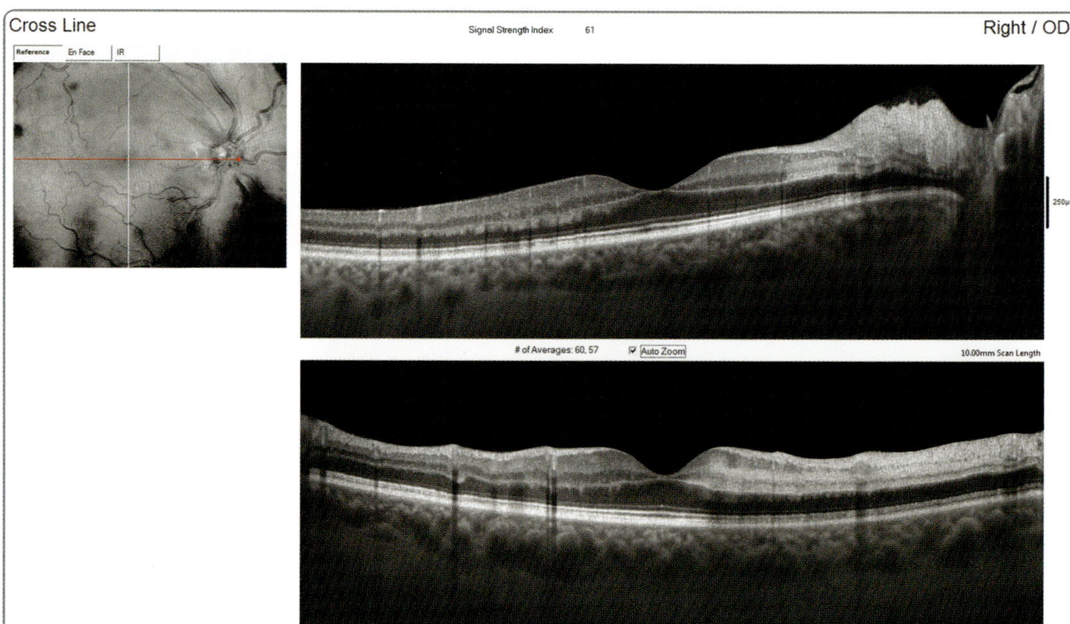

Figure 16 Cross-section optical coherence tomography (OCT) scan showing intense edema of the inner retina, very evident in the foveopapillar zone. The outer retina is normal.

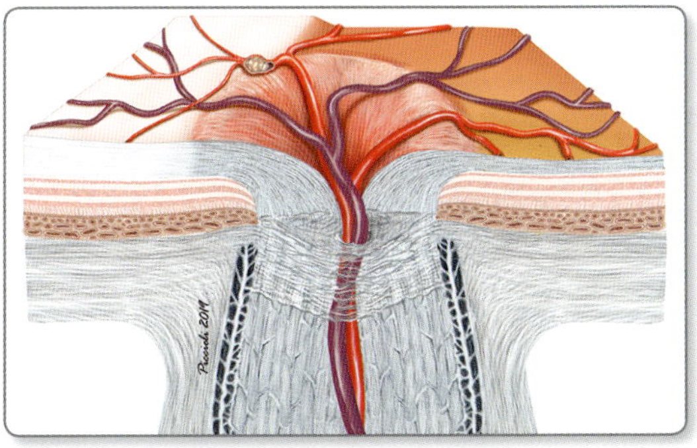

Figure 17 Occlusion by embolus of a retinal artery branch. White ischemia in a retinal area.

Treatment

No treatment has given results. Emergency treatments are ocular massage, anterior chamber paracentesis, and ocular pressure-lowering agents, if the patient is seen few minutes after the event. As the retinal artery occlusion is very frequently followed by cerebral problems, the patient needs to be referred to a specialized department.

23 Retinal microcirculation pathology, DRIL, AMN, PAMM

Dmitrii S Maltsev, Alexei N Kulikov, Maria A Burnasheva

OCT and OCT angiography in the retinal ischemia

The complexity of retinal microcirculation suggests the diversity of retinal vascular pathology, which eventually may vary in volumetric characteristic within two dimensions: of the depth and extension; both of which taken together with the topical presentation define the severity of any retinal vascular event. This structure mostly refers to the central retina, where the microcirculation includes four relatively separated capillary plexuses.[1] The first suggestions for the existence of the isolated retinal ischemic injury appeared with the description acute macular neuroretinopathy (AMN).[2] Later, it was proved in the clinical settings with optical coherence tomography (OCT). Namely, the isolated character of ischemia occupying the middle retina was suggested for paracentral acute middle maculopathy (PAMM), which was identified within the spectrum of AMN.[3,4] However, the undoubtful evidence for the existence of the ischemic retinal conditions varying in the terms of the depth of the injury was obtained only after introduction OCT angiography because optical coherence tomographic angiography (OCTA) allows selective analysis for each of retinal capillary plexuses in clinical circumstances. A reasonable conclusion from a look at the current retinal microcirculation model is a suggestion that the number of the types of isolated retinal ischemia may correspond to the number with potential levels of microcirculatory disturbances. Indeed, there are four capillary plexuses, including radial peripapillary capillary plexus (RPCP), superficial capillary plexus (SCP), intermediate capillary plexus (ICP), and deep capillary plexus (DCP), which may correspond to four types of isolated retinal ischemic injury.

Nerve fiber layer infarct

The affection of RPCP, which supplies nerve fiber layer (NFL) and occupies mostly parapapillary area, one may recognise as NFL infarct. The most clinically relevant cases with acute presentation and visual symptoms are associated with the appearance of peripapillary cotton-wool spots (CWS). Such CWS followed by arcuate or segmental loss of nerve fibers, which get visible after CWS resolution within 2–3 weeks after presentation. The flow signal within the RPCP profoundly inhibited within the affected region and increased when evaluating a thicker SCP slab (which in fact includes two plexuses RPCP and SCP). A CWS itself should not be referred as an ischemic focus since it just reflects the block of axoplasmic transport in ischemic circumstances.[5] This should be bearing in mind because only the actual pattern of circulatory disturbance but not a presence of cotton-wool spots defines if only NFL infarct or a more profound injury occurred in a particular case. However, the size and location of CWS correspond with postischemic RFL loss **(Figure 1)**.

Although in the acute stage, CWS may be interpreted as full-thickness retinal ischemia, the OCT signal block by the CWS tissues is the only reason for such multilevel appearance of flow void. After resolution, the NFL infarct demonstrates no ischemic injuries deeper than RPCP. The NFL infarct may have an idiopathic character and represents the only ocular abnormality in the patients without any other ocular pathology, nevertheless not without systemic cardiovascular risks. Moreover, NFL infarct may accompany more severe retinal vascular conditions such as diabetic retinopathy or retinal vein occlusions where the high prevalence of CWS is well-known. Therefore, the association with retinal vascular diseases as well as possible idiopathic occurrence, association with different systemic cardiovascular risk factors, CWS, and determined ischemic pattern allow defining NFL infarct as a syndrome.

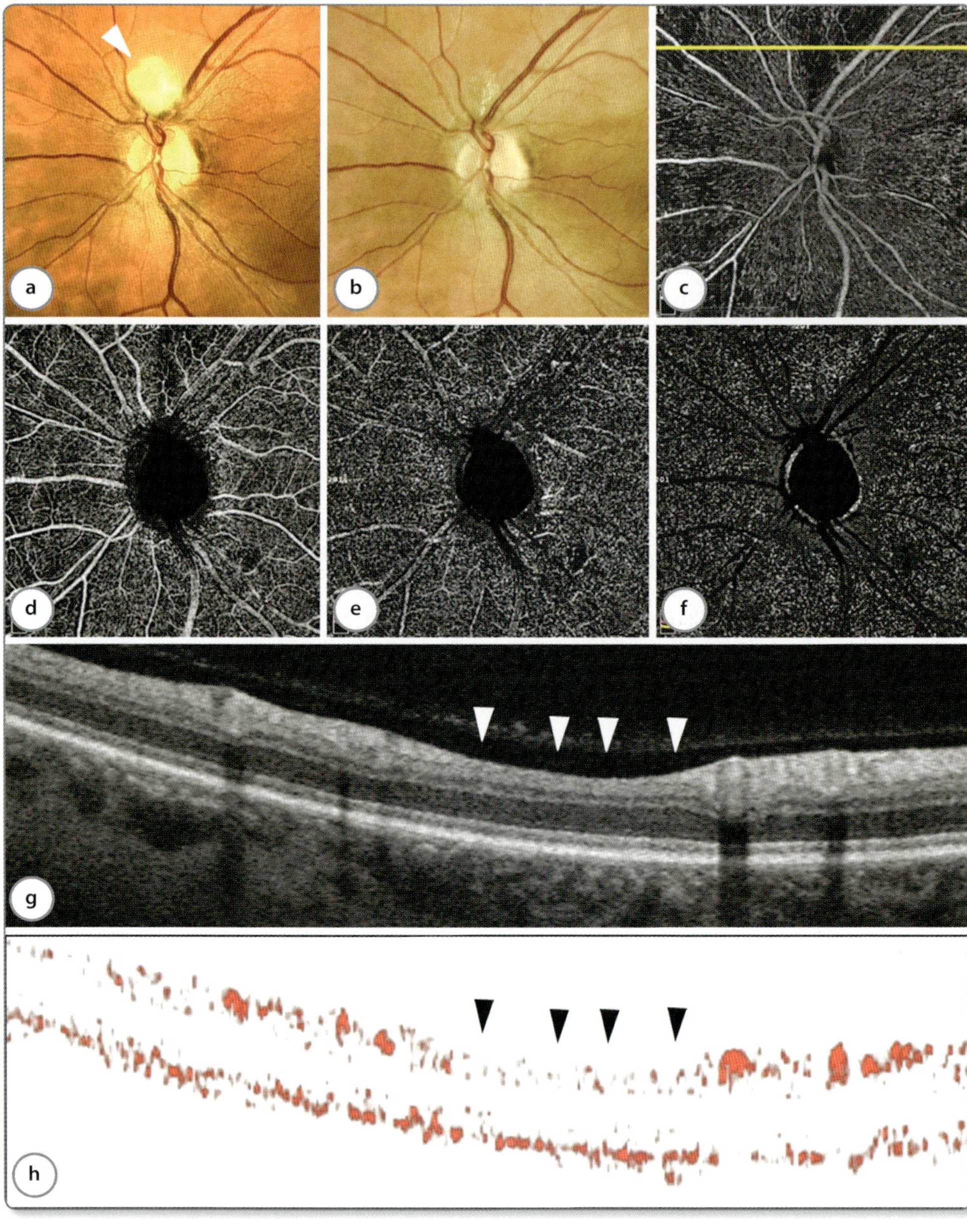

Figure 1 Multimodal imaging of the left eye of a 41-year-old female with infarct of nerve fiber layer (iNFL). (a) Fundus color photography 1 day after onset demonstrates a cotton-wool spot (CWS) (arrowhead). (b) Fundus color photography 3 weeks after presentation showing completer resolution of CWS. (c) Optical coherence tomographic angiography (OCTA) image of radial peripapillary capillary plexus slab after resolution of CWS. Note segmental area of significant flow void corresponding to the area of NFL infarct. The yellow line represents the position of the cross-sectional scan. (d) OCTA image of superficial capillary plexus slab demonstrates minimal changes of perfusion. (e) OCTA image of intermediate capillary plexus demonstrates no changes of perfusion. (f) OCTA image of deep capillary plexus demonstrates no changes of perfusion. (g) Cross-sectional OCT scan showing focal loss on NFL (arrowheads). (h) Distribution of flow signal within cross-sectional scan. The lesion (arrowheads) demonstrates flow void mostly in the innermost retinal layers while deeper retinal circulation is preserved.

Disorganisation of retinal inner layers

The next potential level of ischemic retinal injury is superficial capillary plexus with its structural equivalent of disorganization of retinal inner layers (DRILs). DRIL mostly refers to diabetic retinopathy where, if occupying the macular center, it represents a negative prognostic factor for the restoration of visual acuity in the course of antivascular endothelial growth factor (VEGF) therapy.[6] The analysis of cross-sectional images within the disorganization of retinal inner layers area shows a loss of inner retinal layers from the ganglionar complex to the inner nuclear layer, while NFL and outer retina remain unaffected. These structural changes correspond to the distribution of retinal hypoperfusion on OCT angiography. The maximum of flow signal void lies within superficial capillary plexus, but ICP and DCP also demonstrate hypoperfusion **(Figure 2)**. As NFL infarct, the disorganization of retinal inner layers may be an idiopathic condition when found in generally healthy individuals. On the other hand, disorganization of retinal inner layers may be identified as a component of more severe and complex retinal pathology including diabetic retinopathy, sickle-cell disease, and retinal veins occlusions. Therefore, the association with ocular vascular pathology and systemic conditions as well as possibility to be idiopathic condition, specific structural pattern, and prognostic meaning also make the disorganization of retinal inner layers a syndrome-like condition.

Paracentral acute middle maculopathy

The PAMM was firstly described as a relatively rare idiopathic condition; however after the introduction of spectral-domain OCT and OCTA and with growing awareness of clinicians regarding this entity, the frequency of reporting on the PAMM progressively increases. Concomitantly, appeared the wide spectrum of systemic and ocular conditions associated with PAMM.[7-15] In fact, PAMM looks like a universal indicator reflecting alteration of retinal microcirculation in different circumstances and several other facts confirm this suggestion. First, the resolved asymptomatic PAMM lesions may be found in generally healthy individuals as well as in patients with cardiovascular risk factors.[16] This increases the prevalence of PAMM, which considered to be quite rare in its idiopathic form. Second, quantitative analysis of retinal microcirculation in acute and resolved PAMM showed alteration not only of DPC (which normally occurred in PAMM)[16] but also of SCP.[17] Additionally, some changes were also found in foveal avascular zone (FAZ) parameters. These general changes of retinal microcirculation indicate that it is affected by systemic risk factors, and deep retinal ischemia in such case is just an early ocular manifestation of microvascular alteration resulting from those risk factors.

Another support for this suggestion is the high prevalence of resolved PAMM lesions in fellow eyes of unilateral retinal vein occlusion (RVO) patients[18] highly likely resulting from the systemic cardiovascular risk factors. Small resolved PAMM lesions, therefore, may be considered as a surrogate biomarker for RVO risk.

Analysis of capillary plexuses in idiopathic PAMM cases, even where the lesion occupies a large area, typically shows no substantial local alteration of SCP. At the same time, capillary loss becomes apparent at the level of ICP and DCP (deep vascular complex) and explains thinning of inner nuclear layer in the chronic stage. Therefore, relatively high prevalence and association with a number of systemic risk factors as well as specific structural and vascular changes justify considering of PAMM as a syndrome **(Figure 3)**.

However, there is a substantial difference between classic large symptomatic PAMM, which also may be found as a component of retinal vascular diseases and small resolved asymptomatic lesions. The latter demonstrates a specific spatial distribution, uniformly small size, and completely asymptomatic nature allowing for considering them as a distinct phenomenon or may be as a syndrome of asymptomatic deep retinal ischemia.

Acute macular neuroretinopathy

The next, deepest level for retinal ischemia takes place in DCP with the clinical equivalent referring as AMN. In acute phase, AMN appears as hyper-reflectivity of the outer nuclear layer with its consecutive thinning. Indeed, the analysis of some resolved AMN cases demonstrates

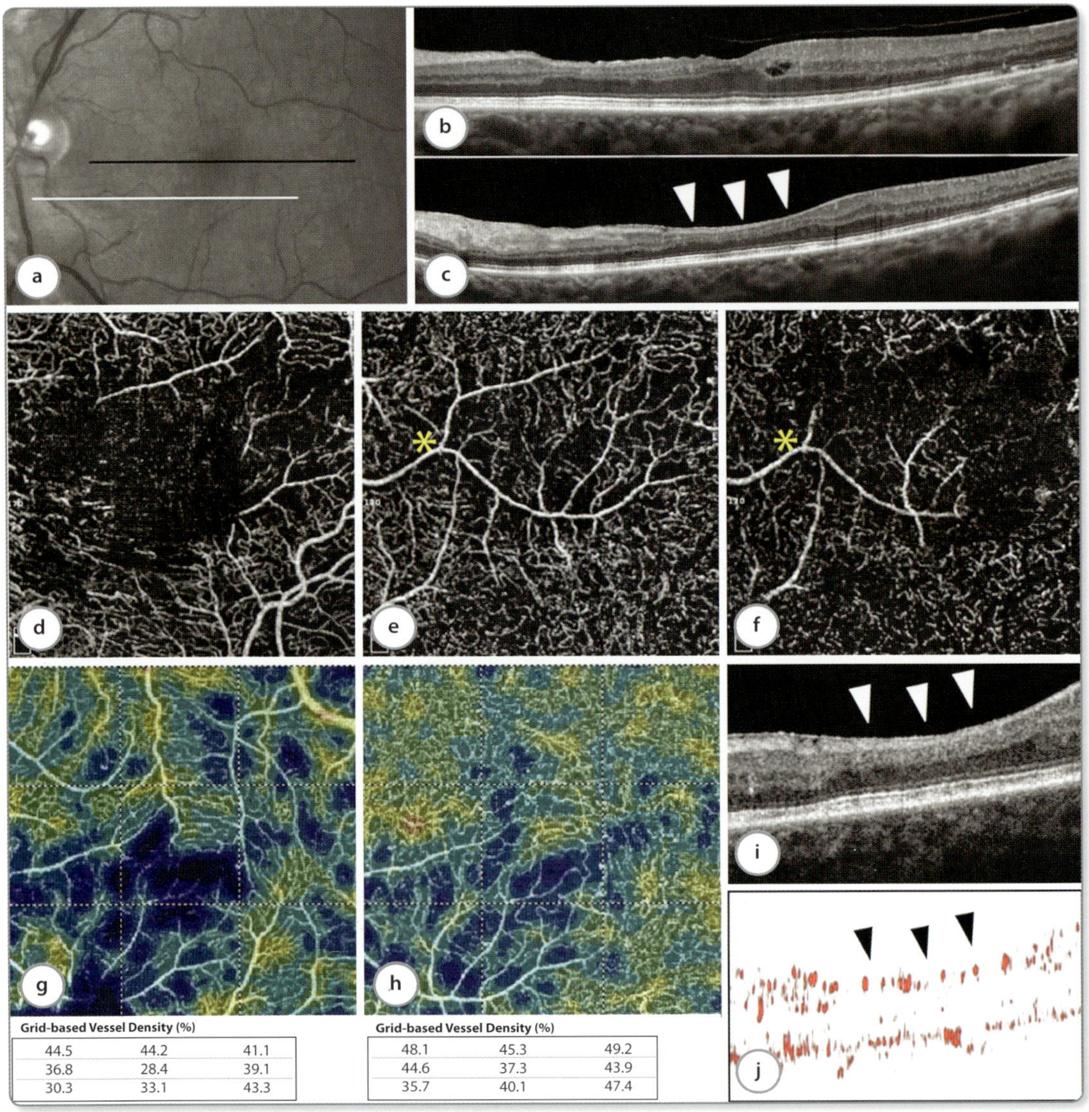

Grid-based Vessel Density (%)

44.5	44.2	41.1
36.8	28.4	39.1
30.3	33.1	43.3

Grid-based Vessel Density (%)

48.1	45.3	49.2
44.6	37.3	43.9
35.7	40.1	47.4

Figure 2 Multimodal imaging of the left eye of a 65-year-old female with diabetic retinopathy. (a) Scanning laser ophthalmoscopy image obtained with 532 nm wavelength. The black line represents the position of cross-sectional scan through the center of the macula. The white line represents the position of cross-sectional scan trough the disorganization of retinal inner layers (DRIL) lesion. (b) Cross-sectional scan through the center of the macula. (c) Cross-sectional scan through the area of DRIL (arrowheads). (d) Optical coherence tomographic angiography (OCTA) image of superficial capillary plexus (SCP) demonstrates substantial loss of perfusion. (e) OCTA image of intermediate capillary plexus (ICP) demonstrates hypoperfusion. (f) OCTA image of deep capillary plexus (DCP) demonstrates hypoperfusion. Note the large retinal vessel (asterisk) of SCP appearing in ICP and DCP due to loss of retinal tissue. (g) Vessel density map of SCP. (h) Vessel density map of deep vascular complex. Note a more substantial loss of vessel density in SCP than in deep vascular complex. (i) Cross-sectional scan through the area of DRIL (arrowheads). Note the preservation of nerve fiber layer. (j). Distribution of flow signal within cross-sectional scan. The lesion (arrowheads) demonstrates flow void mostly in the inner and middle retinal layers while the innermost retinal vessels are preserved.

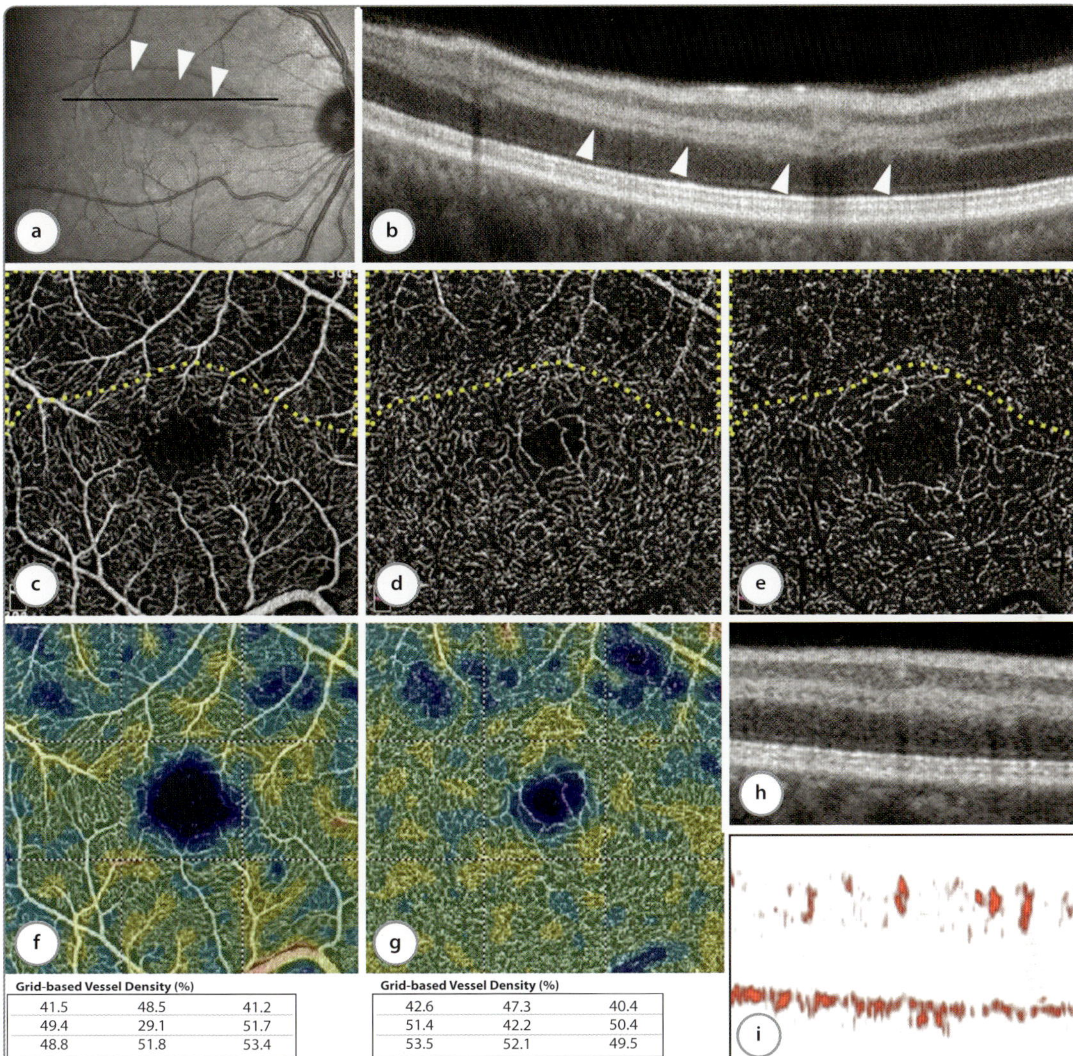

Grid-based Vessel Density (%)

41.5	48.5	41.2
49.4	29.1	51.7
48.8	51.8	53.4

Grid-based Vessel Density (%)

42.6	47.3	40.4
51.4	42.2	50.4
53.5	52.1	49.5

Figure 3 Multimodal imaging of the right eye of a 24-year-old male with paracentral acute middle maculopathy (PAMM) presented 7 days after the onset. (a) Infrared scanning laser ophthalmoscopy image demonstrates a hyporeflective area corresponding to the PAMM area (arrowheads). The black line represents the position of the cross-sectional scan. (b) Cross-sectional scan through the area of the PAMM lesion. (c) Optical coherence tomographic angiography (OCTA) image of superficial capillary plexus (SCP) demonstrates minimal alteration. (d) OCTA image of intermediate capillary plexus demonstrates substantial loss of perfusion. (e) OCTA image of deep capillary plexus demonstrates substantial loss of perfusion. (f) Vessel density map of SCP. (g) Vessel density map of deep vascular complex. Note a more substantial loss of vessel density in deep vascular complex than in SCP. (h) Cross-sectional scan through the PAMM lesion. (i) Distribution of flow signal within cross-sectional scan demonstrates flow void mostly in the middle retinal layers, however, outer and innermost layers also affected.

the maximum of flow voids in DCP while changes of microcirculation absent in SCP and only moderately present in ICP. An important characteristic of AMN at least in some cases is alteration of photoreceptors appearing as attenuation of ellipsoid **(Figure 4)**. On the one hand, photoreceptor damage suggests involvement of choriocapillaris in ischemic injury and, in fact, flow voids within choriocapillaris can be found in AMN eyes. On the other hand, this

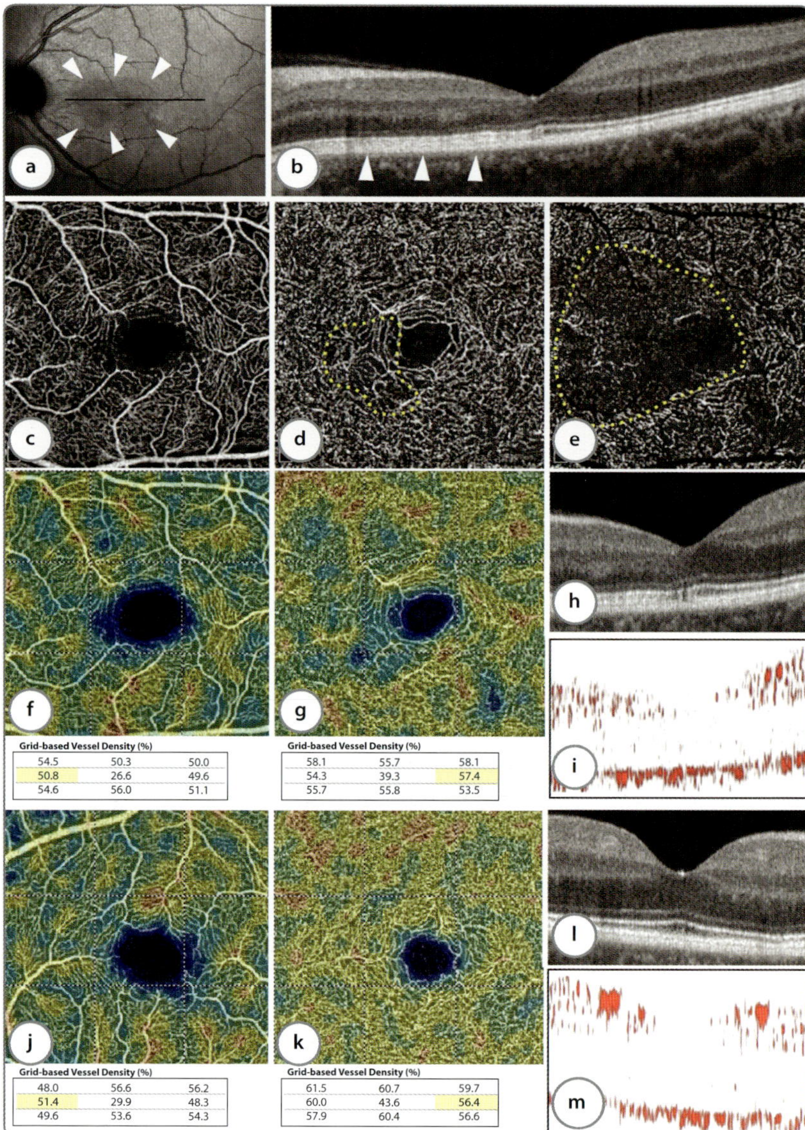

Figure 4 Multimodal imaging of both eyes of 38-year-old patient, 3 months after the onset of acute macular neuroretinopathy (AMN) in the left eye. (a) Infrared scanning laser ophthalmoscopy image demonstrates a hyporeflective area corresponding to the AMN lesion (arrowheads). The black line represents the position of the cross-sectional scan. (b) Cross-sectional scan through the area of the AMN lesion. Note attenuation of photoreceptors (arrowheads). (c) Optical coherence tomographic angiography (OCTA) image demonstrates no changes in superficial capillary plexus (SCP). (d) OCTA image demonstrates mild alteration of intermediate capillary plexus (dashed line). (e) OCTA image demonstrates substantial loss of perfusion in deep capillary plexus (DCP) (dashed line). (f) Vessel density map of SCP in the left eye. (g) Vessel density map of deep vascular complex in the left eye. (h) Cross-sectional scan through the area of AMN demonstrates thinning of outer nuclear layer and attenuation of photoreceptors. (i) Distribution of flow signal within cross-sectional scan demonstrates inhibition of flow signal of DCP within the lesion. (j) Vessel density map of SCP in the right eye. (k) Vessel density map of deep vascular complex in the right eye. (l) Cross-sectional scan through the macula in the right eye. (m) Distribution of flow signal within cross-sectional scan in the right eye. Note that in the left eye vessel density within the area occupied by the lesion is decreased in DCP but not in SCP. This difference is apparent when comparing corresponding areas of the left and right eye (highlighted in yellow in the table).

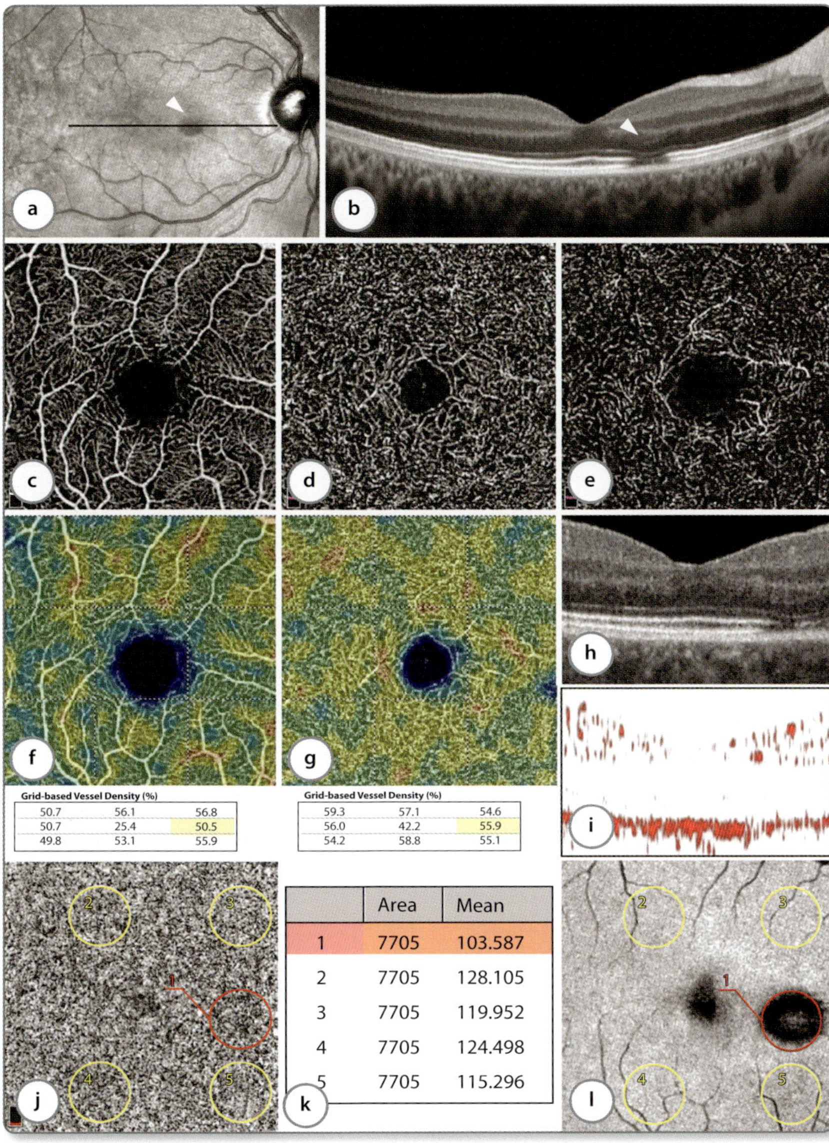

Figure 5 Multimodal imaging of the right eye of 25-year-old female 1 month after onset of acute macular neuroretinopathy (AMN). (a) Infrared scanning laser ophthalmoscopy image demonstrates a small AMN lesion (arrowhead). (b) Cross-sectional scan through the AMN lesion (arrowhead) demonstrates thinning of outer nuclear layer and loss of photoreceptors. (c) Optical coherence tomographic angiography (OCTA) image of superficial capillary plexus (SCP) showing no vascular abnormalities. (d) OCTA image of ICP showing no vascular abnormalities. (e) OCTA image of deep capillary plexus showing no vascular abnormalities. (f) Vessel density map of SCP demonstrates no changes in vessel density, including the AMN region (the vessel density value corresponding to the AMN region highlighted in yellow). (g) Vessel density map of the deep vascular complex demonstrates no changes in vessel density (the vessel density value corresponding to the AMN region highlighted in yellow). (h) Cross-sectional image through the AMN lesion. (i) Distribution of flow signal within cross-sectional scan demonstrates inhibition of flow signal of choriocapillaris within the lesion. (j) Choriocapillaris slab shows no apparent changes in flow signal. The circles represent the areas selected for the quantitative analysis with Image k. (k and l) Quantitative analysis with Image k demonstrates reduction of flow signal (calculated as mean gray value) within the lesion (red circle, position 1) compared to control regions (yellow circles, position 2–5). (l) *En face* image of photoreceptor slab demonstrating location of the areas included in analysis in relation to the AMN lesion.

finding does not conflict with the role of retinal microcirculation in AMN, since previous studies showed association of retinal ischemia and outer retinal damage in diabetic retinopathy.[19] It is also worth noting that not all AMN cases demonstrate changes of retinal microcirculation in resolved stage. This phenomenon can be explained by reperfusion.

Interestingly, a number of AMN studies, as for PAMM, have been shown an association between the incidence of AMN and different systemic and ocular pathologies.[20-24] The AMN, therefore, expands beyond an individual disease and can be considered as a syndrome. However, the relationships between deep retinal circulation and choriocapillaris flow, if any, remains unclear. The existence of a regulatory mechanism unifying these two poles of retinal blood supply could explain the observed combination of DCP and choriocapillaris involvement in AMN **(Figure 5)**.

Taking all the above into account, one cannot conclude that inhibition of perfusion in distinct capillary plexuses is clearly isolated except for the infarct of NFL, which is associated with isolated alteration of RPCP **(Figure 6)**. In fact, in DRIL, perfusion loss occupies not only SCP but ICP and DCP as well. In PAMM, SCP is minimally affected, and the maximum of flow voids can be found in ICP and DCP. Finally, in AMN, SCP remains unchanged, and DCP is mostly affected, but ICP and CC also demonstrate hypoperfusion. The distribution of ischemic retinal changes may follow the same way from RPCP to ICP in the line of ischemic conditions from NFL infarct to DRIL, to PAMM, and AMN.

Interestingly, that described patterns of isolated retinal ischemia agree with the simplified model of retinal microcirculation suggested earlier by Fouquet S and co-authors **(Box 1)**.[25] In that model, the highest level of disturbance

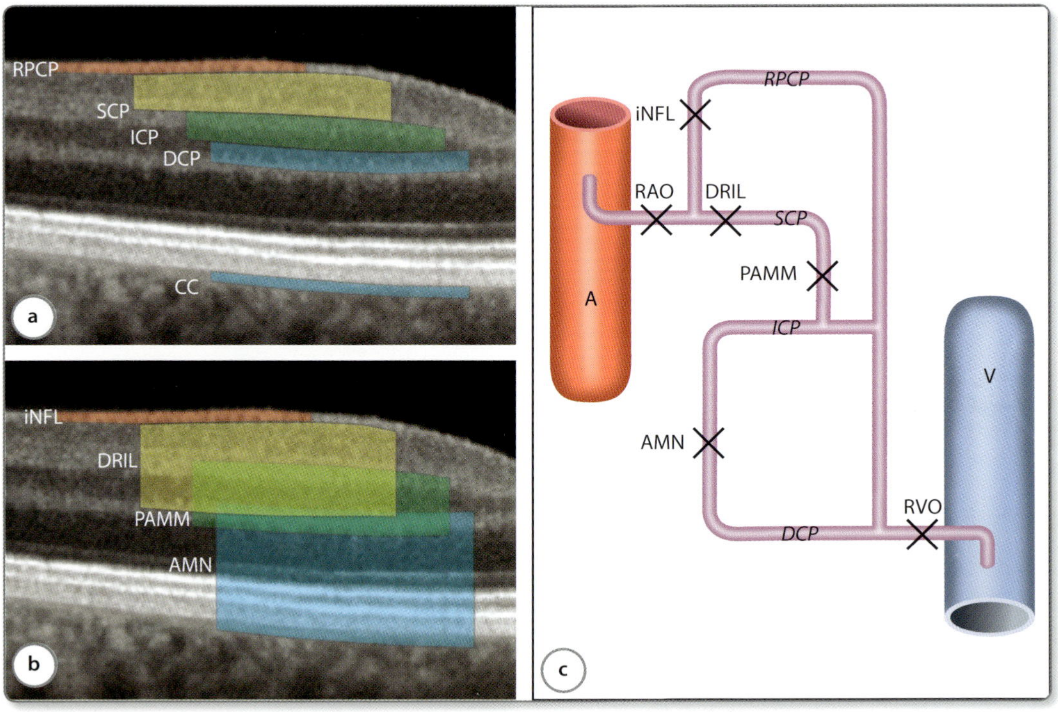

Figure 6 Correspondence between capillary plexuses (a) and different types of isolated retinal ischemia (b) regarding the current model of retinal microcirculation (c).
(A: arteria; AMN: acute macular neuroretinopathy; CC: choriocapillaris; DCP: deep capillary plexus; DRIL: disorganization of retinal inner layers; iNFL: infarct of nerve fiber layer; ICP: intermediate capillary plexus; PAMM: paracentral acute middle maculopathy; RAO: retinal arterial occlusion; RPCP: radial peripapillary capillary plexus; RVO: retinal vein occlusion; SCP: superficial capillary plexus; V: vein)

Box 1: Patterns of isolated retinal capillary ischemia

- Nerve fiber layer (NFL) infarct
- Disorganization of retinal inner layers (DRIL)
- Paracentral acute middle maculopathy (PAMM)
- Acute macular neuroretinopathy (AMN)

corresponds to severe vascular events such as RAO **(Figure 6c)**. An isolated character of NFL infarct, in such cases, is explained by independent blood supply for NFL with the branches, which do not supply deeper plexuses. At the same time, when the primary level of hypoperfusion taking place at the SCP and ICP, the ischemia also occupies deeper retina which supplied from SCP in consecutive manner. The ischemic BRVO with loss of inner retina may be considered as a combination of ischemia in RPCP and ascending ischemia along the DCP–SCP axis.

In conclusion, according to the main patterns of alteration, one may define four distinct patterns of isolated retinal capillary ischemia, which can be considered as syndromes NFL infarct, DRIL, PAMM, and AMN. Each of these syndromes encompasses a specific level of retinal microcirculation and associated with specific ischemic changes of the retina. Each syndrome may manifest as a distinct idiopathic condition or accompany severe retinal vascular disorders. An isolated character of ischemia in these syndromes is not complete and ischemia, except for infarct of NFL, invade neighboring retinal microcirculatory levels although less extensively.

References

1. Campbell JP, Zhang M, Hwang TS, et al. Detailed Vascular Anatomy of the Human Retina by Projection-Resolved Optical Coherence Tomography Angiography. Sci Rep 2017; 7:42201.
2. Bos PJ, Deutman AF. Acute macular neuroretinopathy. Am J Ophthalmol 1975; 80:573–584.
3. Fawzi AA, Pappuru RR, Sarraf D, et al. Acute macular neuroretinopathy: long-term insights revealed by multimodal imaging. Retina 2012; 32:1500–1513.
4. Sarraf D, Rahimy E, Fawzi AA, et al. Paracentral acute middle maculopathy: a new variant of acute macular neuroretinopathy associated with retinal capillary ischemia. JAMA Ophthalmol 2013; 131:1275–1287.
5. McLeod D. Why cotton wool spots should not be regarded as retinal nerve fibre layer infarcts. Br J Ophthalmol 2005; 89:229–237.
6. Sun JK, Lin MM, Lammer J, et al. Disorganization of the retinal inner layers as a predictor of visual acuity in eyes with center-involved diabetic macular edema. JAMA Ophthalmol 2014; 132: 1309–1316.
7. Chen X, Desai SJ, Baumal CR. Paracentral acute middle maculopathy in pregnancy. Retin Cases Brief Rep. 2017. [Epub ahead of print]
8. Aribas YK, Aktas Z, Bayrakceken K, et al. Paracentral acute middle maculopathy in primary congenital glaucoma. Retin Cases Brief Rep. 2017. [Epub ahead of print]
9. Cohen MN, Dang S, Liang MC. Paracentral acute middle maculopathy after cardiac arrest. Ophthalmology 2017; 124:511.
10. Niyousha MR, Hassanpoor N, Eftekhari A, et al. Simultaneous paracentral acute middle maculopathy and Purtscher-like retinopathy after acute febrile illness. Can J Ophthalmol 2018; 53:184–186.
11. Sebastiani S, Pellegrini M, Giannaccare G, et al. Paracentral acute middle maculopathy associated with phosphodiesterase-5 inhibitor therapy. Retin Cases Brief Rep. 2018. [Epub ahead of print]
12. Nakamura M, Katagiri S, Hayashi T, et al. Paracentral acute middle maculopathy after endovascular coil embolization. Retin Cases Brief Rep. 2018. [Epub ahead of print]
13. Chen X, Rahimy E, Sergott RC, et al. Spectrum of retinal vascular diseases associated with paracentral acute middle maculopathy. Am J Ophthalmol 2015; 160:26–34.
14. Rivera-De La Parra D, Fromow-Guerra J. Paracentral acute middle maculopathy in Purtscher retinopathy. Retin Cases Brief Rep. 2017. [Epub ahead of print].
15. Ilginis T, Keane PA, Tufail A. Paracentral acute middle maculopathy in sickle cell disease. JAMA Ophthalmol 2015; 133:614–616.
16. Nemiroff J, Kuehlewein L, Rahimy E, et al. Assessing deep retinal capillary ischemia in paracentral acute middle maculopathy by optical coherence tomography angiography. Am J Ophthalmol 2016; 162:121–132.
17. Kulikov AN, Maltsev DS, Leongardt TA. Retinal microvasculature alteration in paracentral acute middle maculopathy and acute macular neuroretinopathy: a quantitative optical coherence tomography angiography study. Retin Cases Br Rep. 2018. [Epub ahead of print]

18. Maltsev DS, Kulikov AN, Burnasheva MA, et al. Prevalence of resolved paracentral acute middle maculopathy lesions in fellow eyes of patients with unilateral retinal vein occlusion. Acta Ophthalmol. 2019. [Epub ahead of print]
19. Scarinci F, Jampol LM, Linsenmeier RA, et al. Association of Diabetic Macular Nonperfusion with Outer Retinal Disruption on Optical Coherence Tomography. JAMA Ophthalmol 2015; 133:1036–1044.
20. Saurabh K, Roy R, Mishra S, et al. Acute macular neuroretinopathy after blunt ocular trauma : a rare association. Indian J Ophthalmol 2019; 67:566–568.
21. Dedania VS, Ghodasra DH, Kay CN, et al. Ciliochoroidal effusion and acute macular neuroretinopathy associated with cervical traction therapy. Retin Cases Brief Rep 2018; 12:24–28.
22. Vujosevic S, Testi I, Nacci E, et al. Terson syndrome associated with acute macular neuropathy type 2. Ophthalmic Surg Lasers Imaging Retina 2017; 48:764–767.
23. Yang YS, Zhang L, Asdaghi N, et al. Acute macular neuroretinopathy in Susac syndrome: a new association. Retin Cases Br Rep. 2018. [Epub ahead of print]
24. Li M, Zhang X, Ji Y, Ye B, et al. Acute macular neuroretinopathy in dengue fever: Short-term prospectively followed up case series. JAMA Ophthalmol 2015; 133:1329–1333.
25. Fouquet S, Vacca O, Sennlaub F, et al. The 3D retinal capillary circulation in pigs reveals a predominant serial organization. Investig Ophthalmol Vis Sci 2017; 58:5754–5763.

24 Macular telangiectasia type 1 and 2

Bruno Lumbroso, Marco Rispoli

Clinical features, classification

Idiopathic macular telangiectasia (MacTel) refers to retinal capillary ectasia restricted to the perifoveal area without a specific cause. In 2006, the classification of MacTel was revised by Yannuzzi et al. using the optical coherence tomography (OCT).[1]

Idiopathic macular telangiectasia is classified into three categories **(Box 1)**:

1. *MacTel 1*: Aneurysmal telangiectasia. Frequently unilateral and divided in subgroup **(Figure 1)**:
   - Group 1A, based on the clinical detection of the aneurysmal and telangiectatic exudative vessels in the juxtafoveolar area.
   - Group 1B is defined as focal exudative telangiectasia limited to 2 clock hours or less in the juxtafoveal areas. Vascular dilatations, exudates, and edema cysts **(Figure 2)**.
2. *MacTel 2*: Perifoveal telangiectasia is generally bilateral and on the temporal side of the fovea. Pigment epithelium hyperplasia and pigment deposits may appear **(Figure 3)**. Local disruption of retinal pigment epithelium (RPE) and ellipsoid. Hyporeflective, rare angular cavities are normally seen. Neovascularization networks are a complication not rare after a few years' evolution **(Box 2)**.
3. *MacTel3*: Occlusive telangiectasia.

Box 1: Idiopathic macular telangiectasia (MacTel) classification

Revised by Yannuzzi et al. using the OCT. Three categories:

1. *MacTel 1*: Aneurysmal telangiectasia. Frequently unilateral—
   - Group 1A, aneurysmal and telangiectatic exudative vessels in the juxtafoveolar area.
   - Group 1B, focal exudative telangiectasia in the juxtafoveal areas. Vascular dilatations, exudates, and edema cysts.
2. *MacTel 2*: Perifoveal telangiectasia generally bilateral on the temporal side of the fovea. Pigment epithelium hyperplasia and pigment deposits. Disruption of RPE and ellipsoid. Rare angular cavities. Neovascularization is a late complication.
3. *MacTel 3*: Occlusive telangiectasia.

(OCT: optical coherence tomography; RPE: retinal pigment epithelium)

Pathophysiology

MacTel 2 pathogenesis has been these last years the subject of thorough studies, and it is still not well known. Müller cells lesions and

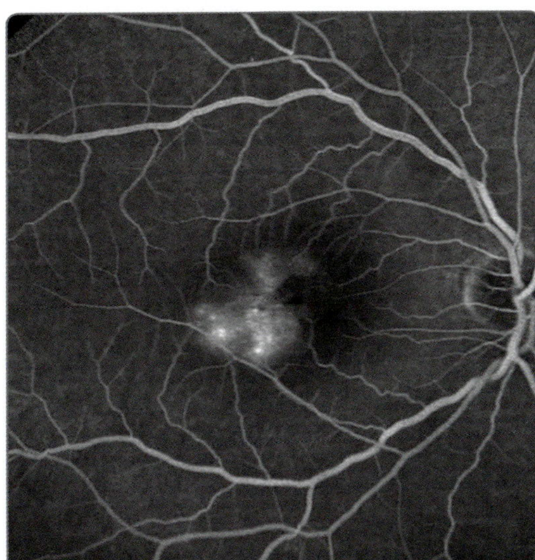

Figure 1 Macular telangiectasia 1 (MacTel 1) fluorescein angiography: aneurysmal telangiectasia. Frequently unilateral: telangiectatic exudative vessels are seen in the juxtafoveolar area.

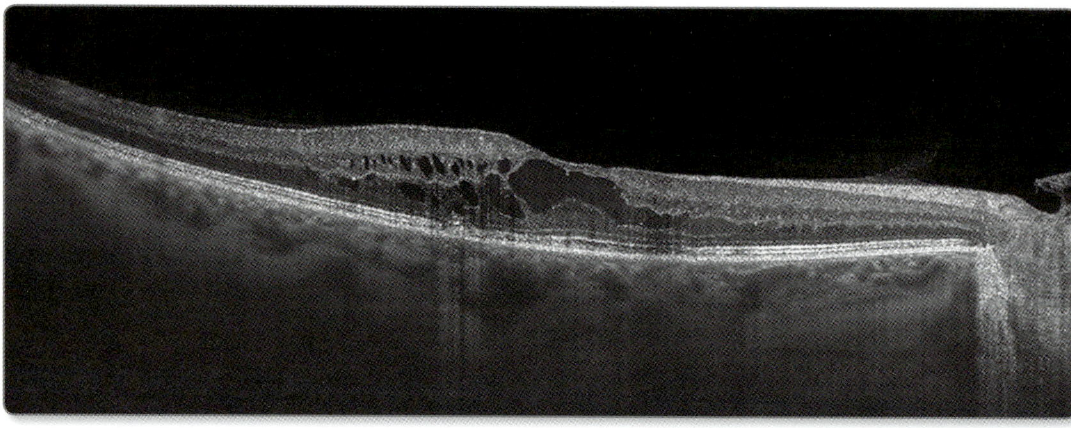

Figure 2 Macular telangiectasia 1 (MacTel 1) cross-section scan. Vascular dilatations, exudates, and various size edema cysts.

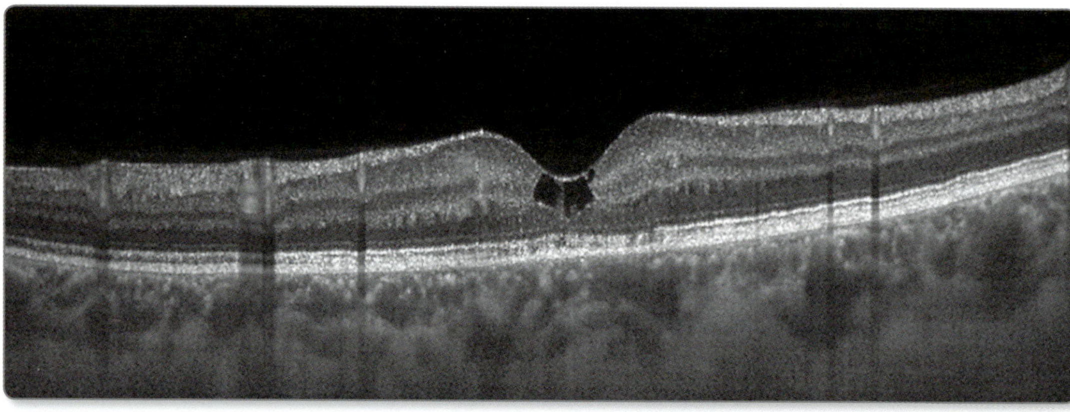

Figure 3 Macular telangiectasia 2 (MacTel 2) cross-section scan. Perifoveal telangiectasia type 2 are generally bilateral and on the temporal side of the fovea. Pigment epithelium hyperplasia and pigment deposits may appear with local disruption of retinal pigment epithelium and ellipsoid. Hypo-reflective, rare angular cavities are normally seen. Angular cavities are typical of MacTel 2.

Box 2: Macular telangiectasia 2 (MacTel 2) classification

MacTel 2 features are generally classified into four grades:

1. *Grade 1:* A break in outer limiting membrane and the ellipsoid, and inner and outer retinal cysts, at the temporal side of the fovea.
2. *Grade 2*: A larger break in the ellipsoid that reaches the foveal center, central outer cysts, and inner cysts, with disorganized retinal layers. The outer plexiform layer and the inner layers collapse toward the choroid. Pigment deposits.
3. *Grade 3*: Retinal cysts persist, the ellipsoid break involves the nasal and the temporal area center, and retinal layers 'collapse' extensively.
4. *Grade 4*: A neovascularization network is frequent after a few years' evolution.

macular pigment play definitely an essential role. MacTel 2 is presumed to be a glio-neurovascular disease conditioned by genetic terrain. Müller cell lesions have unquestionably an important part in MacTel 2 evolution. They form a scaffold for retina and their alteration seems to be an essential and may be primary element in the pathophysiology. Müller fibers also convey the light and their alteration is related with retinal loss of transparency.[2]

Proliferation of capillaries from the deep plexus of neuroretina goes before cellular alterations. Müller cells lesion appear, then photoreceptors lesion followed by dilation and proliferation of capillaries from the deep vascular network. In late stages, a retinochoroidal anastomosis may appear that progresses to fully developed neovascularization. Retinal neovascular networks link with a pigment epithelium detachment with a 'kissing' sign that connects directly the outer plexiform layer with pigment epithelium detachment.

Nevertheless, we do not know yet if MacTel 2 is a primarily vascular or neurosensory syndrome nor why it is mainly localized in central macula and temporal side.[3,4]

Imaging

Structural cross-section OCT

B-scan shows a loss of foveal depression and remodeling of retinal tissue. Retinal layers are disarranged. Hypo-reflective, angular cavities are seen at fovea level, under a thin unbroken retinal layer. Cellular alterations precede the dilation and proliferation of normal capillaries from the deep plexus of neuroretina. In OCT, these proliferations appear in relation to irregularities of the ellipsoid zone, which are an indicator of the progression of MacTel that leads to an extensive macular involvement in a few years. In late stages, retinochoroidal anastomosis may appear that progresses later to neovascularization. Indocyanine green (ICG) and OCT angiography established that the neovascular net communicates with both retinal and choroidal flow. Retinal neovascular networks grow to connect with a pigment epithelial detachment (PED). At this level, the cross-sectional angio-scan shows a flow signal that starts from the OPL going towards a little breach in the RPE located immediately below. In this place, there is a 'kissing' sign that connects directly the OPL with RPE resulting in a retinochoroidal anastomosis that will evolve in full-fledged neovascularization.

OCT angiography

The *en face* images show typical vascular distortion in the superficial and deep capillary complex **(Figure 4)**.

The MacTel 2 features are generally classified in four grades:

1. *Grade 1*: A break in outer limiting membrane and the ellipsoid (IS/OS junction line), and occurrence of inner and smaller outer retinal cysts, restricted to the temporal side of the fovea.
2. *Grade 2*: A larger break in the ellipsoid that reaches the foveal center, central outer cysts, and inner cysts involving also the nasal area, temporal side, with the retinal layers disorganized.
   The outer plexiform layer and the inner layers collapse towards the choroid. Pigment deposits cause hyperreflective intraretinal lesion.
3. *Grade 3*: Minor retinal cysts persist, the ellipsoid break involves the nasal and the temporal area center, and retinal layers 'collapse' extensively. Hyper-reflective intraretinal lesion due to pigment plaques can be seen.
4. *Grade 4*: A neovascularization network is frequent after a few years' evolution **(Figure 5)**. Any of the signs of grade 1 to 3 associated with a neovascularization is comparable to classic NV with hyper-reflective lesion located in the outer retinal layers associated to subretinal fluid and intraretinal edema. The outer retina segmentation displays *a small star-shaped flow that confirms a retinochoroidal anastomosis* with loss of small neighboring vessels.

Management

In MacTel type 1, aneurysmal telangiectasia laser treatment of the vascular anomalies is the preferred treatment of macular edema, while anti-vascular endothelial growth factor (VEGF) injections provide short-term advantage.

In MacTel type 2, no present treatment gives results in the non-proliferative stage. In case of choroidal neovascularization, anti-VEGF treatment gives positive outcome. It is advisable to treat as early as possible, when the neovascular membrane is small.

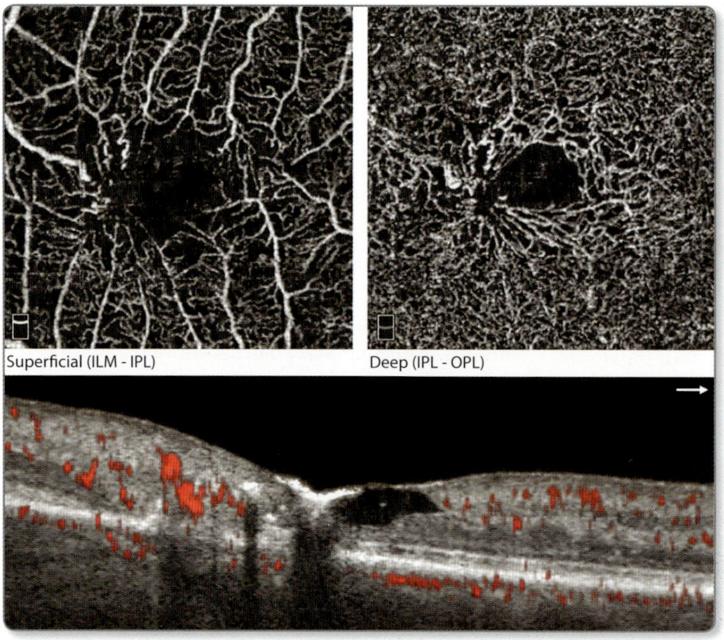

Figure 4 Macular telangiectasia 2 (MacTel 2) cross-section scan with angular cavity. The '*en face*' angioscans show distorted vascular superficial and deep networks.

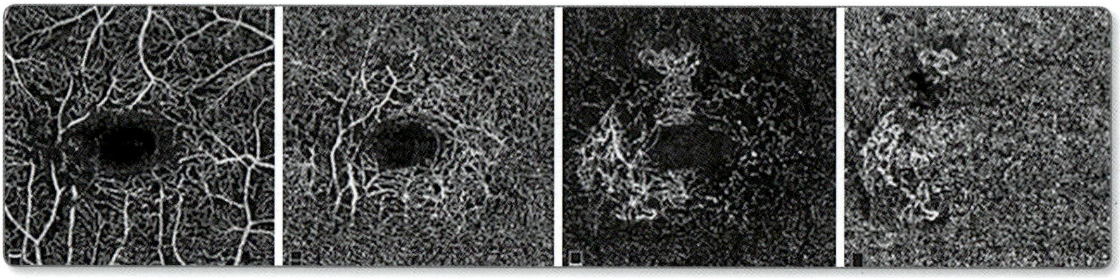

Figure 5 Macular telangiectasia 2 (MacTel 2) with neovascularization. Neovascularization networks are a complication not rare after a few years' evolution. In this figure, the '*en face*' angioscans show some alteration of the vascular superficial and deep networks where vessels are irregular and thickened. In the deeper retinal layers, the new vessels are seen: here two separate NV networks.

References

1. Yannuzzi LA, Bardal AM, Freund KB, et al. Idiopathic macular telangiectasia. Arch Ophthalmol 2006; 124:450–60.
2. Charbel Issa P, Gillies MC, Chew EY, et al. Macular telangiectasia type 2. Prog Retin Eye Res 2013; 34:49–77.
3. Roisman L, Rosenfeld PJ. Optical Coherence Tomography Angiography of Macular Telangiectasia Type 2. Dev Ophthalmol 2016; 56:146–158.
4. Charbel Issa P, Kupitz EH, Heeren TF, et al. Treatment for Macular Telangiectasia Type 2. Dev Ophthalmol 2016; 55:189–195.
5. Toto L, Di Antonio L, Mastropasqua R, et al. Multimodal Imaging of macular telangiectasia type 2: focus on vascular changes using optical coherence tomography angiography. Invest Ophthalmol Vis Sci 2016; 57: OCT268–276.

25 Hereditary macular dystrophies, Stargardt disease

Bruno Lumbroso, Marco Rispoli

Photoreceptors genetic disorders

They are the most common forms of ocular genetic disorders.

Cone dystrophy (Figures 1 to 3)

In the cone dystrophy, the primary defect involves the cones, leading to a central thinning of photoreceptor layer with conservation in the perifoveal portions.

Clinically a central bull's eyes maculopathy is most typical. Signs include loss of visual acuity, colour vision alteration, and hemeralopia. Optical coherence tomography (OCT) shows damage of the outer retina and photoreceptor progressing to atrophy at fovea level. The peripheral retina appears normal. Electroretinogram (ERG) shows abnormal cone function. However, the rod-isolated scotopic ERG is normal.

If the defect involves rod-cells (rod dystrophy), there is thinning of the photoreceptor layer in the extrafoveal area with conservation of foveal photoreceptors.

In the advanced phases, secondary modifications appear: pigmentations, inner limiting membrane thickening, fibrovascular proliferations hemorrhages, cysts, edema, and retinal schisis. Retinal detachment with macular involvement occurs infrequently, as in X-linked retinoschisis.

Pattern dystrophies

Fundus clinical examination shows frequently a pigmented central deposit surrounded by pigment loss. The lesions form a typical pattern on OCT. There is a subretinal accumulation of dystrophy material, with a dense hyper-reflective central part corresponding to the pigmented core of the lesion seen on examination. Drusen-like deposits arranged in various patterns include adult-onset foveomacular pigment epithelial dystrophy, butterfly and reticular pattern dystrophy material. Fundus autofluorescence

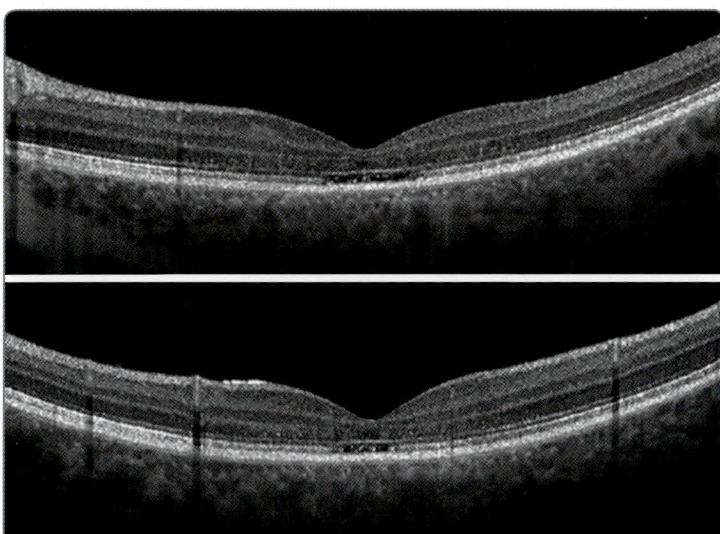

Figure 1 Early cone dystrophy. Cross-section optical coherence tomography (OCT) showing alteration and fading of cone cells in the central retina, leaving a dark area where cones have disappeared.

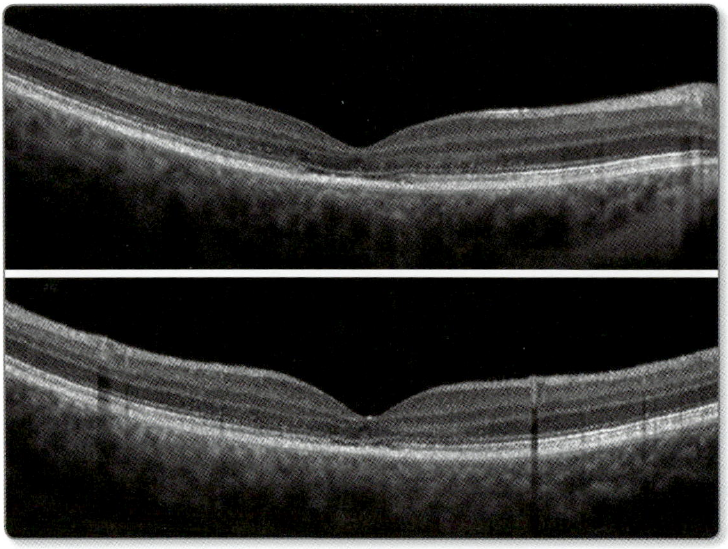

Figure 2 More advanced cone dystrophy. Cross-section optical coherence tomography (OCT). Evident thinning of central macula with alteration of the cone layer.

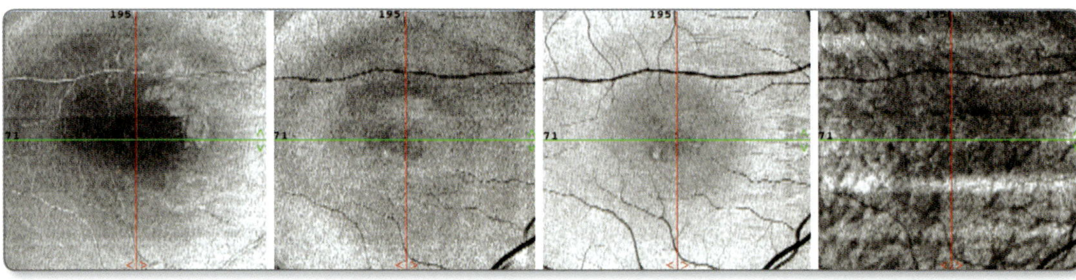

Figure 3 Cone dystrophy *en face* optical coherence tomography (OCT). The *en face* scans show bull's eyes typical features.

reveals hyperfluorescence corresponding to the deposit; however, it is usually not as bright as in true vitelliform maculopathies such as Best disease.

Pathophysiology

Macular dystrophies show a large loss of the photoreceptors and retinal pigment epithelium (RPE) irregularities, leading to vascular alterations and transformation of the vascular networks with decreased flow, and atrophy of retinal layers and choriocapillaris. Lipofuscin accumulates and hyaline deposits between the RPE and Bruch's membrane bring fluid circulation decrease and choriocapillaris atrophy. Progressive pigment epithelium damage leads to reduced production of vascular endothelial growth factor (VEGF) and other factors necessary for choriocapillaris function. Choriocapillaris damage ensues with total atrophy in more late stages. Large choroidal vessels and atrophy margins are neatly evident.[1]

Stargardt disease

Stargardt disease is an autosomal, generally recessive genetic disorder. Its onset is juvenile. The macular dystrophy is characterized by a rapid central visual damage, progressive bilateral atrophy of the macular RPE. In Europe, Stargardt disease is one of the most common causes of inherited low vision and legal blindness in children and young adults **(Figure 4)**.

Pathophysiology

The clinical picture of Stargardt disease has become even more intricate and composite since

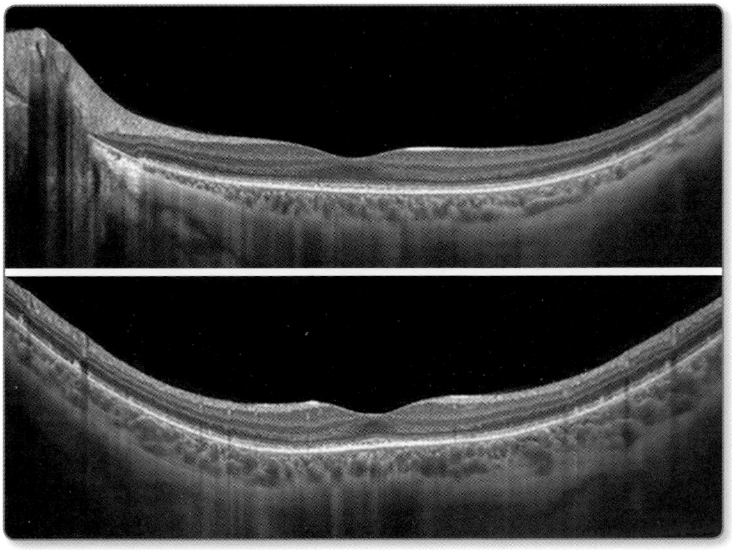

Figure 4 Stargardt disease cross-section. There is disruption of the outer retina, ellipsoid zone, and retinal pigment epithelium (RPE) in a parafoveal ring and hyper-reflective intra-RPE and/or sub-RPE deposits.

the generalized use of genetic testing. Actually, Stargardt, at the moment, is not thought to be a single disease. One phenotype covers at least three different diseases, each related to a different hereditary variation.

Stargardt disease is caused by defects in the *ABCA4* gene, but different combinations of *ABCA4* genes will result in widely different age of onset and retinal pathology. *ABCA4* gene has also importance, in other inherited syndromes, as retinitis pigmentosa, cone-rod dystrophies, and age-related macular degeneration.

Currently, Stargardt disease is subdivided into three categories:

1. *Stargardt 1*—is the most common form of Stargardt disease, both phenotypically and genetically highly heterogeneous. It is recessive, caused by mutations in the *ABCA4* gene. In Stargardt 1, major advances have been made in our ability to identify the disease at the earliest stages, to understand of underlying disease pathophysiology
2. *Stargardt 2 and Stargardt 3*—are rare dominant forms of Stargardt disease caused by mutations
3. *Stargardt 4*—shows a butterfly pattern of dystrophy.

Clinical evolution

Fundus examination shows macular bull's eye features in a child or young adult with vision decrease. A foveal area of yellowish atrophy is surrounded by yellow flecks around the macula and/or in the central and near-peripheral areas of the retina. Fundus autofluorescence shows a central macular hypo-autofluorescence. Evolution is very slow with constant damage increase for years. Final vision after years of progress ranges from 20/70 to 20/200.[2]

OCT and OCT angiography

In Stargardt patients, alterations are located at the deep capillary plexus level and choriocapillaris. Different degrees of choriocapillaris impairment occur leaving no residual choriocapillaris inside area of retinal epithelium pigment atrophy in late stages. Large choroidal vessels and borders of the atrophy are well visualized **(Figure 5; Box 1)**.

Management

In Stargardt 1, major advances have been made in our ability to identify the disease at the earliest stages, to understand of underlying disease pathophysiology.

Many clinical drug trials are being developed. They attempt to decrease lipofuscin accumulation. Gene therapy hopes to slow or avoid further retinal degeneration by replacing the diseased gene. A complement (C5) inhibitor called Zimura (Ophthotech) is being investigated intravitreally in Stargardt patients with mutation STDG1 (autosomal recessive Stargardt). The idea

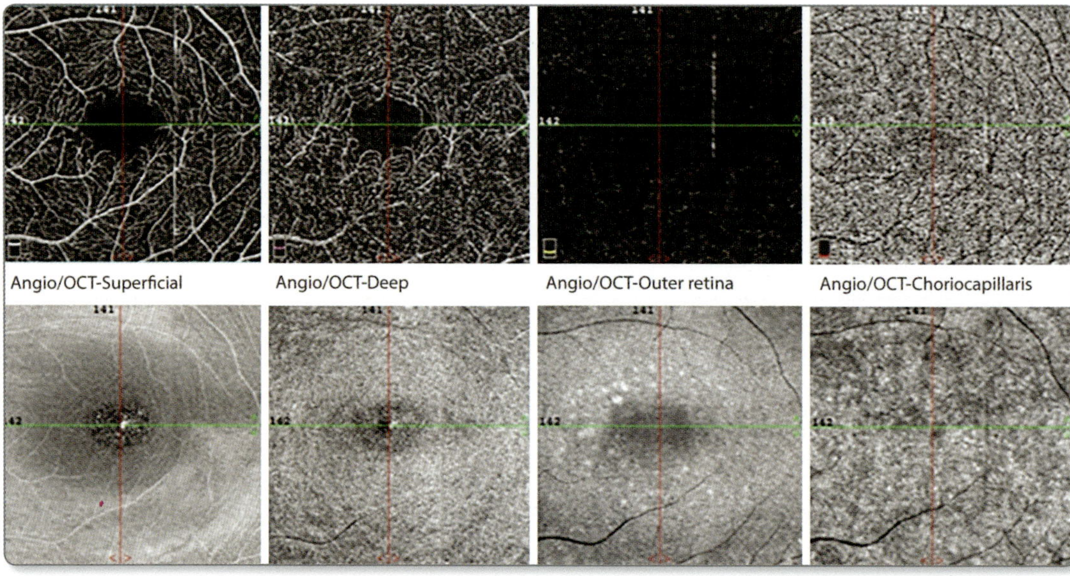

Figure 5 Optical coherence tomography (OCT) in a patient with Stargardt disease *en face* 2 and OCT angiography in a patient with early Stargardt disease show a bull's-eye maculopathy with conservation of the central fovea.

> **Box 1: Stargardt disease**
>
> - *Stargardt 1:* Most common form, recessive, due to mutations in the *ABCA4* gene
> - *Stargardt 2 and Stargardt 3:* Dominant form caused by mutations
> - *Stargardt 4:* Butterfly pattern of dystrophy

is that the final phase of the processes leading to retinal atrophy in Stargardt disease is supported by the activation of vitamin A (A2E) dimers of the alternative complement pathway with activation of MAC by C5.

Adeno-associated virus vectors are generally used. This study conveys potentials of treatment in a not too far future.

Best disease

Pathophysiology

Best disease is an autosomal dominant maculopathy caused by mutations in the *BIST1* gene. Genetic testing is necessary in detecting carriers. There is also variable phenotype, where in some cases, multifocal vitelliform lesions are scattered between or outside the vascular arcades.

Other mutations can generate autosomal recessive bestrophinopathy.

This recessive disorder is associated with progressive retinal function modification, with vision decrease, RPE abnormality, and yellowish flecks.

Pseudovitelliform macular degeneration

Pseudovitelliform macular degeneration in adults is a dominant autosomal genetic disease. Evolution is very slow and leads from the vitelliform stage to the pseudohypopyon stage and then to the atrophic stage. In pseudohypopyon stage, we observe a subretinal deposit, bright orange surrounded by a ring of retinal detachment.

Cross-section OCT shows a hyper-reflective, nodular formation, probably lipofuscin, in tight contact with pigment epithelium at the fovea. Retina is thinned above the nodular formation. During evolution, choroidal neovascularization (CNV) may appear. Optical coherence tomography angiography enables diagnosis, quantification, and monitoring of neovascularization in patients with retinal dystrophies despite distorted retinal architecture. It may assess, if CNV are active or quiescent **(Box 2)**.

Box 2: Pseudovitelliform macular degeneration, stages

1. Vitelliform stage
2. Pseudohypopyon stage
3. Atrophic stage

References

1. Patel RC, Gao SS, Zhang M, et al. Optical Coherence Tomography Angiography of Choroidal Neovascularization in Four Inherited Retinal Dystrophies. Retina 2016; 36:2339–2347.
2. Tanna P, Strauss RW, Fujinami K, et al. Stargardt disease: clinical features, molecular genetics, animal models and therapeutic options. Br J Ophthalmol 2017; 101:25–30.

26 Cystoid macular edema after surgery: Irvine–Gass syndrome

Bruno Lumbroso, Marco Rispoli

Clinical features

A few weeks or months after cataract or other ocular surgery, the operated eye may present a decrease in vision. Ophthalmoscopy shows macular edema. In some cases of postsurgical cystoid macular edema (CMO), acute onset of foveomacular subretinal deposits in the absence of have been seen.

Pathophysiology

The pathogenesis of post-surgery CMO (Irvine–Gass syndrome) is multifactorial. Three possible mechanisms are involved, separately or together.

Inflammation

The main etiology is most probably inflammatory. After surgery, inflammatory mediators increase in the aqueous and vitreous. Many inflammatory mediators such as prostaglandins, cytokines, and other play a decisive role in the genesis of postoperative edema. These mediators are probably released by invasive manoeuvers and handling of iris tissue during intraocular surgical procedure. Other elements secreted by ischemic tissues are also suspected to participate in the genesis of edema. Vascular endothelial growth factor (VEGF) and insulin-like growth factor-1, mediators secreted by ischemic tissues, are suspected to participate in postsurgical edema. Inflammation breaks the blood-aqueous and blood–retinal barriers, leading to increased vascular permeability. Transudation accumulates in the outer plexiform and inner nuclear layers to create cystoid cells that later merge to form larger fluid collections. In chronic macular edema evolution, lamellar macular holes, and subretinal fluid may also appear.

Phototoxicity

Light trauma to the pigment epithelium can cause blood–retinal barriers rupture and results in edema. Two mechanisms are advanced: thermal lesions by absorption of light by the pigment epithelium during surgery and/or photochemical lesions caused by the light of the operating microscope. This supposition is not recognized by all.

Vitreoretinal traction

Vitreomacular traction is possible during surgeries, especially in cases of capsular tears with vitreous incarceration. Vitreous is dragged on macula with decompensation of Müller cells. Optical coherence tomography (OCT) confirms this mechanism in some cases.

Imaging

Fluorescein angiography

Fluorescein angiography shows a cystoid macular edema and optic disc hyperfluorescence.

Cross-section structural OCT and '*en face*' OCT

Structural OCT shows a conical swelling of the retina and cystoid intraretinal edema with cells very regularly placed around the fovea, in the inner nuclear layer. Retinal thickness is increased. Cystoid cavities can also be seen in the outer layers of the retina. The inner retinal layers show increased thickness, the outer limiting membrane and the ellipsoid are normal. After a few weeks, the central edema cells enlarge to the full thickness of the retina reaching the junction between inner and outer segments of the photoreceptors that are fragmented and disrupted. They create cystic spaces that coalesce to form larger pockets of fluid. This syndrome responds normally well to treatment. The efficacy of non-steroidal anti-inflammatory drugs (NSAIDs) in primary prevention supports mainly the inflammatory hypothesis. Foveomacular subretinal deposits in the absence of drusen or intraretinal fluid respond well to standard therapy (**Box 1; Figure 1**).

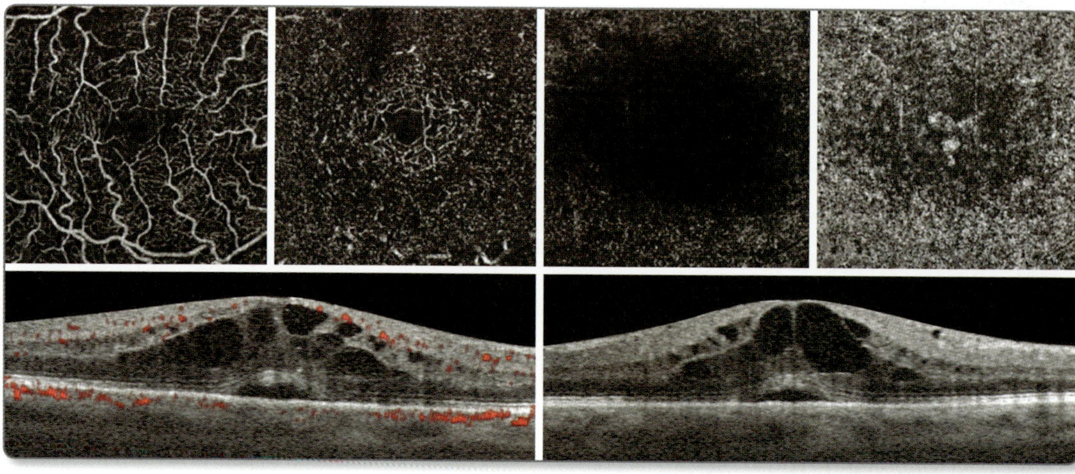

Figure 1 Irvine–Gass syndrome structural cross-section optical coherence tomography (OCT) scan. This patient noticed a decrease in visual acuity 2 months after surgery. The B-scan shows cystoid macular edema involving mainly the inner nuclear layer. There are small, cavities of cystoid edema, mostly in the inner and outer nuclear layers. Retinal thickness is increased, and the ellipsoid/IS/OS junction is normal. (Optovue)

Box 1: Structural OCT signs of edema after surgery

- Retinal conical swelling
- Retinal thickness is increased
- Cystoid intraretinal edema cells very regularly placed around the fovea, in the inner and outer nuclear layer
- Inner retinal layers have increased thickness
- Outer limiting membrane intact
- Ellipsoid normal

After a few weeks:

- Central edema cells expand to the full thickness of the retina
- Ellipsoid fragmented and disrupted

Management

Prevention of post-surgery Irvine–Gass syndrome may be obtained by co-administration of nepafenac or bromfenac and steroids in patients who are operated for routine cataract surgery. It is associated with a lower incidence of CMO compared with steroid monotherapy. Local treatment comprises nonsteroidal anti-inflammatory and corticosteroid drops.

General treatment consists in intravitreal anti-VEGF injections. Anti-VEGF plays an important role in the inflammation and capillary permeability that causes CMO.

Intravitreal dexamethasone injection may improve quickly visual acuity and macular thickness. A second injection is necessary after 6 months.

Presently, accepted treatment of post-surgical edema is the association of intravitreal triamcinolone, intravitreal anti-VEGF, and topical NSAIDs. It has obtained good results.

27 Dome-shaped macula

Bruno Lumbroso, Marco Rispoli

Introduction

Dome-shaped macula is a frequent anomaly of the myopic eye where a forward scleral and retinal bulge is observed at macula level. A forward scleral swelling is observed at the posterior pole and is secondary to excessive scleral thickening. This is not generally associated with choroidal neovascularization. A serous foveal detachment is frequently seen. This serous detachment, when it exists, is persistent and obstinate, showing fluctuating changes over time, with alternating active and inactive phases. It rarely regresses naturally or with treatment.

Pathophysiology

Serous retinal detachment in dome-shaped macula is probably caused by choroidal vascular changes, similar to central serous chorioretinopathy, but specifically confined in the inward bulge of the staphyloma and secondary to excessive scleral thickening. Serous subretinal fluid shows fluctuating oscillations over time, with increasing active and decreasing inactive periods. According to Viola, Staurenghi, et al., angiographic findings in dome-shaped macula suggest the choroid as a target for possible treatment strategies. Staurenghi et al. observed that dome-shaped macula eyes with serous retinal detachment have thicker choroid and thicker sclera and greater bulge height.[1]

Imaging

Fluorescein angiography indocyanine green angiography

Sometimes, a pinpoint leakage is seen on fluorescein angiography. Choroid, normally very thin, in the high myopic eye shows a greater subfoveal choroidal thickness and punctate cyanescence on indocyanine green (ICG) angiography. These features simulate morphological changes occurring in the choroid of central serous chorioretinopathy (CSC) patients and may make it difficult to differentiate these disorders.[2]

Structural optical coherence tomography

A serous retinal detachment is the most common anomaly associated with dome-shaped macula, detected by optical coherence tomography (OCT) in about half the cases. Macula protrudes where OCT shows a localized scleral thickening.

Management

There is no known effective treatment. Intravitreal bevacizumab and laser photocoagulation have been tried with no results. Half-fluence photodynamic therapy (PDT) has given good results in a few cases.

On the hypothesis that mineralocorticoid receptors may be implicated in the choroidal remodeling associated with dome-shaped macula, two cases of chronic serous retinal detachment (SRD) treated with oral spironolactone during 3 and 6 months with maintained efficacy until 3 and 12 months have been reported. More investigations are needed to determine the management of these cases.[3]

References

1. Daruich A, Matet A, Dirani A, et al. Central serous chorioretinopathy: Recent findings and new physiopathology hypothesis. Prog Retin Eye Res 2015; 48:82–118.
2. Viola F, Dell'Arti L, Benatti E, et al. Choroidal findings in dome-shaped macula in highly myopic eyes: a longitudinal study. Am J Ophthalmol 2015; 159: 44–52.
3. Dirani A, Matet A, Beydoun T, et al. Resolution of foveal detachment in dome-shaped macula after treatment by spironolactone: report of two cases and mini-review of the literature. Clin Ophthalmol 2014 20; 8:999–1002.

28 Epiretinal membranes

Maria Cristina Savastano, Bruno Lumbroso

Introduction

Epiretinal membrane (ERM) is represented by avascular semitranslucent, fibrocellular membranes that are generated on the inner surface of the retina. ERMs commonly cause minimal symptoms and can be simply observed, but in some cases can result in vision loss and metamorphopsia appearance. Generally, ERMs are most symptomatic when affecting the macula and cause deformation of retina profile.

Although several potential risk factors for the development of an ERM have been identified, including race, ethnicity, sex, smoking, diabetes, arteriolar narrowing, and hypercholesterolemia, the most consistently identified risk factor is the age.

Clinically, an ERM can be classified as either cellophane macular reflex or preretinal macular fibrosis based on severity of the disease.

The introduction of optical coherence tomography (OCT) devices more than two decades ago dramatically changed the landscape of vitreoretinal interface (VMI) diagnosis with greater consistency and accuracy than ever before. The capabilities afforded by new imaging technologies, together with the introduction of new therapies, made essential to define and classify the diseases affecting the VMI.

The International Vitreomacular Traction Study Group, few years ago, proposed a classification for several disorders of the VMI based completely on OCT findings.[1]

Vitreomacular adhesion (VMA) was defined as perifoveal vitreous separation with residual vitreomacular attachment and normal foveal morphology. VMA was subclassified as isolated or concurrent based on the absence or presence of associated macular abnormalities. Vitreomacular traction (VMT) was defined as anomalous posterior vitreous detachment (PVD) in association with an anatomic distortion of the normal foveal morphology, and VMT was subclassified as isolated or concurrent and focal or broad in the same manner as VMA. Full-thickness macular hole (FTMH) was defined as a foveal lesion that interrupts all layers of the macula from the inner limiting membrane (ILM) to the retinal pigment epithelium. FTMH was subclassified based on the presence or absence of VMT. FTMH was also subclassified as primary, if it was initiated by VMT, or secondary, if it was associated with a disorder known to cause macular hole in the absence of prior VMT (**Table 1; Box 1**).

Table 1: From the classification of the International Vitreomacular Traction Study Classification System for vitreomacular adhesion, traction, and macular hole[1]

Classification	Sub-classification
Vitreomacular adhesion (VMA)	Size: Focal (≤1,500 mm) or broad (>1,500 mm) isolated or concurrent
Vitreomacular traction (VMT)	Size: Focal (≤1,500 mm) or broad (>1,500 mm) isolated or concurrent
Full-thickness macular hole (FTMH)	Size: Small (≤250 mm), medium (>250e ≤ 400 mm), or large (>400 mm) Status of vitreous: With or without VMT Cause: Primary or secondary

Box 1: Risk factors for the development of an epiretinal membrane (ERM)

- Age
- Race
- Ethnicity
- Sex
- Smoking
- Diabetes
- Hypercholesterolemia

Physiopathology

The origin of epiretinal membranes formation is debated.

Separation of the posterior vitreous seems to be necessary for the formation of epiretinal membranes. Part of the posterior cortical vitreous allows glial cells to proliferate on the retinal surface.

Histologic study highlights mainly RPE cells and retinal glial cells (astrocytes and Müller cells), but also myofibroblasts, fibroblasts, hyalocytes, and macrophages. The precise identification of the cells involved in the pathogenesis of idiopathic ERMs has been hindered by the ability of the cells involved to transdifferentiate during the pathological disease.

However, glial cells are thought to predominate in early idiopathic ERMs; there is evidence that Müller cells plays a key role in this process.[2,3]

Inflammation is a central component of many of the disorders associated with secondary ERMs, as evidenced by the increased expression of cytokines. These cytokines support the inflammatory cells that have been identified in ERMs.

Activation of Müller cells is characterized by:

- Reactive gliosis
- Hypertrophy with increased expression of filament proteins intermediates: nestin, vimentin, and glial fibrillary acidic protein (GFAP)
- Proliferation and migration[4]

Epiretinal membranes can be observed as consequence of inflammation, hemorrhages, and retinovitreal adherences.

Secondary epiretinal membranes are more likely to be characterized by focal retinal adhesion than are primary epiretinal membranes. Primary epiretinal membranes tend to be globally adherent. This finding may contribute to understand the underlying mechanisms of epiretinal membranes formation in different clinical settings.

Epiretinal membranes retraction gives a large range of features from slight cellophane maculopathy to dense macular pucker. Epiretinal membranes grow causing parallel or radial retinal folds inducing retinal distortion and metamorphopsia. Increased traction causes flat macular detachment, diffuse retinal oedema, or cystoid macular edema.

Predictability of vision function recovery

The ellipsoid zone (EZ) and external limiting membrane (ELM) are more sensitive of the hyper-reflective retinal bands on OCT in ERM disorders. Their band integrity is the preoperative OCT finding that has been most consistently associated with postoperative visual acuity recovery. A majority of studies have reported that intact preoperative EZ and ELM are associated with a better postoperative VA than a disrupted preoperative EZ and ELM.

The visual loss associated with ERM has also been suggested to be caused by retinal ganglion or inner nuclear layer cell damage due to the inner retinal layer wrinkling, which is represented as an increase in inner-retinal thickness or ganglion cell–inner plexiform layer thickness. The development of inner-retinal thickness thicker has been recognized as ectopic inner foveal layers (EIFLs) development (**Figures 1a** to **c**).[5]

The presence of EIFL should be considered as a negative prognostic factor for postoperative anatomical and functional recovery.

The introduction of OCT angiography (OCTA) allowed to assess preoperative and postoperative vascular changes after surgery. The capability of some algorithms to measure the vascular density permitted to quantify the onset of possible vascular defect. In ERMs generally, the superficial vascular plexus seems elongated and stretched; sometimes there is the disappearance of the foveal avascular zone (FAZ). Deep vascular plexus, on the other hand, is almost more compromized and the vessels are sometimes not visible. The deep vessels reappear only after the surgery when retinal layers appear relaxed although extremely damaged (**Figure 2**).

Assessing macular capillary plexuses via OCTA may be useful to quantify structural changes of the inner retinal layer and predict visual function in patients undergoing ERM removal surgery.

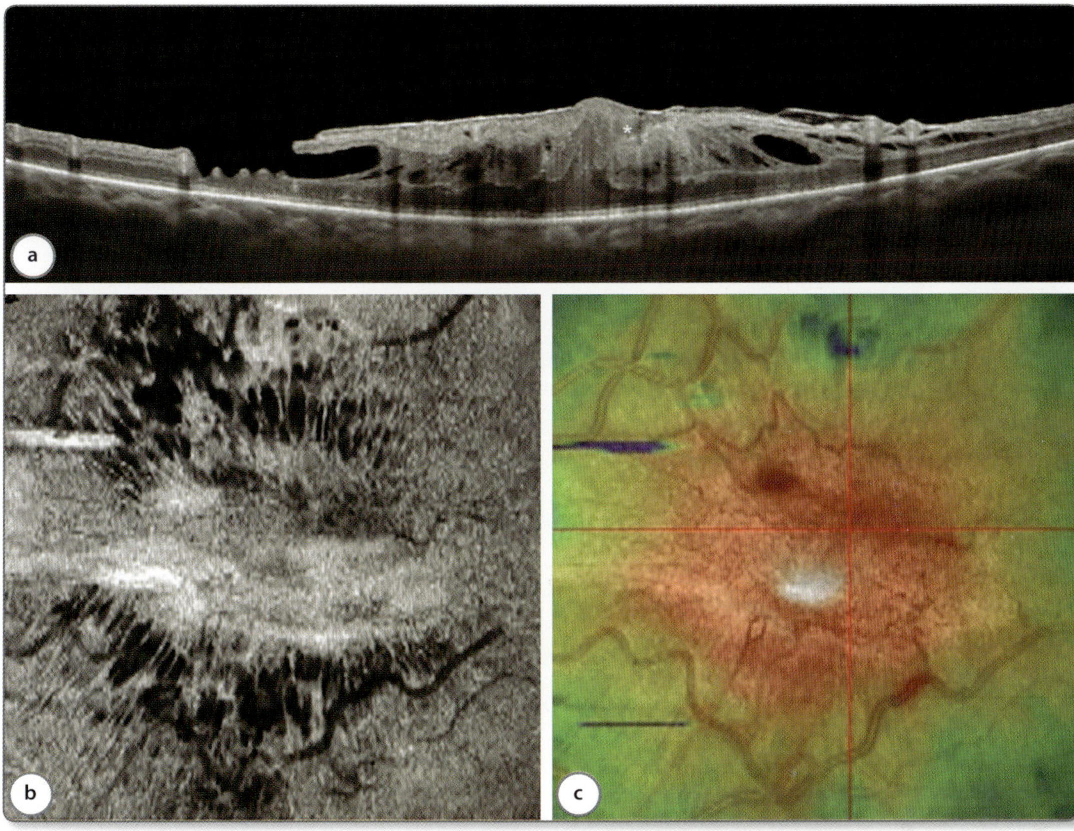

Figure 1 Epiretinal membrane with significant alteration of retinal profile and inner retinal reflectivity. (a) B-scan shows the ectopic inner foveal layers (EIFLs) (asterisk) that correspond to chronic inflammation signs. (b) *En face* optical coherence tomography (OCT) reveals the topographic distribution of epiretinal membrane with star shape. The relative thickness map (c) shows the higher thickness in white central apex.

Treatment

The management options for ERM are currently limited and consist of either observation or surgical intervention.

Surgical intervention includes pars plana vitrectomy with ERM removal with ILM removal. Surgical peeling of the ILM may help to decrease the risk of ERM recurrence. The surgical techniques used in the treatment of ERM generally afford excellent postoperative visual outcomes. However, ILM removal has potentially more extensive damage that can be observable as the dissociated outer nerve fiber layer (DONFL) visualization.[6]

The introduction of *en face* OCT scans provides an easy-to-understand global overview of the retinal surface. It can detect and classify tiny progressive morphologic changes in the texture of the retinal surface occurring after internal limiting membrane peeling and in particular the DONFL. DONFL appearance is reported to be caused by dimples on the retina, their depth limited to the thickness of the retinal nerve fiber layer (**Figures 3** and **4**).

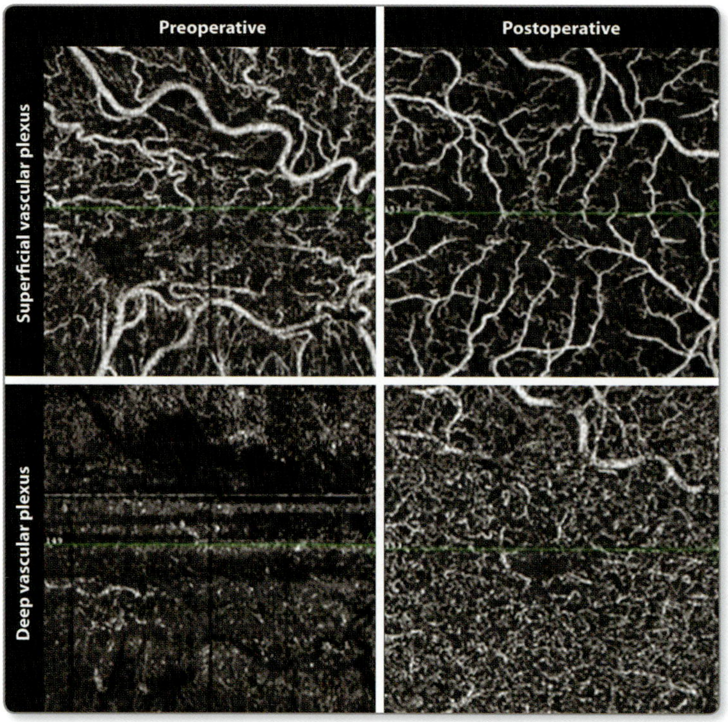

Figure 2 Optical coherence tomography (OCT) angiography preoperatory and postoperatory epiretinal membrane (ERM) removal. In ERMs generally, the superficial vascular plexus seems elongated and stretched with foveal avascular zone (FAZ) disappear. Deep vascular plexus is almost more compromized and the vessels are sometimes not visible. The deep vessels become visible only after the surgery although extremely damaged.

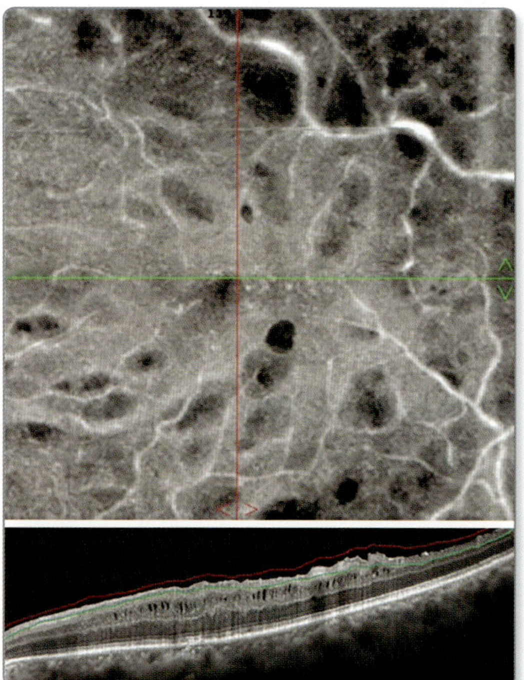

Figure 3 Postoperative epiretinal membrane removal. (Upper) *En face* scan shows the presence of dissociated outer nerve fiber layer (DONFL) after peeling of inner limiting membrane (ILM). DONFL correspond to Muller cells damage during the ILM removal. These DONFLs remain observable for several years after the surgery. (Bottom) DONFL appearance is reported in B-scan as dimples on the retina where their depth is limited into the retinal nerve fiber layer.

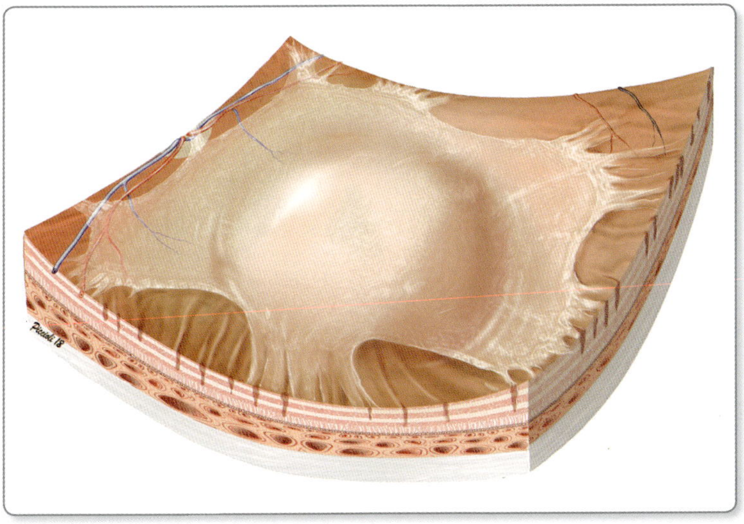

Figure 4 Epiretinal membrane (ERM) is represented by avascular semitranslucent, fibrocellular membranes that are generated on the inner surface of the retina. Generally, ERMs are most symptomatic when affecting the macula and cause deformation of retina profile and retinal folds.

References

1. Duker JS, Kaiser PK, Binder S, et al. The International Vitreomacular Traction Study Group classification of vitreomacular adhesion, traction, and macular hole. Ophthalmology 2013; 120:2611–2619.
2. Bringmann A, Wiedemann P. Involvement of Muller glial cells in epiretinal membrane formation. Graefes Arch Clin Exp Ophthalmol 2009; 247:865–883.
3. Govetto A, Lalane RA 3rd, Sarraf D, et al. Insights Into Epiretinal Membranes: Presence of Ectopic Inner Foveal Layers and a New Optical Coherence Tomography Staging Scheme. Am J Ophthalmol 2017; 175:99–113.
4. Wang M, Ma W, Zhao L, et al. Adaptive Müller cell responses to microglial activation mediate neuroprotection and coordinate inflammation in the retina. J Neuroinflammation 2011; 8:173.
5. Govetto A, Virgili G, Rodriguez FJ, et al. Functional and anatomical significance of the ectopic inner foveal layers in eyes with idiopathic epiretinal membranes: Surgical Results at 12 Months. Retina 2019; 39:347–357.
6. Rispoli M, Le Rouic JF, Lesnoni G, et al. Retinal surface en face optical coherence tomography: a new imaging approach in epiretinal membrane surgery. Retina 2012; 32:2070–2076.

29

Retinitis pigmentosa, inherited retinal dystrophies

Enzo Maria Vingolo, Federico Anselmucci, Lorenzo Casilio

Pathogenesis

Currently, the clinical definition of 'retinitis pigmentosa' commonly used for several retinal rare diseases, thanks to the progress of molecular biology and genetics, has become obsolete; in fact, the usual and commonly known clinical classification referred to an aspect of the fundus oculi has been overcome by the new classification mainly based on the single genetic deficit, so frequently a mutation of the same gene, but in a different site, can cause diseases with different clinical appearance and definition (phenotypic). The term actually widely used that has a clear significance of these clinical conditions is 'inherited retinal dystrophies' (IRDs).

More than 2,000 proteins are expressed in the retina and most of them are involved in the phototransduction and transmission of the bioelectric signal to the retina. The characteristic pathogenetic mechanism of IRD is cellular death by apoptosis. Despite the genetic defect is present since birth, the cell death occurs in a more or less long period depending on the importance of the genetic defect; therefore, we will have very early forms of IRDs such as the Leber congenital amaurosis (LCA), others affecting childhood age such as Stargardt (SD), or adult onset forms such as some rod dystrophies; then there are forms that do not progress at all like congenital stationary night blindness (CSNB).

While electrophysiology in the past had a primary role in old classification with the genotype-phenotype, knowledge needs to be based on a morphologic tool, and in this view, optical coherence tomography (OCT) represents a very useful task to study the retinal anatomy, sometimes suggesting, a genetic defect or a carrier status and is very useful in monitoring the progression of the disease.

Under the etiopathological point of view, we distinguish genes that are expressed in the different layers of the retina and consequently in the different cells with different outcomes at OCT scan and instrumental examination.

- Genetic defects of the choroid
- Genetic defects of the electron paramagnetic resonance (EPR)-photoreceptor complex
- Genetic defects of the photoreceptor
- Genetic defects of the internal retina

Genetic defects of the choroid, such as choroideremia or gyrate atrophy of choroid , show thinning of small and later of the large choroidal vessels that corresponds to a retinal thinning area with hyper-reflective zones.

In genetic defects of the EPR-photoreceptor complex, such as Stargardt or Best diseases, alterations are mainly seen in the Bruch's membrane with consequent thinning of the EPR and subsequently of the whole retina; sometimes, some fluid can be present (as in Best disease). In some rarer cases, such as the Levantine disease or the Norrie's disease, irregularities can be detected at the Bruch's membrane level.

Genetic defects of the photoreceptor: They are the most common forms of IRDs. It is the classic form of retinitis pigmentosa as we know it. Primary defect involving the cone cells are known as cone dystrophy, leading to a central thinning of photoreceptor layer with conservation in the perifoveal portions. If the defect is expressed in rod cells (rod dystrophy), there is thinning of the photoreceptor layer in the extrafoveal area with conservation of foveal photoreceptors. Obviously, in the advanced phases, secondary alterations may appear: pigmentations, thickening of the ILM, fibrovascular proliferations (as in the Coat's like), and haemorrhages are high reflectivity findings; cysts, edema, lamellar or external retinoschisis (unlike what happens in acquired forms that are localized in the internal retina) are low reflectivity findings. Retinal detachment with macular involvement can rarely occur, as in X-linked retinoschisis.

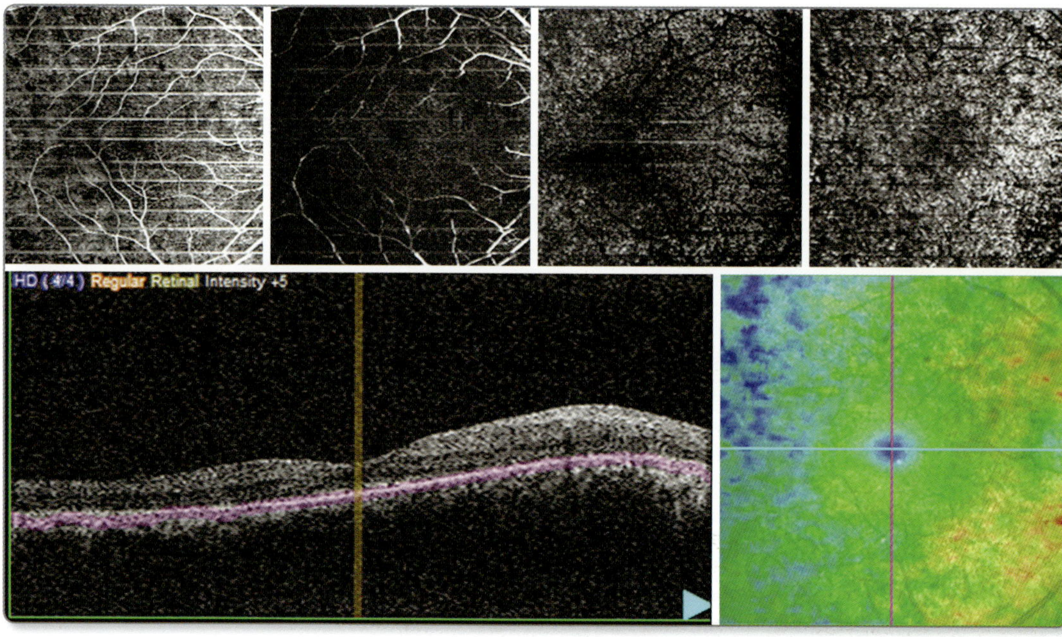

Figure 1 OCT angiography *en face* and B-scan. Superficial vessels, SCP, DCP, choriocapillaris network, and color flow map show the described vascular changes. B-scan shows extrafoveal outer retina thinning.

Genetic defects of the inner retina: As in the S-rod monochromatism, or in Goldmann-Favre syndrome, the defect is present in the inner retinal layers with highly reflective areas referable to fibrous proliferations and cystic spaces often with a columned aspect, these are more evident in external retina; this differs from acquired retinoschisis that shows similar lesions, but involves the inner retina.

Obviously, these findings can be highlighted only with the latest generation OCTs.

The new therapies for IRDs will be increasingly based on the use of viral vectors loaded with wild type genes that can be inserted inside the retina. They deserve a separate chapter. These are currently extremely expensive therapies (about € 850,000.00) whose administration involves the assessment of anatomical conditions through OCT. They require the existence of surviving retinal cells, even if they are not able to perform the phototransduction function due to the lack of a correctly active protein (RPE65). In fact, in many diseases, the genetic defect, especially in the early stages of the disease, does not result in the death of the photoreceptor, but a halt of its activity (to give an example: like an engine without fuel). The supplying of the wild-type gene causes the photoreceptor (at least in part) to restart as when the petrol is refuelled and the engine starts again. Therefore, the crucial point is to assess the presence of surviving photoreceptors. OCT with the support of electrofunctional examinations is the test accepted by scientific committee and is inclusion criterion for administered therapies. It is thus important to become increasingly familiar with these features.

OCT in IRD

Optical coherence tomography alterations in patients with IRD can be summarised according to the anatomic retinal layer involved.

Photoreceptors

One of the first histopathological modifications of the disease is the thinning of the photoreceptor layer due to the degeneration of the photoreceptors themselves. The death of the rods leads to a subsequent alteration of the EPR which, in a centripetal manner, leads to alteration of the cones.

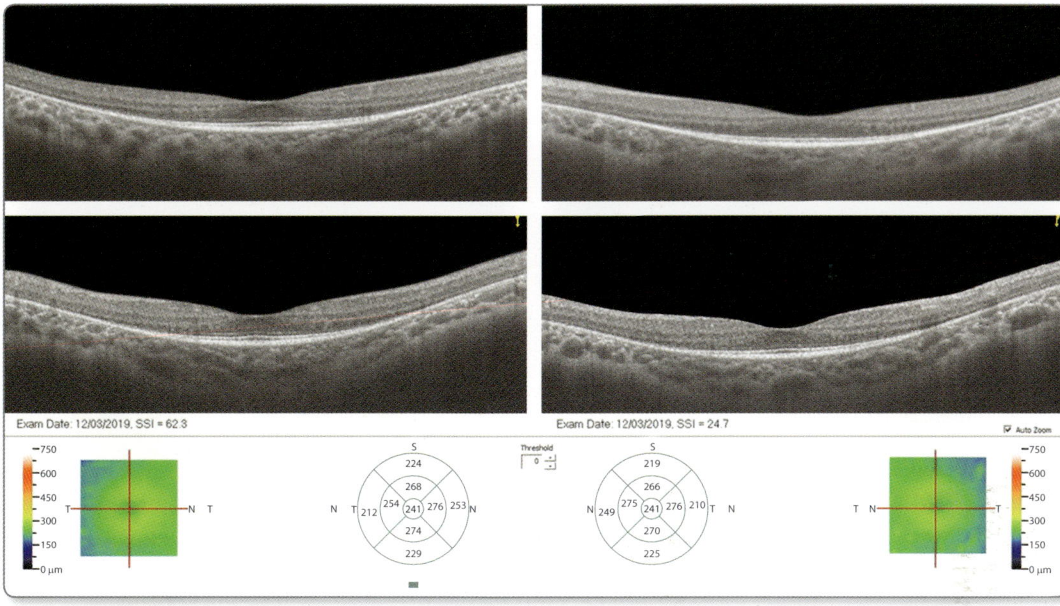

Figure 2 Cross-sectional scans. In all these cases of retinitis pigmentosa central retinal fovea level is normal. There is a major retinal thinning outside the central zone. Retina thickness map shows most important retinal thinning outside the central zone.

A thinning of the photoreceptors has been observed related to a decrease in thickness of the outer nuclear layer. The correlation between a lower visual function and a peripheral visual field contraction in patients with thinning of the outer nuclear layer of the photoreceptors has been demonstrated.

This shows that OCT can be used for monitoring visual field and visual acuity evolution of patients with IRD. Especially the IS/OS junction line (ellipsoid zone) seems to be the best OCT rating index of visual acuity (**Figures 1** to **3**).

Inner retina

Compared to the outer nuclear layer that is thinned, the inner retina (including the inner nuclear layer and the ganglion cell layer) is unchanged or in any case much less thinned. A thinning of the inner retinal layers has been observed only in the advanced stages of the disease and only in the most external retinal portions, above all in the inferonasal quadrant.

Hyper-reflective foci

Small hyper-reflective foci composed of macrophages, migrated EPR cells, and lipoprotein deposits have been observed in patients with age-related macular degeneration (AMD) and diabetic retinopathy. In the IRD, these foci seem to have a different origin depending on their position.

Outer nuclear layers: Their presence is related to the integrity of the EPR, if EPR is healthy they are not present.

Inner nuclear layers: Foci can be observed also in presence of healthy EPR but close to unhealthy IS/OS line; this proves that these foci correlate to photoreceptors and not to the EPR.

It would seem that the presence of the foci is a negative factor for the patient's visual acuity.

Retinal nerve fiber layer

Both thinning and thickening of retinal nerve fibers were observed in these patients. Specifically, it is thinned in the nasal and inferior sectors and thickened in the temporal and superior sectors.

It was also seen that the thickening is more evident in the horizontal scans more than the vertical ones.

The thickening is thought to be due to a proliferation of astrocytic cells and retinal nerve

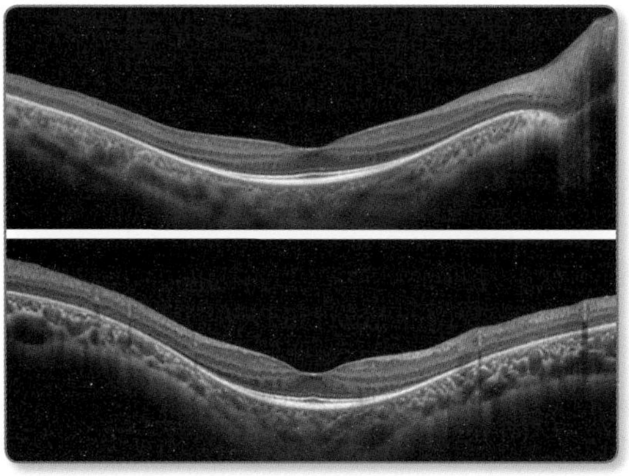

Figure 3 Cross-sectional scans. Similar cases of retinitis pigmentosa showing normal central retinal fovea level and retinal thinning outside the central zone.

fiber layer (RNFL) edema itself. As the astrocytic cells proliferate closer to the optic nerve, an increase in thickness was observed at the optic nerve, inducing the typical yellow-wax colour.

It has also been seen that the increase in thickness of the RNFL was greater in young patients even though in the late stages of the disease a general thinning was observed.

Macular area and thickness

In patients with advanced IRD, it is difficult to identify the boundary between the various retinal layers; however it is useful to evaluate the extent and macular thickness as an index of the retinal health status.

The normal macular area is 6 mm wide and has been observed to be very small in patients with IRD, especially in the outer segments.

The retinal thickness can be both increased and decreased; this thickening seems to be caused by retinal edema. However, on average, visual acuity is greater in thickened macula than in thinning. The presence of cysts in the retinal layers is a marker of worse visual acuity.

Choroidal vessels layer

In the IRDs, chorioretinal, EPR, and photoreceptors atrophies can be observed.

The choroid appears irregular and the boundaries between choroid and sclera appear less defined than healthy subjects. Vascular atrophy involves mostly small vessels leading to a prevalence of medium and large vessels. Choroid thickness is another important parameter for staging disease.

Macular abnormalities

In IRD patients, the most common macular alteration is macular edema followed by epiretinal membranes, vitreomacular traction syndrome, and macular hole.

These deviations cause a significant decrease of the visual acuity at any stage of the disease. It is important thus to diagnose them in time to treat them.

Optical coherence tomography is much more sensitive than fluorescein angiography (FA) to diagnose cystoid macular edema; for this reason, OCT screening is highly recommended.

Macular edema is similar to the diabetic one with the difference that in the retinitis pigmentosa, cysts are found in the inner nuclear layer while in diabetics, macular edemas are in the external one. This difference is probably due to the EPR function: healthy in diabetic edema; unhealthy in retinitis pigmentosa.

The most suitable intravitreal therapy for oedema in these patients seems to be aflibercept.

The presence of cystic spaces as well as edema is also associated with the epiretinal membranes, which are the second most important macular complication.

Development of epiretinal membranes appears to be supported by the proliferation of fibrous astrocytes and the remodelling of the RNFL.

In conclusion, the OCT is undoubtedly the most suitable technique for the study of this pathology.

OCT angiography in IRD

The reduction of the retinal vascular network is a characterising finding in IRD. Over time, the study of this alteration has stimulated more and more interest in the scientific community for its still uncertain pathogenesis, for its pathological significance, and for its prognostic role.

Since 1994, it was observed in subjects suffering from retinitis pigmentosa, the reduction of the calibre of the superficial retinal vessels associated with a thickening of the perivascular extracellular matrix probably supported by the local migration of retinal pigment epithelial cells; this condition leads to a reduction in the superficial retinal flow with resulting suffering of the inner retinal layers. However, other studies suggest a totally inverted pathogenesis; it would be, in fact, the atrophy of the inner retina and in particular of the ganglion cells, subsequent to the destruction of the photoreceptor tissue, to cause a decrease of the metabolic requirement with consequent vascular remodelling. A third theory sees at the centre of the pathogenesis the atrophy of photoreceptors that would involve a relative hyperoxia of the inner retina that would lead to a compensatory vasoconstriction of the retinal circulation.

The reduction in retinal flow was demonstrated over the years through the instruments that were available at the moment. In the seventies, fluorescein angiographic studies showed the reduction of the calibre of arterioles and venules associated with flow decrease; in addition, a delay in choroidal filling was shown, characterized by non-perfused areas. The main limitation of FA was, in addition to the invasive examination technique, in the impossibility of studying the retinal capillary network due to the low vascular flow and the poor spatial resolution.

Optical coherence tomography angiography is currently part of the daily practice of the study of retinal and non-retinal diseases. The main advantages of this technique compared to classical dye angiography methods consist in the speed of acquisition, in non-invasiveness, in repeatability, and in the great resolution of the acquired images, as well as in the possibility to locate the findings on a three-dimensional model.

Typically, IRD subjects show changes in superficial capillary (SCP) and deep (DCP) plexuses from the early stages of the disease. In particular, greater involvement of the DCP and a foveal avascular zone (FAZ) enlargement in the DPC are featured. This finding correlates to the pathogenesis, consisting in atrophy of the outer retinal layers, partially perfused by the DPC.

However, further studies show a strong correlation between reduction of visual acuity and flow in foveal SCP, supporting the hypothesis of a role of Müller cells in the anatomical-functional maintenance of retinal neuroepithelium, especially in some forms of IRD. Furthermore, a correlation between visual acuity and perfusion of the superficial and deep plexuses of the parafoveal area has been demonstrated too.

In addition to the foveal and parafoveal flow, reduction in the superficial and deep capillary plexus and FAZ enlargement, in the last few years several studies focussed on the optic nerve head (ONH) and peripapillary perfusion. In particular, vascular flow reduction in the ONH and in the peripapillary area (RPC) appears frequent. There is also a correlation between the hypoperfusion of the RPC and the RNFL thickness and the functional perimetric damages.

Optical coherence tomography angiography, thanks to its features, is useful for an effective follow-up of patients affected by IRD. In particular, it has been observed that, over time, the perfusion of SCP and DCP tend to decrease equally. Instead, the FAZ area at the DCP level increases at twice the rate of the FAZ measured at the SCP level; however, the progressive decline in visual acuity shows the strongest association with the FAZ measured in the SCP.

However, OCT angiography has some limitations, similar to that identified in FA. In fact, the angio-OCT technology estimates the flow through a decorrelation signal obtained from the interpolation of two consecutive retinal B-scans. Therefore, each software has a preset threshold value below which the decorrelation signal is not analyzed. Capillaries, with a flow so low that is unable to generate a signal that reaches the threshold value, will not be shown. This prevents us from discriminating whether the capillary network gradually depleted at the SCP and DCP level is extremely low or has actually disappeared.

In conclusion, we can confirm that OCT angiography is a valid tool for the diagnosis and staging of the IRDs, allowing an effective follow-up, and having a prognostic predictability.

30 Glaucoma

Luca Di Antonio, Luca Agnifili, Lorenza Brescia, Barbara Scatena, Leonardo Mastropasqua

Introduction

Glaucoma is a worldwide leading cause of irreversible visual loss. It is a multifactorial disease caused by disequilibrium in the hydrodynamics of the aqueous humor which is mainly reflected in two aspects: increase in intraocular pressure and change in the microcirculation of the optic nerve head (ONH) with consequent degeneration of retinal ganglion cells (RGC) and their axons. Because glaucomatous damage is irreversible, its management required a precise 'micron-scale' quantification of ocular structures [i.e. retinal nerve fiber layer (RNFL), ganglion cell complex (GCC), and vessel density of radial peripapillary capillaries measurements] that improves both detection and progression of the disease.

Epidemiology

Glaucoma is the second leading cause of blindness that affects more than 70 million people worldwide. In industrialized countries, the statistics report age-related macular degeneration (AMD) as a major cause of blindness (26%), followed by glaucoma (20.5%), and diabetic retinopathy (8.9%).[1]

Predictions are that glaucoma will affect almost 80 million people by 2020 and 112 million people by 2040, mainly in Asian and African people.[2,3]

Risk factors

Main risk factors are age (the prevalence of the disease grows in the most advanced age, especially over 55 years),[4] black race (the African-Caribbean Eye Survey has shown a risk of development of 3.9 times greater open-angle glaucoma in the black race compared to the Caucasian),[5] familiarity (those who have affected relatives are more likely to develop glaucoma), diabetes, systemic vascular alterations, myopia, prolonged use of topical or systemic corticosteroid, and high intraocular pressure as listed in the **Box 1**.

Box 1: Main risk factors for glaucoma

- Age
- Black race
- Family history
- Use of systemic or topical corticosteroids
- Ocular hypertension

Pathophysiology

Glaucoma encompasses different clinical entities characterized by specific areas of injured optic nerve axons and retinal ganglion cell loss that finally match the peripheral vision damage.

Although pathophysiology of the glaucoma in not well understood, it seems to be multifactorial. Multiple factors lead to the death of retinal RGC and their axons. Elevated intraocular pressure and vascular dysregulation were considered as the first factors that contribute to both axoplasmic flow blockage within RGC axons and altered ONH circulation at the level of lamina cribrosa. The secondary factors are excitotoxic damage of glutamate released from injured neurons, and oxidative damage due to nitric oxide over-production.[6] Besides raised IOP, a low ocular perfusion (the difference between intraocular and systemic blood pressures) could be associated with glaucomatous changes in individuals with normal IOP.[7]

Recently it was been discussed on the relationship between the difference of the pressure inside the brain and glaucoma (translaminar pressure gradient). If the pressure inside the brain is lower than normal and the pressure in the eye is normal, the difference between these two pressures may damage the ONH.

Further data suggested that glaucoma could be included in the neurodegenerative process such as Alzheimer's and Parkinson's disease. The retina is like a window open into the brain and RGC share structural morphology with other central nervous system (CNS) neurons. So retinal microvascular changes may represent similar pathophysiological events within cerebral microvasculature. Conversely glaucoma patients also have CNS degenerative alterations of ONH, lateral geniculate bodies, and visual cortex. Recently it was been speculated that patients with low tension glaucoma were at significantly greater risk of developing Alzheimer's disease compared with subjects without glaucoma. Moreover glaucomatous-like neuropathy can be highlighted in patients with vascular disease (i.e. hypertension, atherosclerosis, etc.). It seems due to an impaired ocular perfusion pressure.[7]

It is clear that the intraocular pressure alone does not cause development of glaucomatous optic neuropathy. It was been evidenced that both blood pressure and blood flow abnormalities may play a role in glaucoma pathogenesis. It would be important to avoid both under or overtreatment of systemic hypertension in order to achieve an optimal range of ocular perfusion. For the suspected optic neuropathy, it should be mandatory to follow a specialist referral (**Figure 1**), in order to improve the assessment and minimize any kind of misdiagnosis.

Classification

According to European Glaucoma Society (EGS),[8] glaucoma is classified into different types—primary glaucoma, which encloses two main subtypes such as primary open-angle glaucoma (POAG) and primary angle-closure glaucoma (PACG), as listed in **Table 1**.

Primary open-angle glaucoma

Primary open-angle glaucoma is a chronic and progressive ONH disease mainly due to increased IOP, and in absence of other ocular or systemic diseases. The gradient of IOP is determined by the balance between the secretion of aqueous humor by the ciliary body and its drainage through both

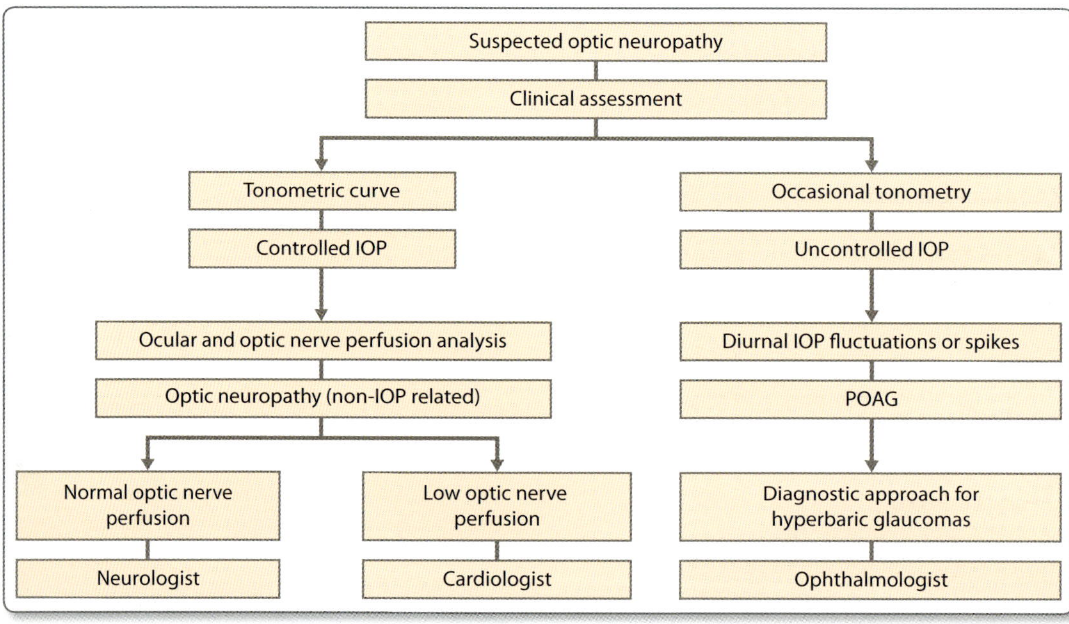

Figure 1 Optic neuropathy assessment.
(IOP: intraocular pressure; POAG: primary open-angle glaucoma)

Table 1 Primary glaucoma classification (According to EGS Guidelines, 4th edition)

Primary glaucoma	
Primary open-angle glaucoma (POAG)	**Primary angle-closure glaucoma**
• Primary open-angle glaucoma	• Primary angle-closure glaucoma
• Primary juvenile glaucoma	• Acute angle-closure with plateau iris configuration
• POAG suspect	• Intermittent angle-closure glaucoma
• Ocular hypertension	• Chronic angle-closure glaucoma

trabecular meshwork and uveoscleral outflow pathways. In POAG, usually there is an increase of resistance to aqueous outflow through the trabecular meshwork.[8] The POAG represents the most common type of glaucoma (about 75%). The prevalence of POAG is highest in Africa (4.20%).[3]

Primary angle-closure glaucoma

- In the primary angle-closure glaucoma, conversely to PAOG, there is an obstruction of the drainage pathways mainly due to pupillary block caused by disorders of the iris, the lens, and retrolenticular structures. The PACG represents the 25% of glaucoma and its prevalence is highest in Asia (1.09%).[3]
- Secondary glaucoma, based on different pathophysiological mechanisms,[8] also includes two types as listed in **Table 2**
- Normal tension glaucoma (NTG) is a chronic and multifactorial disease which differs from high-tension glaucoma because its pathophysiology is not influenced by high IOP. Several factors as vascular dysregulation, low diastolic blood pressure, and altered endothelial reactivity might impair ocular blood flow, leading to a chronic ischemia of the ONH and resulting in RGC and axons damage.[9]

Diagnosis

The diagnosis of glaucoma is generally clinical and requires an accurate ocular examination, including a slit-lamp biomicroscopy, applanation tonometry, gonioscopy, stereoscopic fundus, photography evaluation, and pachimetry.[10] Also the visual field (VF)

Table 2 Secondary glaucoma classification (According to EGS Guidelines, 4th edition)

Secondary glaucoma	
Secondary open-angle glaucoma	**Secondary angle-closure glaucoma**
	1. *Anterior 'pulling' without pupillary block*
• Exfoliative glaucoma	• Neovascular glaucoma
• Pigmentary glaucoma	• Iridocorneal endothelial syndrome
• Lens-induced glaucoma	• Posterior polymorphous dystrophy
• Corticosteroid glaucoma	• Inflammatory membranes
• Iatrogenic glaucoma, not induced by corticosteroids	• Peripheral anterior synechiae
• Uveitic glaucoma	• Aniridia
• Glaucoma associated with intraocular hemorrhage or intraocular tumors	• Epithelial or connective in-growth (post-traumatic, postsurgical, post-inflammatory)
• Post-traumatic glaucoma	
• Postsurgical glaucoma	
• Glaucoma caused by increased episcleral venous pressure	
	2. *Posterior 'pushing' without pupillary block*
	• Aqueous misdirection
	• Iris, ciliary body or intraocular tumors
	• Silicon oil/other tamponading gas or fluids in vitreous cavity
	• Uveal effusion
	• Retinopathy of prematurity (V stage)
	• Congenital anomalies (neurofibromatosis, Marfan syndrome, etc.)
	3. *With pupillary block*
	• Lens-induced (cataract, traumatic cataract, lens dislocation)
	• Posterior synechiae, pupil seclusion or occlusion
	• Aphakia
	• Miotic-induced pupillary block
	• IOL-induced pupillary block (anterior chamber IOL, phakic IOL, dislocated posterior chamber IOL)

testing is required in the diagnosis and follow-up of glaucomatous ONH damage. The introduction of newer, faster, and high-resolution techniques for imaging anterior segment, retina, and ONH improved the quantitative assessment of glaucoma by using optical coherence tomography (OCT) measurements of iridocorneal angle width, GCC, and RNFL thickness, respectively.[11,12] Furthermore, functional information such as blood flow index (defined as the average flow signal intensity or the average decorrelation value) and the radial peripapillary capillary (RPC) vessel density (defined as the ratio or the percentage of the area occupied by vessels in a region of interest) by means of OCT angiography (OCTA) can be complementarily used for assessing glaucomatous changes.[13] A hypothetical diagnostic approach to be taken for a suspected glaucoma patient is shown in the diagnostic (**Figure 2**).

Evolution of the optic nerve head imaging

In the last 30 years, we have witnessed to an ONH imaging revolution (**Figure 3**). VF testing represents the gold standard for the diagnosis and follow-up of glaucoma.

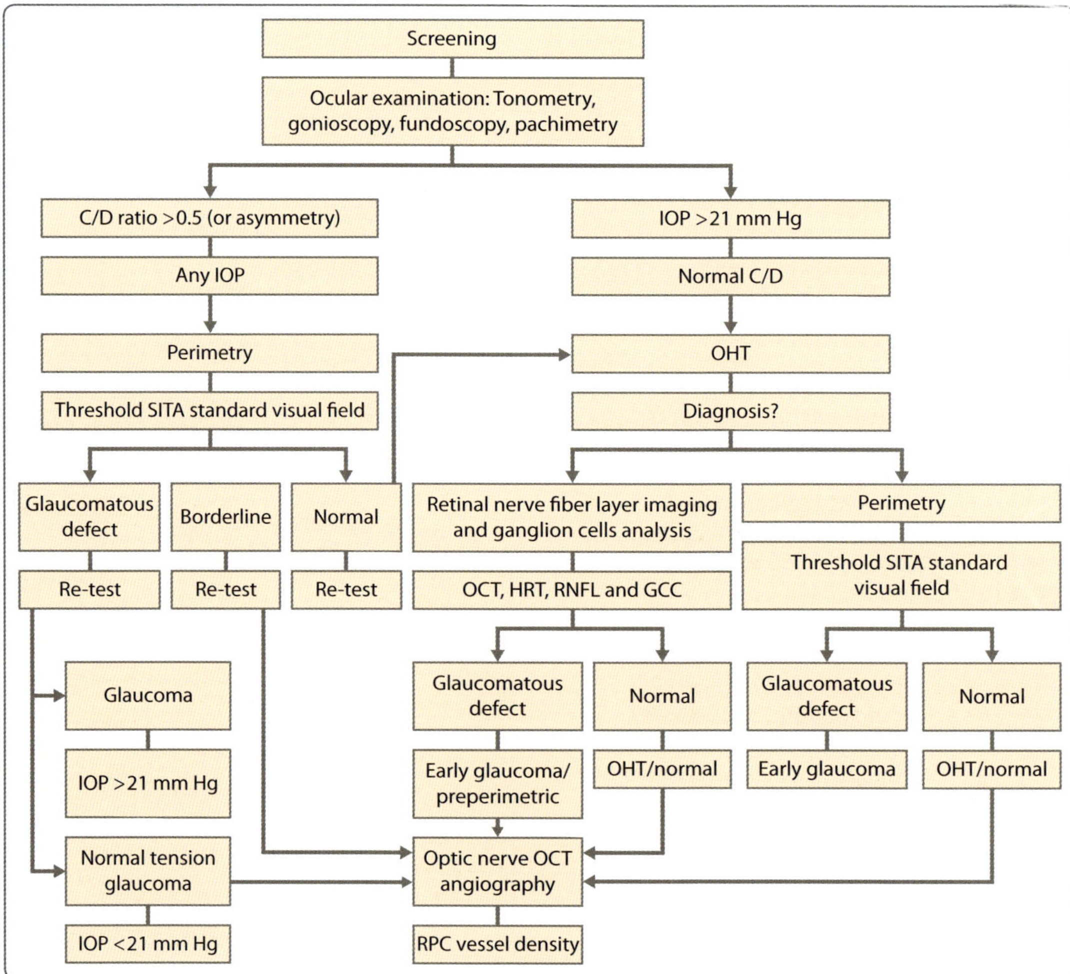

Figure 2 Diagnostic approach for glaucoma.
(IOP: intraocular pressure; OHT: ocular hypertension; OCT: optical coherence tomography; GCC: ganglion cell complex; RPC: radial peripapillary capillary)

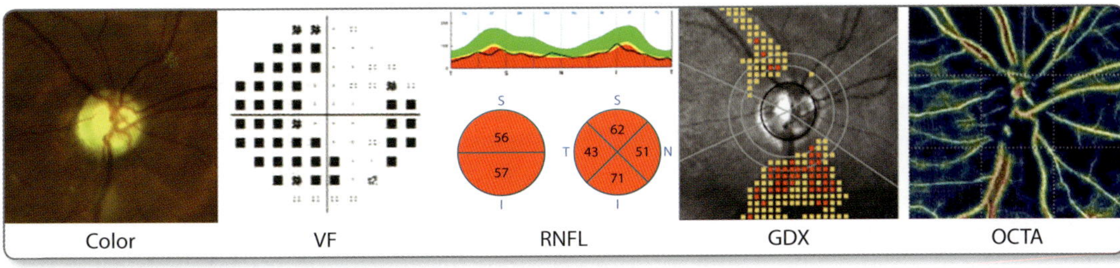

Figure 3 Optic nerve head imaging evolution: Color fundus photography (color), visual field (VF) testing, retinal nerve fiber layer thickness (RNFL), scanning laser polarimetry (GDx), and optical coherence tomographic angiography (OCTA).

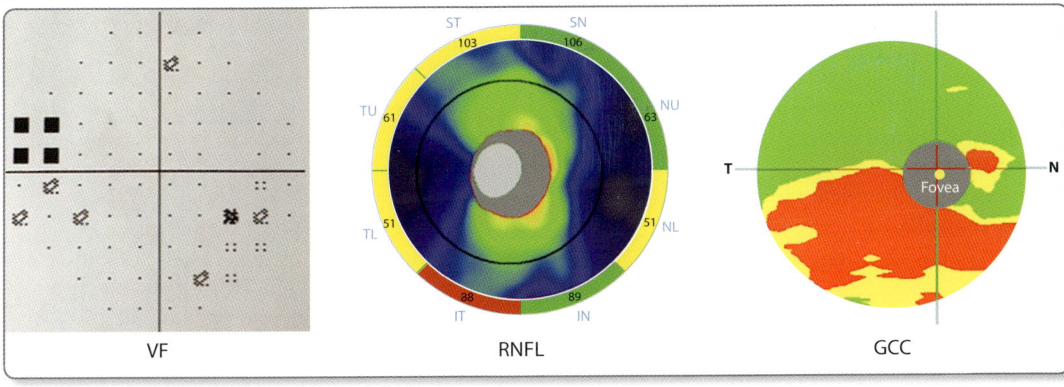

Figure 4 Functional (visual field testing) and structural (RNFL and GCC thickness) tools showing a focal defect in a 49-year-old man with early glaucoma.

Combining functional information from VF testing with other ONH structural imaging is useful for the clinical assessment and monitoring patients with glaucoma (**Figure 4**). Several high-resolution imaging techniques have improved the detection of structural changes:

- Anterior segment OCT (AS-OCT) is able to assess both anterior chamber depth and the anterior iridocorneal angle width (**Figure 5**, top and bottom, respectively) with more accuracy, and correlates well with the information provided by standard gonioscopy.[11] Moreover AS-OCT may give more insight into the pathophysiology of the angle closure (**Figure 5**, bottom)
- Optical coherence tomography is able to detect early RNFL and GCC thinning that correlate well with VF defect (**Figure 4**).

These latter occur as consequence of the loss of RGC axons. Although the reliability of OCT measurement of RNFL,[14] and GCC[15] thickness has given more insight into the diagnosis of

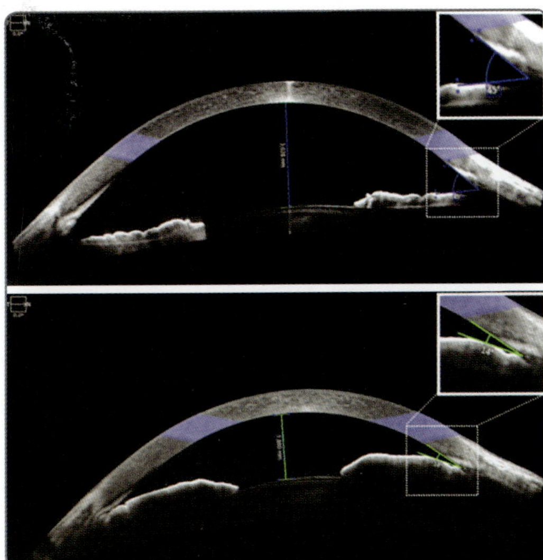

Figure 5 Anterior segment optical coherence tomography (AS-OCT) assessment showing both anterior chamber depth and iridocorneal angle width measurements (squared magnification) in healthy subject (top) and in primary angle-closure glaucoma (bottom), respectively.

glaucoma, the relationship between structural and functional changes is still debated.[16] Several studies stated that structural damage (RNFL thinning) might precede VF defect in case of ocular hypertension (OHT),[17] and in preperimetric glaucoma.[18] On the other hand, structural tests alone are not sensitive and specific for the diagnosis of glaucoma, because of measurement errors (i.e. in high myopia, astigmatism, tilted disc, or tilted OCT scan acquisition) that might falsify the thickness values.

More recently, the OCT technology has introduced the Bruch's membrane opening minimum rime width (BMO-MRW) as a new structural biomarker that improved the sensitivity (81%) for the detection of the glaucoma compared to RNFL thickness (70%).[19] The BMO-MRW is a parameter more reliable for measuring the optic disc size than clinical examination **(Figure 6)**.

The glaucomatous damage is better visualized on the *en-face* OCT images than on the RNFL thickness map. It appears as a focal or diffuse (**Figure 7**) less reflective and/or missing RNFL bundles[20] compared to healthy subjects. OCTA is a development of *en-face* OCT technology based upon motion contrast imaging that uses red blood cells movement to distinguish flow in the vessel from the static tissue. It is a safe, fast, and dyeless imaging technique that provides 'in vivo' detailed visualization of the retina[21] and ONH microcirculation,[13] and enabled both the qualitative and quantitative evaluation of these structures in different disease involving ONH.[13,22,23] The blood flow of the ONH is supplied by two main sources: the central retinal artery supplies the superficial layer (nerve fiber layer on the surface of the optic disc), and the posterior ciliary arteries (PCA), with a minor contribution of the central retinal artery branches, supplies the deep layer (the prelaminar, lamina cribrosa, and retrolaminar regions) (**Figure 8**).[24]

The impairment of these two vascular networks may lead to different forms of ischemic ONH diseases. In glaucoma, optic disc ischemia (or reduced ocular blood flow) may be a causative factor for the development and progression of the RGC loss either by itself (due to chronic ischemia or postreperfusion damage) or in conjunction with the elevated IOP. There is a growing body of evidence suggesting that vascular alterations are a major contributor in the pathophysiology of POAG and in PACG, as the reduction of RPC microcirculation.[25-28]

Overall, several OCTA studies have reported reduced values of both ONH perfusion and RPC vessel density in patients with glaucoma.[25-30]

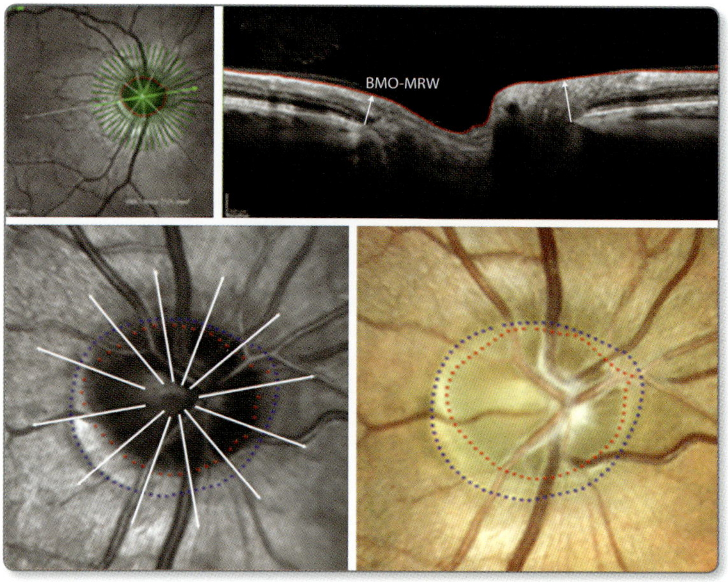

Figure 6 Bruch's membrane opening (BMO) assessment based on minimum rim width (BMO-MRW), determining the minimum distance between BMO and ILM (cyan arrow, top). Clinical (color funds photography, bottom right) and retinal imaging (infrared SD-OCT, bottom left) of BMO measurement of a healthy subject. Note the mismatch between the clinically visible disc margin (blue dots) and BMO (red dots) indicating a significant overestimation of the neuroretinal rim width disc margin.

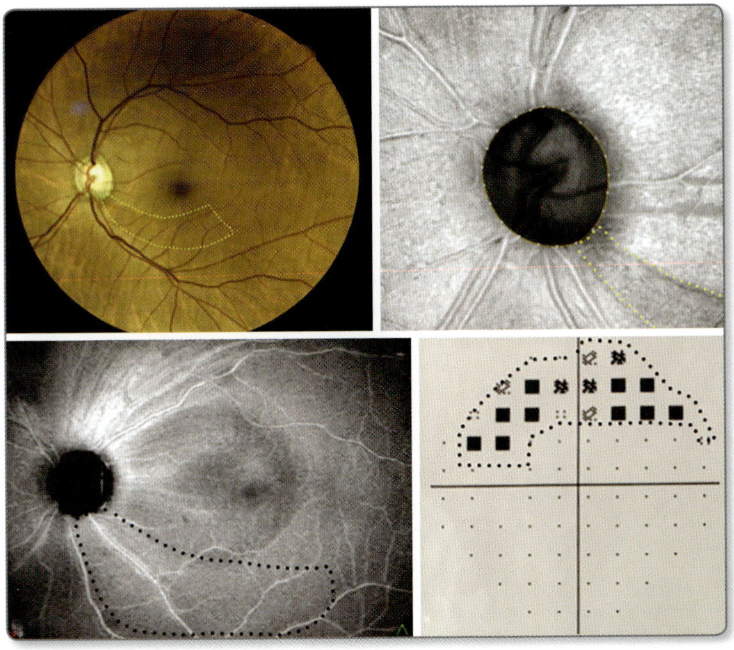

Figure 7 Multimodal ONH imaging showing both focal (yellow dots in both color picture, top left, and *en face* OCT image, top right) or diffuse (black dots in both widefield *en face* OCT image, bottom left, and VF testing, bottom right) RNFL bundles defect. (OCT: optical coherence tomography; ONH: optic nerve head; RNFL: retinal nerve fiber layer)

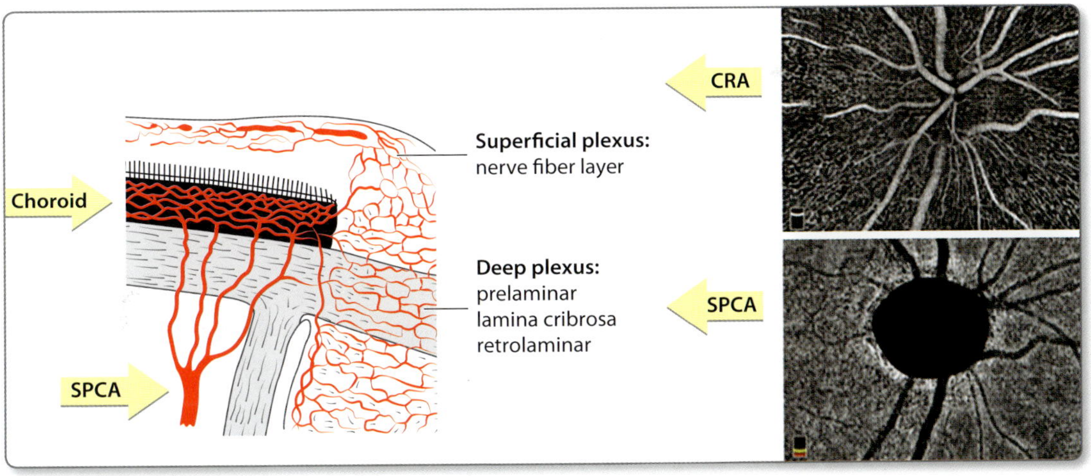

Figure 8 Blood supply of the optic nerve head microcirculation (Modified according Hayreh SS). (CRA: central retinal artery. SPCA: short posterior ciliar arteries; RPC: radial peripapillary capillary)

In particular they stated that:

- There was a decrease of RPC vessel density in patients with OHT (**Figure 9**), preperimetric glaucoma (**Figure 10**), and POAG compared with healthy subject[25,26]
- The decrease in structural parameters, such as RNFL thickness, and functional parameters, such as VF defects, were strongly correlated with RPC vessel density reduction (spatial correlation) in both early (**Figures 11** and **12**) or advanced (**Figure 13**) glaucoma[31]
- RPC vessel density was not affected by 'floor effect' like RNFL thickness (**Figure 14**)[32]
- Retinal superficial capillary plexus (SCP) vessel density in the glaucomatous eyes was lower than in the healthy eyes (**Figure 15**), independently of the ONH[26]

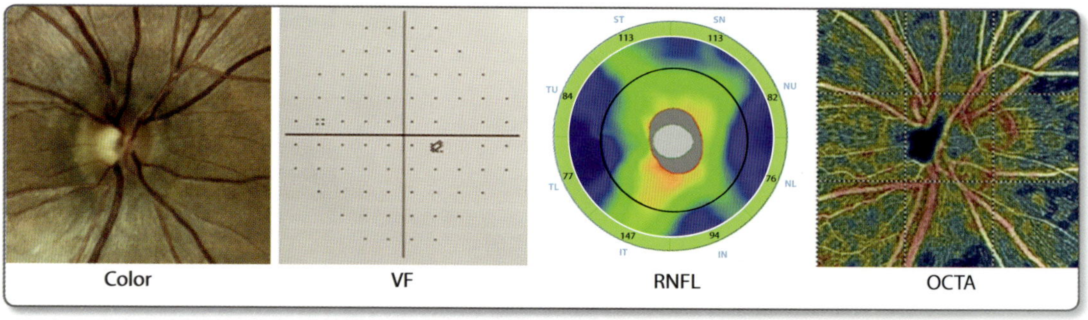

Figure 9 Multimodal optic nerve head imaging of a 47-year-old man with ocular hypertension (OHT): Color fundus photography (color), visual field (VF) testing, retinal nerve fiber layer (RNFL) thickness appeared normal. Optical coherence tomographic angiography (OCTA) depicted a reduction of retinal peripapillary capillary (RPC) vessel density.

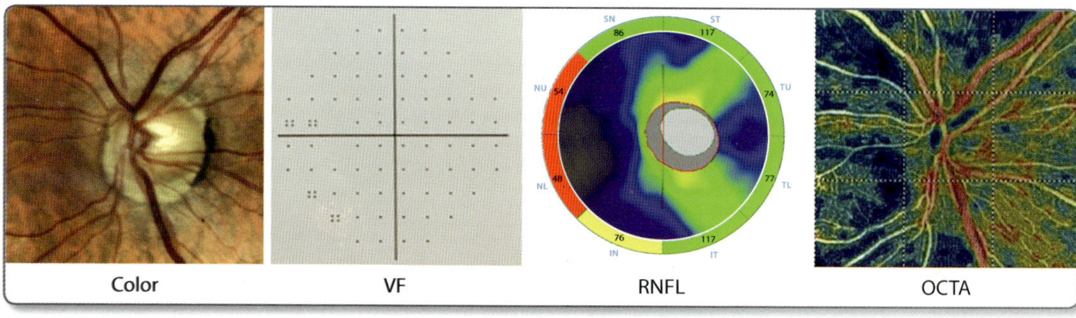

Figure 10 Multimodal optic nerve head imaging of a 54-year-old man with preperimetric glaucoma: Color fundus photography (color) and visual field (VF) testing appeared normal. Retinal nerve fiber layer (RNFL) showed a thinning, and optical coherence tomographic angiography (OCTA) examination highlighted a reduction of retinal peripapillary capillary (RPC) vessel density.

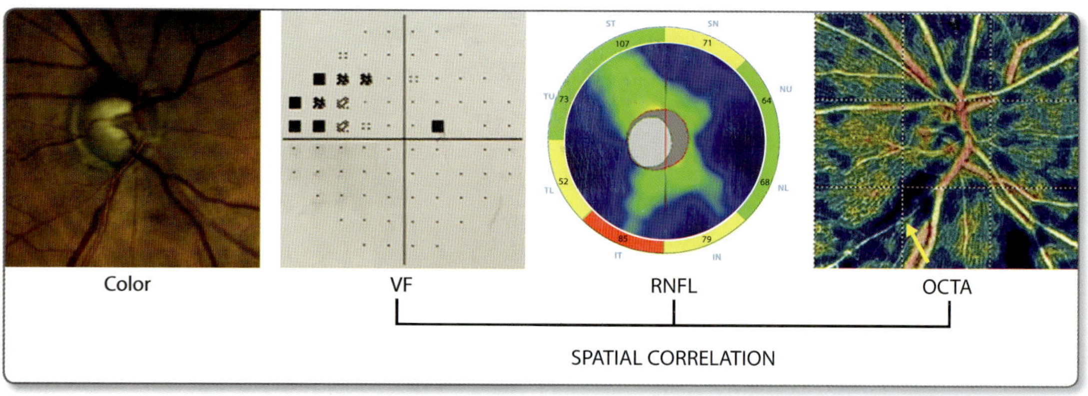

Figure 11 Multimodal optic nerve head imaging of a 63-year-old man with early glaucoma. Note the spatial correlation between functional and structural parameters: Color fundus photography (color) showed an inferotemporal notching. Visual field (VF) testing showed a superotemporal defect. Retinal nerve fiber layer (RNFL) showed an inferotemporal thinning, and optical coherence tomographic angiography (OCTA) examination highlighted a focal reduction of retinal peripapillary capillary (RPC) vessel density (yellow arrow).

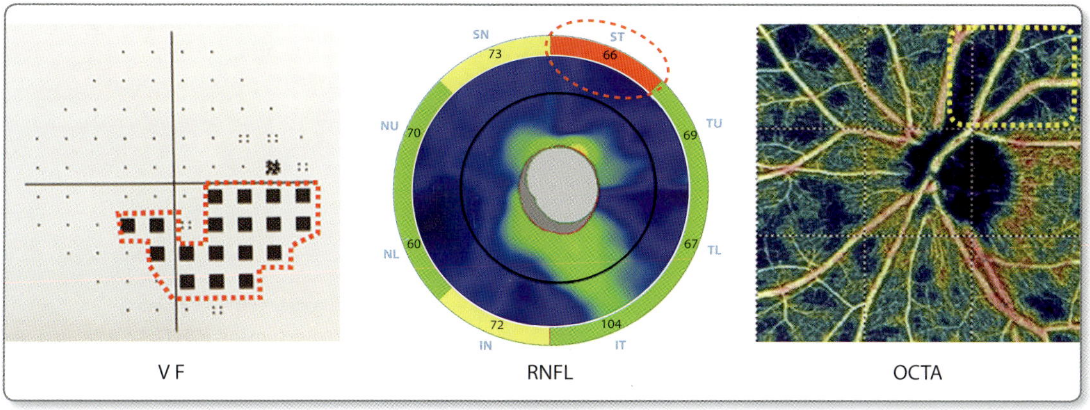

Figure 12 Spatial correlation between functional and structural parameters of a 59-year-old woman affected by early glaucoma. Visual field (VF) testing showed Bjerrum scotoma (red dots); Optical coherence tomography (OCT) showed focal RNFL thinning (red dotted circle); and OCT angiography (OCTA) depicted a focal reduction of RPC vessel density (yellow dotted square).

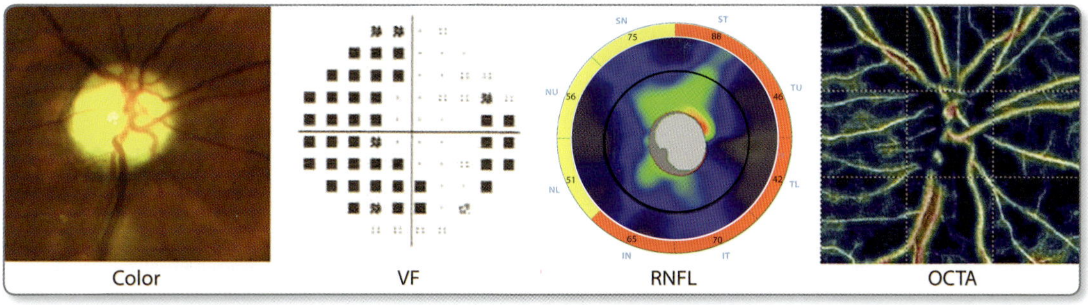

Figure 13 Multimodal optic nerve head imaging of a 72-year-old man with advanced glaucoma. Note the diffuse reduction of functional and structural parameters: Color fundus photography (color), visual field (VF) testing, and retinal nerve fiber layer (RNFL) thickness. Optical coherence tomographic angiography (OCTA) examination highlighted a diffuse reduction of retinal peripapillary capillary (RPC) vessel density.

- Choroidal microvasculature dropout was associated with VF defects (**Figure 16**)[33]
- Peripapillary perfused capillary density was decreased in exfoliation glaucoma compared with POAG, and in exfoliation syndrome compared with controls (**Figure 17**)[34]
- In NTG, there was a greater vascular impairment than in nonarteritic ischemic optic neuropathy (NAION) probably due to the chronicity of the disease (**Figure 18**)[35]

Nevertheless, as for structural parameters (RNFL and GCC thickness), OCTA may have limitations for detecting vascular changes in early stage of glaucoma. It cannot be used alone to diagnose or to follow-up the glaucomatous damage progression, or to change therapeutic strategy.

The use of retinal and ONH multimodal imaging and/or the more recently deep learning (artificial intelligence)[36] might help clinicians to obtain detailed structure-function maps in order to enhance sensitivity for the diagnosis and the progression rate of the glaucoma, so we could treat something besides IOP.

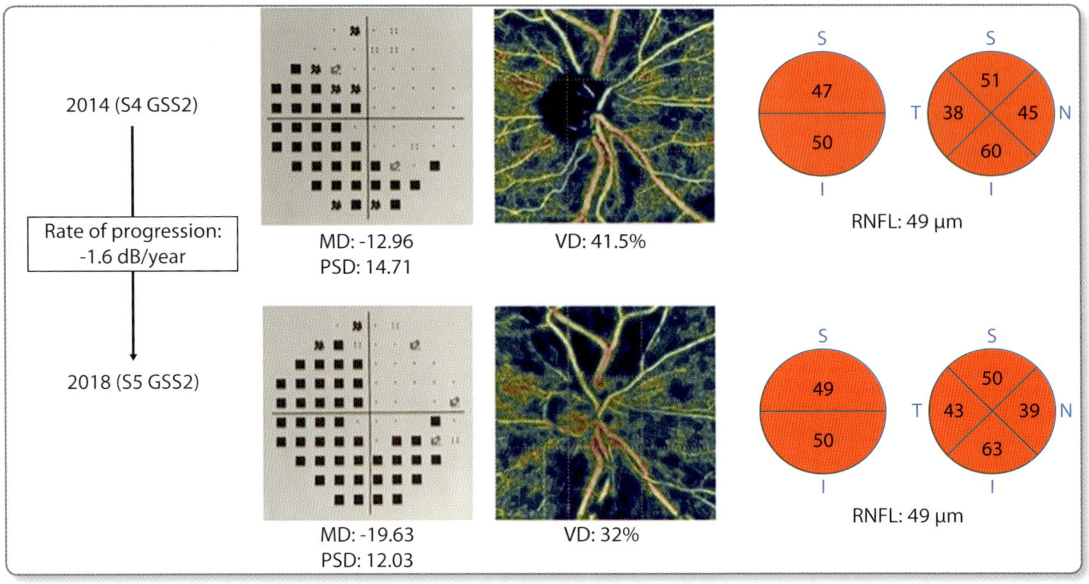

Figure 14 Glaucoma staging system (GSS) rate of progression (from stage 4 to stage 5) in a 58-year-old man with advanced glaucoma. The progression of visual field defect well correlates with overtime retinal peripapillary capillary vessel density impairment, but not with the retinal nerve fiber layer thinning that seems to be reach a stable level (approximately 50–70% of RNFL loss). This latter phenomenon is known as 'floor effect'. It can be explained by the presence of non-neural tissue (i.e. glia) that remains even in case of advanced RGC cell loss.

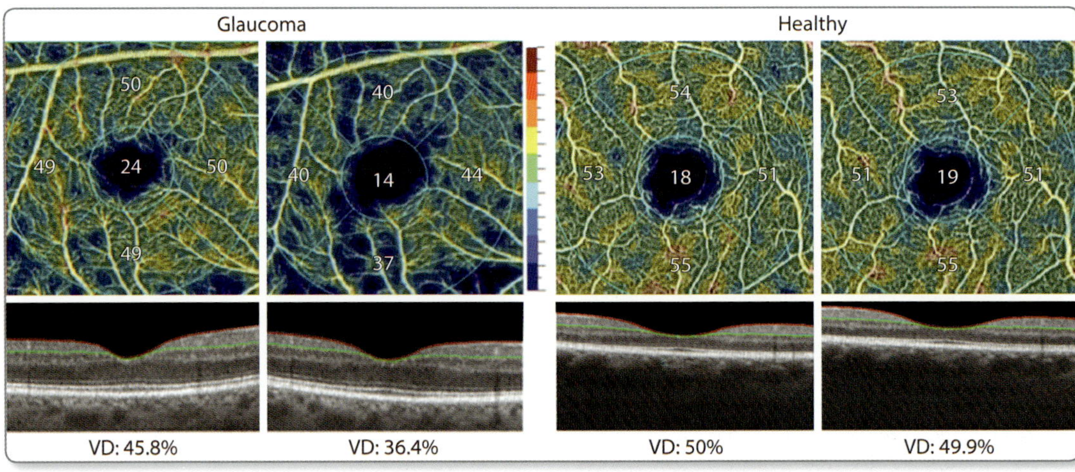

Figure 15 Long-term follow-up (Angio Retina Trend Analysis) of a 63-year-old man affected by glaucoma. The optical coherence tomographic angiography (OCTA) examination showing a progressive impairment of superficial capillary plexus vessel density (VD) compared with a healthy age-matched subject.

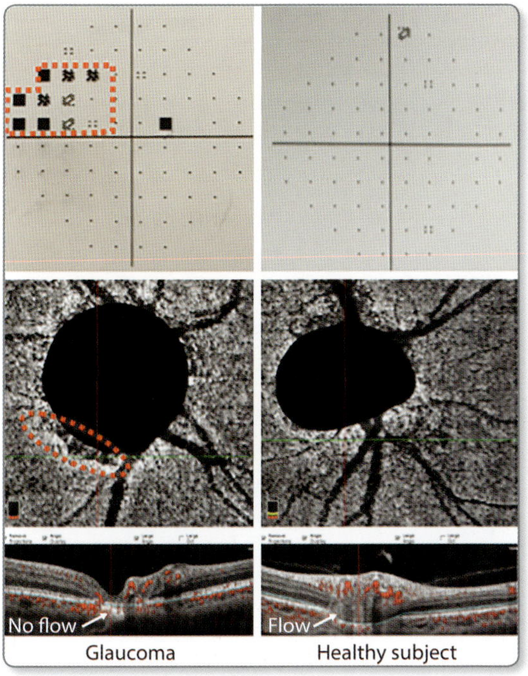

Figure 16 Visual field (VF) defect (red dots, top left) and choroidal microvasculature dropout (red dotted circle, middle left) in optical coherence tomography (OCT) angiography image that appears as no flow signal on the co-localized structural OCT (red arrow, bottom left) in patient with early glaucoma compared with healthy subject (top, middle, and bottom right).

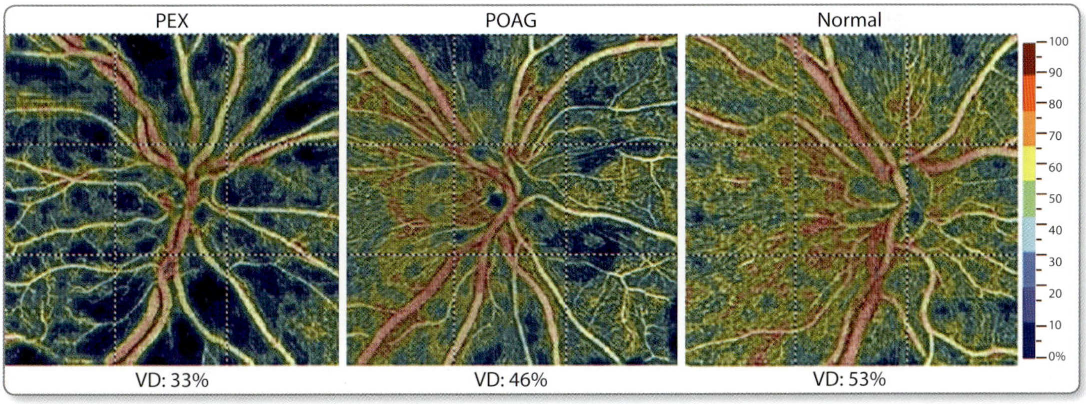

Figure 17 Optical coherence tomography (OCT) angiography assessment of retinal peripapillary capillary (RPC) vessel density (VD). Note the RPC vascular impairment in exfoliation glaucoma (PEX) and in the primary open-angle glaucoma (POAG) compared with healthy subject.

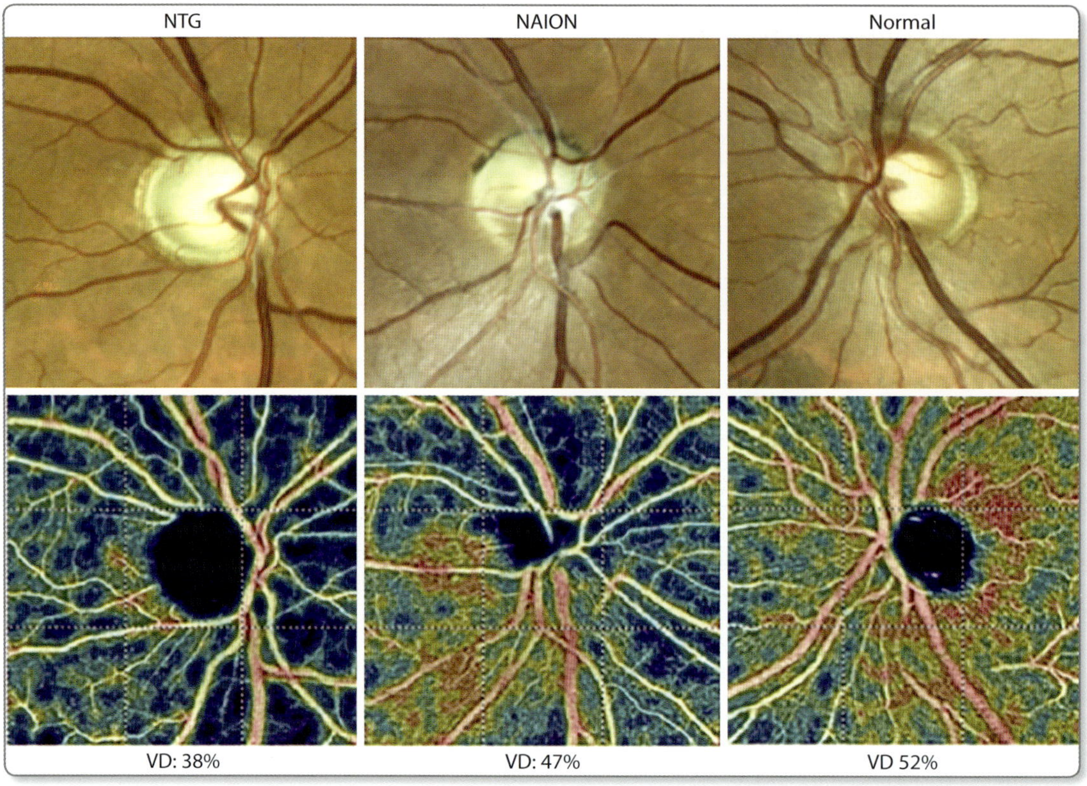

Figure 18 Color fundus photography (top) and optical coherence tomographic angiography (OCTA) analysis of retinal peripapillary capillary (RPC) vessel density (VD) changes (bottom) in normal tension glaucoma (NTG) and nonarteritic ischemic optic neuropathy (NAION) compared with normal subject.

References

1. Prokofyeva E, Zrenner E. Epidemiology of major eye diseases leading to blindness in Europe: a literature review. Ophthalmic Res 2012; 47:171–188.
2. Quigley H, Broman A. The number of people with glaucoma worldwide in 2010 and 2020. Br J Ophthalmol 2006; 90:262–267.
3. Tham Y, Li X, Wong T, et al. Global prevalence of glaucoma and projections of glaucoma burden through 2040: a systematic review and meta-analysis. Ophthalmology 2014; 121:2081–2090.
4. Kass MA, Heuer DK, Higginbotham EJ, et al. The Ocular Hypertension Treatment Study: baseline factors that predict the onset of primary open-angle glaucoma. Arch Ophthalmol 2002; 120:701–713.
5. Wormald RP, Basauri E, Wright LA, et al. The African Caribbean Eye Survey: risk factors for glaucoma in a sample of African Caribbean people living in London. Eye (Lond) 1994; 8:315–320.
6. Agarwal R, Gupta SK, Agarwal P, et al. Current concepts in the pathophysiology of glaucoma. Indian J Ophthalmol 2009; 57:257–266.
7. Zheng Y, Wong TY, Mitchell P, et al. Distribution of ocular perfusion pressure and its relationship with open-angle glaucoma: the Singapore Malay Eye Study. Invest Ophthalmol Vis Sci 2010; 51:3399–3404.
8. European Glaucoma Society terminology and guidelines for glaucoma 4th edition. Br J Ophthalmol 2017; 101:73–127.
9. Park SC, Lee DH, Lee HJ, et al. Risk factors for normal-tension glaucoma among subgroups of patients. Arch Ophthalmol 2009; 127:1275–1283.
10. Jonas JB, Budde WM. Diagnosis and pathogenesis of glaucomatous optic neuropathy: morphological aspects. Prog Retin Eye Res 2000; 19:1–40.
11. Tun TA, Baskaran M, Tan SS, et al. Evaluation of the anterior segment angle-to-angle scan of cirrus

high-definition optical coherence tomography and comparison with gonioscopy and with the visante OCT. Investig Ophthalmol Vis Sci 2017; 58:59–64.
12. Oddone E, Lucenteforte E, Michelessi M, et al. Macular versus retinal nerve fiber layer parameters for diagnosing manifest glaucoma: A systematic review of diagnostic accuracy studies. Ophthalmology 2016; 123:939–949.
13. Jia Y, Wei E, Wang X, et al. Optical coherence tomography angiography of optic disc perfusion in glaucoma. Ophthalmology 2014; 121:1322–1332.
14. Carpineto P, Nubile M, Agnifili L, et al. Reproducibility and repeatability of Cirrus™ HD-OCT peripapillary retinal nerve fibre layer thickness measurements in young normal subjects. Ophthalmologica 2012; 227:139–145.
15. Carpineto P, Aharrh-Gnama A, Ciciarelli V, et al. Reproducibility and repeatability of ganglion cell-inner plexiform layer thickness measurements in healthy subjects. Ophthalmologica 2014; 232:163–169.
16. Malik R, Swanson WH, Garway-Heath DF. Structure-function relationship' in glaucoma: past thinking and current concepts. Clin Experiment Ophthalmol 2012; 40:369–380.
17. Mastropasqua L, Brusini P, Carpineto P, et al. Humphrey matrix frequency doubling technology perimetry and optical coherence tomography measurement of the retinal nerve fiber layer thickness in both normal and ocular hypertensive subjects. J Glaucoma 2006; 15:328–335.
18. Lisboa R, Leite MT, Zangwill LM, et al. Diagnosing preperimetric glaucoma with spectral domain optical coherence tomography. Ophthalmology 2012; 119:2261–2269.
19. Chauhan BC, O'Leary N, Almobarak FA, et al. Enhanced detection of open-angle glaucoma with an anatomically accurate optical coherence tomography-derived neuroretinal rim parameter. Ophthalmology 2013; 120:535–543.
20. Hood DC, Fortune B, Mavrommatis MA, et al. Details of glaucomatous damage are better seen on oct en face images than on OCT retinal nerve fiber layer thickness maps. Invest Ophthalmol Vis Sci 2015; 56:6208–6216.
21. Mastropasqua R, Di Antonio L, Di Staso S, et al. Optical coherence tomography angiography in retinal vascular diseases and choroidal neovascularization. J Ophthalmol 2015; 2015:343515.
22. Mastropasqua R, Borrelli E, Agnifili L, et al. Radial peripapillary capillary network in patients with retinitis pigmentosa: an optical coherence tomography angiography study. Front Neurol 2017; 8:572.
23. Spain RI, Liu L, Zhang X, et al. Optical coherence tomography angiography enhances the detection of optic nerve damage in multiple sclerosis. Br J Ophthalmol 2018; 102:520–524.
24. Hayreh SS. Blood supply of the optic nerve head and its role in optic atrophy, glaucoma, and oedema of the optic disc. Br J Ophthalmol 1969; 53:721–748.
25. Jia Y, Morrison JC, Tokayer J, et al. Quantitative OCT angiography of optic nerve head blood flow. Biomed Opt Express 2012; 3:3127–3137.
26. Chihara E, Dimitrova G, Amano H, et al. Discriminatory power of superficial vessel density and prelaminar vascular flow index in eyes with glaucoma and ocular hypertension and normal eyes. Invest Ophthalmol Vis Sci 2017; 58:690–697.
27. Lévêque PM, Zéboulon P, Brasnu E, et al. Optic disc vascularization in glaucoma: Value of spectral-domain optical coherence tomography angiography. J Ophthalmol 2016; 2016:6956717.
28. Wang X, Jiang C, Ko T, et al. Correlation between optic disc perfusion and glaucomatous severity in patients with open-angle glaucoma: an optical coherence tomography angiography study. Graefes Arch Clin Exp Ophthalmol 2015; 253:1557–1564.
29. Liu L, Jia Y, Takusagawa HL, et al. Optical coherence tomography angiography of the peripapillary retina in glaucoma. JAMA Ophthalmol 2015; 133:1045–1052.
30. Yarmohammadi A, Zangwill LM, Diniz-Filho A, et al. Optical coherence tomography angiography vessel density in healthy, glaucoma suspect, and glaucoma eyes. Invest Ophthalmol Vis Sci 2016; 57:OCT451–459.
31. Sakaguchi K, Higashide T, Udagawa S, et al. Comparison of sectoral structure-function relationships in glaucoma: vessel density versus thickness in the peripapillary retinal nerve fiber layer. Invest Ophthalmol Vis Sci 2017; 58:5251–5262.
32. Rao HL, Pradhan ZS, Weinreb RN, et al. Relationship of optic nerve structure and function to peripapillary vessel density measurements of optical coherence tomography angiography in glaucoma. J Glaucoma 2017; 26:548–554.
33. Kwan J, Shin JW, Lee J, et al. Choroidal microvasculature dropout is associated with parafoveal visual fields defects in glaucoma. Am J Ophthalmol 2018; 188:141–154.
34. Suwan Y, Geyman LS, Fard MA, et al. Peripapillary perfused capillary density in exfoliation syndrome and exfoliation glaucoma versus POAG and healthy controls: an OCTA study. Asia Pac J Ophthalmol (Phila) 2018; 7:84–89.
35. Mastropasqua R, Agnifili L, Borrelli E, et al. Optical coherence tomography angiography of the peripapillary retina in normal-tension glaucoma and chronic nonarteritic anterior ischemic optic neuropathy. Curr Eye Res 2018; 43:778–784.
36. Medeiros FA, Jammal AA, Thompson AC. From machine to machine: an OCT-trained deep learning algorithm for objective quantification of glaucomatous damage in fundus photographs. Ophthalmology 2019; 126:513–521.

31 Neurodegenerative diseases

Gilda Cennamo, Daniela Montorio

Introduction

Increased ageing of the population makes more significant the importance to identify reliable tools in early diagnosis and monitoring of the neurodegenerative diseases.

Different studies have reported the close clinical relationship between the brain and the retina because they are anatomically interconnected and show similar features.

The possibility to evaluate the eye as a 'window' into the central nervous system has attracted great attention in recent years.

Monitoring retinal structures and vascularization may add important information to the pathophysiology of neurological diseases.

Optical coherence tomography (OCT) is a well-established, non-invasive technique that provides high-resolution images for the analysis of the retinal morphology and it can identify retinal abnormalities, useful as potential biomarkers of neurodegenerative disorders.

Ganglion cell layer (GCL) and retinal nerve fiber layer (RNFL) represent important parameters to evaluate the optic nerve damage because they allow to assess neuronal and axonal degeneration.

The introduction of the OCT angiography (OCTA), a novel and non-invasive and highly reproducible technique, has allowed a detailed visualization of the retinal and choroidal microvascular network and a quantitative analysis of the vessel density in the region of the macula and optic disc.

The OCTA has a much higher resolution than angiography fluorescein (FA) and allows to detect small capillaries and microareas of retinal non-perfusion in the different retinal vascular plexus.

Evaluating the structure and flow of the retinal vessels offers the possibility of objective measurements, useful in the field of the neurodegeneration, to obtain more knowledge about the pathophysiological mechanism involved in neurological diseases.[1]

Multiple sclerosis

Multiple sclerosis (MS) is a chronic inflammatory demyelinating disorder of the central nervous system (CNS) associated with progressive neurodegeneration.

Optic neuritis (ON) is a primary manifestation in 25% of patients and occurs in approximately 50% of the patients during the course of the disease.

Different studies report that GCL, RNFL thickness, and macular volume show thinning both in patients with and without ON compared to control eyes, this reduction is more represented in ON eyes.[2]

Some studies report that the inner nuclear layer (INL), which contains the bipolar neurons, reveals a transient slight thickening in ON eyes that may be a possible sign of retinal inflammatory activity.

Regarding the clinical aspects, many correlations have been found between the thickness of GCL–inner plexiform layer (IPL), RNFL, and visual acuity.

Multiple sclerosis is a multifactorial disease in which cerebral hypoperfusion and vascular pathology are gaining interest as possible factors related to disease risk and progression.

The degree of vascular involvement in the retina can be measured by OCTA, a useful tool, which appears to detect and monitor the damages of the retinal vascular network in MS patients.

The possible causative role of cerebral circulation in MS is still being debated but it has been hypothesized that the inflammation leads to a loss of neurons in the inner retina. This reduction causes a reduced metabolic demand resulting in a reduced blood supply.

Moreover, the inflammation can lead to alterations in vascular function, such as endotheliopathy that causes decreased perfusion and neuronal damage.

The blood flow index and vessel density in the macular region (superficial and deep capillary plexus) and in the optic nerve head are significantly lower in MS with or without ON compared to control eyes.[3,4]

The vascular density in the macular region is correlated with RNFL, GCL, while no significant correlations are found between the optic nerve head flow index and structural OCT parameters.

Regarding the clinical aspects, reverse significant correlations are found between the vessel density parameters and expanded disability status scale (EDSS) and between ganglion cell complex (GCC) and multiple sclerosis severity score (MSSS), while no correlation is present with disease duration parameters.

On the basis of the absence of a correlation between all the OCT parameters and the disease duration, it has been hypothesized that vascular alteration precedes neuronal damage (**Figures 1a** to **f**).

The OCTA parameters could represent good markers of disease and disability in MS patients and further studies are needed to evaluate, if the vascular alterations may help in early diagnosis.

Alzheimer's disease

Alzheimer's disease (AD), the most common cause of dementia, is a progressive neurodegenerative disorder characterized by an accumulation of misfolded protein, in particular amyloid-beta (AB) and neurofibrillary tangles (NFTs).

In early stages, the patients can present a mild cognitive impairment (MCI) in which the cognitive functions begins to decline; it is a transitional state between normality and dementia, as a prodromal stage of AD.

The OCT examination reveals an RNFL and GCL thinning in AD suggesting the loss of retinal neurons and their axons.

The GCL and RNFL thickness significantly correlate with mini-mental state examination (MMSE) in AD reinforcing the promising role of OCT in the clinical evaluation of these patients.

Moreover, AD patients show a significant choroidal thinning, probably reflecting the importance of vascular factors in their pathogenesis.

Different evidence indicate that the vascular factors (cerebral hypoperfusion, increased cerebral vascular tortuosity and decreased vascular density), due to an accumulation of amyloid in the walls of the vessels, contribute to cerebral neurodegeneration in AD.

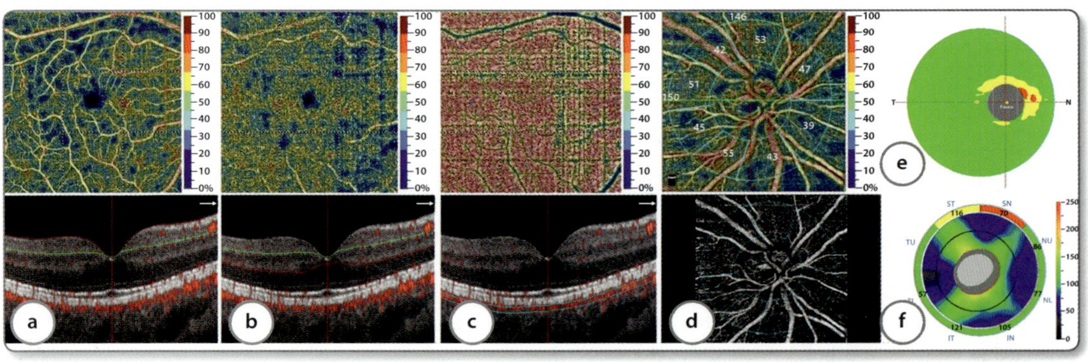

Figure 1 Spectral-domain optical coherence tomography (SD-OCT) and optical coherence tomography angiography (OCTA) analysis in right eye of a patient affected by multiple sclerosis. OCTA of the superficial capillary plexus (a), deep capillary plexus (b), and choriocapillaris (c) shows a reduction in vessel density in some macular sectors. OCTA measurements of the radial peripapillary capillary (RPC) vasculature reveal a decrease in vessel density in several areas (d). SD-OCT shows the presence of focal abnormalities in the ganglion cell complex (GCC) and circumpapillary retinal nerve fiber layer (cpRNFL) thickness (e and f).

It is still being debated whether the cerebral amyloid angiopathy precedes the neuronal loss or whether it is a consequence of a reduced metabolic demand.

These pathological mechanisms can be investigated through the retinal microvasculature because, similar to the brain, AB accumulation was found in the retina in AD.

All regions of the superficial vascular plexus (SVP) and deep vascular plexus (DVP) and choroidal flow rates present a significant reduction in retinal vascular density in AD patients.

There is a trend of vascular density loss from control to MCI then AD.

Only DVP loss has been found to correlate significantly with GCL-IPL (ganglion cell layer–inner plexiform layer) thinning in AD but not in MCI, probably due to more sensibility of the smaller vessels within the DVP to disease progression.[5]

Significant enlargement of the foveal avascular zone (FAZ) is found in AD that may represent a sign of ischemia.[6,7]

Regarding the clinical aspects, all retinal vascular density parameters positively correlate with MMSE in AD and MCI patients.

The OCTA represents a valid method to investigate the retinal microvascular alterations in early diagnosis and to individuate possible predictor biomarkers of conversion from MCI to AD (**Figures 2** and **3**).

Parkinson's disease and Huntington's disease

Parkinson's disease (PD) is one of the most common neurodegenerative disorders; it is characterized by the loss of dopaminergic neurons in the substantia nigra and by well-known movement alterations (i.e. bradykinesia, resting tremor or rigidity).

Patients with PD also suffer from non-motor symptoms, such as dementia, depression, and autonomic and gastrointestinal disturbance.

Visual dysfunction is one of the non-motor systems altered by PD with clinical manifestations including photophobia, diplopia, altered visual acuity, dry eyes, visuospatial dysfunction, and complex visual hallucinations.

Previous studies have demonstrated that retinal dopamine deficiency may play a central role in the pathogenesis of visual dysfunction in PD.

Dopamine is a neurotransmitter released by amacrine cells, which have been found in the human retina and are responsible for the transmission of visual information.

Retinal structures, measured by OCT, show a significative decrease in macular thickness

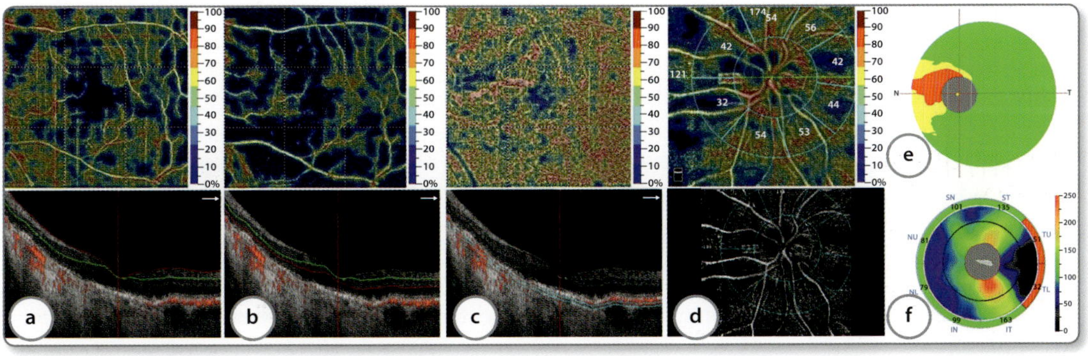

Figure 2 Spectral-domain optical coherence tomography (SD-OCT) and optical coherence tomographic angiography (OCTA) analysis in left eye of a patient affected by Alzheimer disease. OCTA of the superficial capillary plexus (a), deep capillary plexus (b), and choriocapillaris (c) shows significative reduction in vessel density in all macular sectors. OCTA measurements of the radial peripapillary capillary (RPC) vasculature reveal a significative decrease in vessel density in different areas (d). SD-OCT shows the presence of focal abnormalities in the ganglion cell complex (GCC) and circumpapillary retinal nerve fiber layer (cpRNFL) thickness (e and f).

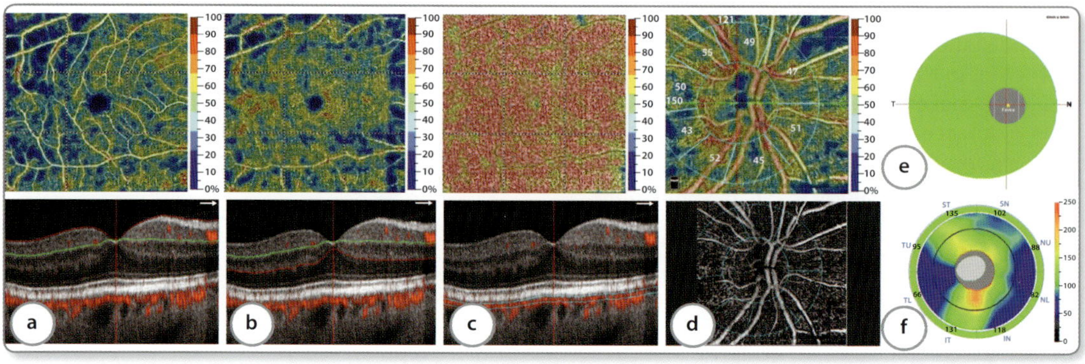

Figure 3 Spectral-domain optical coherence tomography (SD-OCT) and optical coherence tomographic angiography (OCTA) analysis in right eye of a patient affected by mild cognitive impairment. OCTA measurements of the superficial capillary plexus (a), deep capillary plexus (b) choriocapillaris (c), and radial peripapillary capillary (RPC) vasculature (d) reveal some areas of reduction in vessel density. SD-OCT shows the absence of abnormalities in the ganglion cell complex (GCC) and circumpapillary retinal nerve fiber layer (cpRNFL) thickness (e and f).

and volume; GCL and RNFL thickness turnout to be significantly reduced in different sectors compared with controls.[8]

The OCT parameters can be useful for evaluating the progression of PD because they present further decrease in their thickness after about 2–5 years of follow-up.

Moreover, PD patients present worse visual outcomes (visual acuity, contrast sensitivity, and color vision) than controls and a significant progression of visual dysfunction during the follow-up.

Inverse correlations are found between RNFL thickness and visual dysfunction while no correlation is established with Unified Parkinson's disease rating scale (UPDRS) total and motor scores.

Regarding the choroidal thickness, it shows a significant reduction in thickness compared to control eyes.

Choroidal thinning in PD may be the result of the decreased metabolic activity associated with the retinal ganglion cells (RGCs) atrophy or may also be due to vascular changes resulting from levodopa therapy.

Furthermore, irregularities in the choroidal blood flow may cause ischemia in the optic nerve head (ONH) and RGCs regions and may explain the damage in these structures in PD patients.

Different studies report that the vascular degeneration plays a significant role in contributing to neurodegenerative in PD.

Optical coherence tomography angiography could shed light on the pathogenesis of PD and be useful for monitoring the progression of this disease.

The first study, that used this tool, shows that the retinal microvascular density significantly decreases in PD patients compared to controls.[9]

Moreover, the correlation between microvascular impairment in the superficial retinal capillary layer and GCL–IPL thinning reveals that the retinal microvascular abnormality may contribute to the neurodegeneration in PD patients.

The retinal superficial and deep capillary plexuses do not significantly correlate with the disease severity scale or disease duration.

Optical coherence tomography angiography measurements of the retinal microvascular network with quantitative analysis may be useful in the future as objective biomarkers for detecting vessel impairment in early stages and in the management of PD.

Huntington's disease (HD) is an autosomal-dominant progressive neurodegenerative disorder that affects motor functions and leads to cognitive impairment and behavioral symptoms.

In recent years, there have been studies directed at the development of biomarkers, using OCT, in Huntington's disease to identify specific retinal changes as biomarkers that can reliably detect early abnormalities and disease progression.

Temporal peripapillary RNFL, macular RNFL (mRNFL), and GCL–IPL present a lower thickness in HD compared to controls.

Macular thickness and volume are not significantly different between HD patients and controls.

While a significant negative correlation is found OCT parameters (macular volume, GCL, and mRNFL thickness) and disease duration, disease progression score.

Visual acuity and color vision are significantly worse in the HD patient compared to the controls.

Regarding the choroidal measurements, a study shows that the macular choroidal thickness is significantly reduced in patients but is not correlated to the disease severity score suggesting that the choroidal changes occur earlier than the retinal changes.[10]

In the future, OCTA may help clarify a possible vascular involvement and identify choroidal and retinal microvascular abnormalities for monitoring neurodegeneration in this disease.

Conclusion

The introduction of new tools, such as OCT and OCTA, has allowed to study neurological diseases through the retinal tissue.

Optical coherence tomography has contributed to greater insights into the pathophysiology of the neurodegenerative disease.

Loss of RNFL and GCL–IPL thickness allows to follow the neuronal damages and correlates well with the alterations in clinical parameters such as visual and cognitive functions, disability, and magnetic resonance imaging.

The emerging researches have found an interesting role for retinal vascular alterations in the pathogenesis of these diseases.

Moreover, OCTA with quantitative analysis offers a new path of study and an objective biomarker for detecting vessel impairment in early stages of the neurodegenerative processes.

Further analysis with larger sample sizes is needed to evaluate the changes in retinal blood flow and the presence of correlations between the microvascular impairment and the neuronal damage to monitor not only the disease progression but also the effectiveness of therapy.

References

1. Wylęgała A. Principles of OCTA and Applications in Clinical Neurology. Curr Neurol Neurosci Rep 2018; 18:96.
2. Cennamo G, Romano MR, Vecchio EC, et al. Anatomical and functional retinal changes in multiple sclerosis. Eye (Lond) 2016; 30:456–462.
3. Lanzillo R, Cennamo G, Criscuolo C, et al. Optical coherence tomography angiography retinal vascular network assessment in multiple sclerosis. Mult Scler 2018; 24:1706–714.
4. Spain RI, Liu L, Zhang X, et al. Optical coherence tomography angiography enhances the detection of optic nerve damage in multiple sclerosis. Br J Ophthalmol 2018; 102:520–524.
5. Jiang H, Wei Y, Shi Y, et al. Altered Macular Microvasculature in Mild Cognitive Impairment and Alzheimer Disease. J Neuroophthalmol 2018; 38:292–298.
6. Bulut M, Kurtuluş F, Gözkaya O, et al. Evaluation of optical coherence tomography angiographic findings in Alzheimer's type dementia. Br J Ophthalmol 2018; 102:233–237.
7. O'Bryhim BE, Apte RS, Kung N, et al. Association of Preclinical Alzheimer Disease with Optical Coherence Tomographic Angiography Findings. JAMA Ophthalmol 2018; 136:1242–1248.
8. Satue M, Obis J, Alarcia R, et al. Retinal and Choroidal Changes in Patients with Parkinson's Disease Detected by Swept-Source Optical Coherence Tomography. Curr Eye Res 2018; 43:109–115.
9. Kwapong WR, Ye H, Peng C, et al. Retinal Microvascular Impairment in the Early Stages of Parkinson's Disease. Invest Ophthalmol Vis Sci 2018; 59:4115–4122.
10. Andrade C, Beato J, Monteiro A, et al. Spectral-Domain Optical Coherence Tomography as a Potential Biomarker in Huntington's Disease. Mov Disord 2016; 31:377–383.

32 How to write a clinical OCT angiography report

Marco Rispoli, Bruno Lumbroso

Writing an OCT angiography report

Writing a clinical optical coherence tomography angiography (OCTA) report is the concluding part of an OCTA analysis. The quantity of data to evaluate is enormous. It entails a long time to apply, for each case, the logical method of analysis and interpretation. Knowledge of clinical data and confrontation with structural OCT, and *en face* OCT, are essential for an accurate reporting.

An accurate description of an OCTA examination takes more time, and the report is much longer than for fluorescein angiography (FA) or structural OCT. A different interpretation modality is needed when using OCTA imaging.

Fluorescein angiography and OCTA differ greatly in technology and imageries. Structural OCT shows retinal alterations in morphology and structure of retinal layers (**Box 1**). OCTA integrates the structural imaging by showing the blood flow.

First report on structural OCT and *en face* OCT

An OCTA report always has to begin with a short report on the structural OCT and *en face* OCT of the case in question. For each element in structural OCT, we should evaluate:

- Morphology
- Structure
- Segmentation
- Reflectivity
- Abnormal formations

En face OCT layer-by-layer analysis

The images acquired by *en face* OCT require a layer-by-layer retinal analysis from the vitreous to the choroid, we study each *en face* layer.

- *Vitreous and hyaloid*: Evident, partially or totally detached. Likely evidence of internal limiting membrane
- Epiretinal membranes (plaque shape, limits sharp or not), folds (radial or parallel, regular or irregular)
- *Foveolar depression*: Normal or transformed in width and depth
- *Nuclear and plexiform layers*: Evaluation of thickness, reflectivity, and possible abnormal structures
- *External limiting membrane*: Integrity, discontinuity, and abnormal structures
- *Ellipsoid (inner/outer photoreceptor segment junction)*: Reflectivity, integrity, discontinuity, and abnormal structures
- *Retinal pigmented epithelium*: Thickness,

Box 1: How to write an OCTA report

- Optical coherence tomography angiography (OCTA) interpretation requires applying a logical method of analysis and interpretation. First analysis, then synthesis, and then diagnosis
- It is necessary to know the patient clinical history

An OCTA report must cover a structural OCT report.

- OCTA report deals with a huge amount of data that have to be checked, sorted, shifted, and selected to include only the ones necessary to understand the case under study
- OCTA report will incorporate elements from structural OCT and *en face* OCT
- Without general clinical data and comparison with structural OCT, *en face* OCT, reporting properly is not possible
- The images acquired by *en face* and OCTA technology require a layer-by-layer retinal analysis

integrity, reflectivity, and abnormal structures
- *Bruch's membrane*: (If visible) integrity and discontinuity
- *Choroid*: Choriocapillaris, thickness at fovea and at 1,000 μ from it, Sattler's layer, Haller's layer, lamina fusca, and suprachoroidal space.

Continue with OCTA report leaf: Layer-by-layer analysis

Step-by-step analysis:

- *Step 1*: Superficial retinal vascular plexus
- *Step 2a*: Deep capillary plexus (DCP)
- *Step 2b*: Intermediate capillary plexus (ICP)
- *Step 3a*: Avascular retina. Normally no vessel should be seen. If flows are seen, they belong to type 3, type 2 or type 4 choroidal neovascularizations (CNVs)
- *Step 3b*: Neovascular membrane description
- *Step 3c*: Describe signs for CNV activity
- *Step 4*: Choriocapillaris—choroid
- *Step 5*: Optic disc
- *Step 6*: AngioAnalytics data: Quantitative aspect, superficial vascular network, deep vascular network
- *Step 7*: Assessment of changes since last examination and follow-up
- *Step 8*: Conclusion and diagnosis

Add specific features description

Superficial, intermediate, and deep retinal vascular network

In case of vascular problems, the report should describe:

- *Network shape and course*: Shape—regular or irregular; course—winding, stretched out, distorted, and contorted
- Normal anastomoses and abnormal shunts between superficial and deep vascular plexus
- *Capillaries density*: Sparse or dense; capillaries diameter—small, large, regular or irregular
- *Vessels diameter*: Large or small, irregular with dilatations or without dilatations
- *Vascular abnormalities*: Irregular diameter, microaneurysms, and dilatations
- *Cystoid edema cysts*: Large or small, irregular, rounded, and angular
- New vessels intraretinal, preretinal
- *Foveal avascular zone (FAZ)*: Normal, increased or decreased, shape normal or irregular dimension increased or dimension decreased
- *Perifoveal arcade*: Complete, broken and lacking
- AngioAnalytics software

Avascular retina

Normally no vessel should be seen. If flows are seen, they are CNVs. To find flows in the avascular zone is not normal: it may mean there are abnormal vessels. It is important to locate exactly Bruch's membrane, to classify CNVs.

OCTA terminology for neovascular membranes

Exudative CNV:

- Location (depth and offset):
  - Intraretinal (type 3)
  - Subretinal, preretinal pigmented epithelium (RPE) (type 2)
  - Sub-RPE (type 1)
  - Macular
  - Extramacular—parapapillary
- CNV morphology
- Neovascular membranes features:
  - *Branching*: Dense or sparse—secondary branches present or lacking
  - *Fractal*: Great or small
  - *Capillary density*: Dense or sparse
  - *Loops*: Present or lacking
  - *Peripheral anastomoses*: Present, lacking, broken, partially present
  - *Afferent vessel*: Single trunk or bundle
- CNV morphology:
  - Bush, bicycle wheel, coral bush, medusa head, fan-shaped and tangled
  - *Filament like*: Dead tree; naked tree—star shaped, tuft, and glomerular
  - *Branched structure*: Tangled structure
- CNV arterialization: After long-term evolution and repeated recurrences—vessels thicker and straighter, rigid in aspect, lacking thin capillaries
- *Peri-CNV dark halo:* A halo or dark circle is always seen around the new vessels; report halo variation after treatment
- Flow area/CNV area (AngioAnalytic data).

Nonexudative CNV:

- Choroidal neovascularization: Location (depth and offset)
  - Sub-RPE (type 1)
  - *Macular:* Extramacular–parapapillary
  - Inside or outside vascular main arcades

- CNV morphology
- Neovascular membranes features:
  - *Fractal*: Great or small
  - *Afferent vessel*: Single trunk or bundle
- CNV morphology:
  - *Filament like:* Dead tree, naked tree, branched structure, tangled structure

Angio-OCT terminology for active or quiescent CNV

- *CNV activity:* Active
  - Lesion shape; branching structure—dense; secondary branches—present; loops—mainly in periphery; fractal—small; arcade—present; anastomoses of vessels at the periphery of the lesion; wide dark halo surrounding the lesion
- *CNV activity:* Quiescent
  - Lesion shape; branching structure sparse; dead tree or tangled; secondary branches lacking; few loops; fractal great
  - No anastomoses of vessels at the periphery of the lesion
  - Small or no dark halo surrounding the lesion

Choriocapillaris—choroid

The report should describe:

- *Fine microlobular background:* Normal or damaged (describe)
- Sattler and Haller layers dark and big vessels
- It is important to locate exactly Bruch's membrane, to classify CNVs, type 1 or type 2. If flows are seen, they are type 1, type 2 or type 4 CNVs
- Classify CNV, type 1 exudative or non-exudative

Optic disc

The report should describe:

- Superficial vascular complex (SVC)
- Radial peripapillary capillary plexus (RPCP)
- All of NFL

Angioanalytic data: Quantitative features

The report should describe:

- Flow area shows flows in the vascular structures of the segmented volume; follow-up of CNV; study of preretinal and prepapillary new vessels in proliferative diabetes and venous occlusion
- *Nonflow area and vascular dropout area:* In nonflow area, the blood flow is lower or lacking completely; study separately at the superficial vascular network and at the deep vascular network
- *Flow density map:* Differentiate the areas where flow can be recorded from those where there is no flow - scale of false colors. The warm colors show high density vascular areas, cold colors indicate low flow or no density at all
- Flow speed map—scale of false colors. The warm colors high speed and cold colors low speed
- Thickness of retina and choroid

Attach selected scans to the report

- At least two orthogonal cross-section scans that cross the anatomic fovea
- At least one scan outside macula if the disease does not interest the foveal region
- A macular map
- One or more coronal (C-scan) analysis of the lesion
- The OCTA imaging comprises four segmentation slabs:
  - Superficial vascular network
  - Deep vascular network
  - Avascular retina
  - Choriocapillaris
- *AngioAnalytic data:* Quantitative aspect
  - *Flow area*: Superficial vascular network and deep vascular network
  - *Nonflow area*: Superficial vascular network and deep vascular network
  - *Flow density map*: Superficial vascular network and deep vascular network
  - Soon flow speed will be available

Box 2: Check and verify the correct segmentation borders placing

- The automated segmentation system is not always able to place properly all boundaries
- In some cases, it will be necessary to change, move or redraw some boundary in order to make a correct segmentation

Box 3: Steps in writing an OCTA report

- First report on structural OCT and *en face* OCT
- Then continue with OCTA report sheet: Layer-by-layer analysis report
- Add specific features' description
- Attach to the report a few selected scans
- Comparison with successive examinations and follow-up
- Conclusion and diagnosis

Comparison with successive examinations and follow-up

The report should describe measurements and compare it with successive examinations during the follow-up. Data should be saved for comparison.

Conclusion and diagnosis

The last step is the result of the synthesis of all elements you have separately analyzed. Writing the diagnosis is the final part of the report and requires carefulness and caution (**Boxes 2** and **3**).

33 The future

Bruno Lumbroso

OCT angiography new developments and advances in imaging and interpretation

Optical coherence tomography (OCT) angiography advances develop swiftly. Automating OCT image detection will significantly decrease the dull part of clinician work and achieve a correct pre-diagnosis from the analysis of retinal elements. The performance of the automated approach shows comparable results to that of human experts with significant clinical experience. It will find promising applications in an automatic diagnosis and classification of common retinal diseases.

Diagnosis and image analysis assisted by artificial intelligence

Artificial intelligence (AI) gives to the computer the human capability of thought and conception, and bonds it with the superior memory of the machine. The current main application of AI is image reading through deep learning. Ophthalmology is the medical specialty where AI applications are already most developed. Many applications will soon find their place in the clinical devices as AI achieves tasks quicker and better than a trained man. The machine algorithm progresses itself without human intervention during a learning period. Deep learning has numerous benefits: a large database, a learning reliable period, and final results superior to that of the human. The forthcoming major change will be in the diagnostic field and in personalizing management. Diagnosis and treatment scheduling will be improved and considerably automatized. It will free up time for the physician who will not need to evaluate data himself.

OCT and OCT angiography analysis and synthesis

Artificial intelligence will help ophthalmologists to make a better OCT diagnosis. Automated OCT and OCT angiography (OCTA) interpretation assisted by AI will support possible treatment. OCT analysis will speed up the treatment decision: treat or not treat, or select another diagnosis and help the specialist to a fast evaluation, and to immediate action.[1,2]

Surveys and mass screening

In these initial moments of AI, it may help clinician for surveys and mass screening—a panel of experts chooses and classifies a series of images; the machine studies the images, learns, and commits to memory. The algorithm is confirmed on a second series of images. It is then used for surveys and mass screening.

Clinical work, diagnosis, and personalized management

In everyday clinical work, AI will undoubtedly change the OCT interpretation process. It will suggest the specialist a range of possible diagnosis, leaving to human mind the decisive option. It will help determine several options and help choose the best treatment options. The machine assesses thousands of ocular OCT and OCTA scans to appreciate the earliest changes that man cannot distinguish.

Diagnosis and treatment of diabetic retinopathy

Diabetic retinopathy is the disease where most AI clinical work is starting to take hold. Deep learning was first used to detect diabetic retinal lesions in color photos of the fundus and differentiate between proliferative or non proliferative retinopathies and edematous or non edematous maculopathies. The machine needs at least 100,000 images for training. The machine algorithm progresses itself without human involvement during a learning period. Currently machine sensitivity and specificity are 90%; which is more than what the ophthalmologist can do. Nurse or technician can perform the screening, with automated AI interpretation and excellent approximation.[1]

Diagnosis and treatment of AMD

AI will diagnose with precision the type of choroidal neovascularization and will assess and quantify intra- and subretinal fluid, guiding treatment choice. Then it will choose a specific treatment, forecasting efficacy of a treatment in a definite patient. It will assess with big data the profile of the patients who could most benefit from a definite therapy and forecast the disease evolution by integrating personal data and personal situation.

Diagnosis and treatment of glaucoma

Deep learning is already used in glaucoma mass screening. The machine indicates the probability of glaucoma based on optic disc images. Their sensitivity and specificity exceed the possibilities offered by man.

New biomarkers discovered

Ursula Schmidt-Erfurth and her team in Vienna work on algorithms that will discover new, previously unimagined biomarkers that will help ophthalmologists in diagnosis and treatment, as deep learning systems notice details that are not seen by man. They search by themselves and identify entirely new biomarkers. And this unsupervised learning will really help us to understand disease beyond the already conventional knowledge (Ursula Schmidt-Erfurth).[5]

Deep choroid and choriocapillaris segmentation

Deep learning approach will also be used to automatically segment out the choroid layer, using morphological operations and convolutional neural networks. The acquired segmentation results are quite equivalent to the segmentation performed by specialists. This technology will improve present techniques and will help observe choroidal and retinal abnormalities as pachychoroid, uveitis, macular edema, hypertensive retinopathy, and glaucoma.

Flow density quantification

Vessel density will be provided by the OCTA machine. An automatic algorithm will classify the image (as healthy, DR, AMD, or RVO) and provide quantitative information obtained from the angiograms, including global vessel density, global fractal dimension, and fovea avascular zone (FAZ) area. Classification results were compared with the diagnosis made by a retina specialist. The algorithm will improve vessel density values assessment and omit false vessels.[3]

Flow speed quantification

VISTA new technology using variable interscan time analysis (Jay Duker)[4] has allowed to assess CC alteration and to differentiate varying degrees of choriocapillaris flow impairment. OCTA using VISTA can distinguish varying degrees of choriocapillaris alteration and flow impairment and may be useful for elucidating disease pathogenesis, progression, and response to therapy. A color scale shows flow speed.

Automated vascular detection

Deep transfer learning method shows significant effectiveness on classification of retinal OCT images and diagnosis of new vessels. The method can provide assistant support for medical decision-making.

Leakage detection in OCT images in diabetic retinopathy and inflammatory diseases

José Cunha-Vaz localized and measured by OCT leakage in eyes that were classified as having well-defined sites of seepage on fluorescein angiography (FA). His method of OCT leakage detection showed a sensitivity of 95.9% and a specificity of 75.4% regarding agreement between these sites of alteration of the blood–retinal barrier. The areas of abnormal extracellular fluid increase were larger than the areas of fluorescein leakage and included the well-defined leakage sites identified by FA.[6]

Leakage measured by OCT did better than FA in identifying abnormal retinal fluid than FA and showed good sensitivity and specificity for identification of sites of alterations of the blood–

retinal barrier. This methodology will develop in clinical work.

Widefield OCT: Study of peripheral retina

For the moment, OCT of retinal periphery is limited. Image montage already provides detailed information over a wide area. However, it is time-consuming and takes significant efforts to create montaged images. Lately, commercial widefield OCT has become available. Many systems have been developed and put on the market. Widefield OCT offers significant aid in the imaging of retinal disorders.

Wide field will increase our information of outlying diseases and will give us a global assessment of retina. OCT study of retina periphery will facilitate diagnosis and follow-up of peripheral disorders leading to earlier and more precise management. It will increase knowledge of disorders that cover larger areas than those covered by regular scans. Distinction of retinal detachments and retinoschisis will be greatly facilitated. Lesions can be multifocal and far from each other, giving us an incomplete understanding of the disorder. For instance, pseudo vitelliform maculopathy or choroiditis may have multiple peripheral foci. Vitreomacular traction or proliferative diabetic retinopathy may be difficult to delineate with regular OCT scans. Widefield will show the framework of these connections better.

One important improvement in retinal imaging is the ultra-widefield (UWF). It reaches the retinal periphery at 200°, covering most of the retina in one image. It consents highlighting and quantification of peripheral retina diseases.

To these advances in OCTA, I add a short summary of a future innovation in retinal disorders management that will have to be considered by the new technologies.

Gene therapy

Many studies worldwide investigate on cell therapy in various areas that range from hereditary or degenerative retinal diseases to neurodegenerative diseases such as multiple sclerosis, Alzheimer's disease, Parkinson's disease to diabetes. OCT angiography will have an important place in field of research. The eye is an organ of choice for the development of gene and cellular biotherapies, because it is the seat of very few immunological reactions, it is easily reachable, and easy to observe.[7]

References

1. Li F, Chen H, Liu Z, et al. Fully automated detection of retinal disorders by image-based deep learning. Graefes Arch Clin Exp Ophthalmol 2019; 57:495–505.
2. Masood S, Fang R, Li P, et al. Automatic choroid layer segmentation from optical coherence tomography images using deep learning. Sci Rep 2019; 9:3058.
3. Aharony O, Gal-Or O, Polat A, et al. Automatic characterization of retinal blood flow using OCT angiograms. Transl Vis Sci Technol 2019; 8:6.
4. Ploner SB, Moult EM, Choi W, et al. Toward quantitative optical coherence tomography angiography: Visualizing blood flow speeds in ocular pathology using variable interscan time analysis. Retina 2016; 36:S118–S126.
5. Schmidt-Erfurth U, Klimscha S, Waldstein SM, et al. A view of the current and future role of optical coherence tomography in the management of age-related macular degeneration. Eye 2017; 31:26–44.
6. Cunha-Vaz J, Santos T, Alves D, et al. Agreement between OCT leakage and fluorescein angiography to identify sites of alteration of the blood–retinal barrier in diabetes. Ophthalmol Retina 2017; 1:395–403.
7. Szilard K. 24-week results of phase 1 study of intravitreal gene therapy with ADVM-022 for neovascular AMD (OPTIC trial). American Academy of Ophthalmology Annual Meeting; 2019.

Suggested reading

To study in depth the matters debated in this Handbook, we suggest the following books:

1. Freund KB, Sarraf D, Miele WE, et al. Retinal Diseases. In: Retinal Atlas. Amsterdam: Elsevier; 2017.
2. Lumbroso B, Rispoli M. Structural OCT. In: Practical Handbook of OCT. New Delhi: Jaypee Brothers Medical Publishers (P) Ltd.; 2012.
3. Huang D, Duker JS, Fujimoto JG, et al. Imaging the eye from front to back with RTVue Fourier Domain OCT. New Jersey: Slack Inc.; 2010.
4. Lumbroso B, Huang D, Romano A, et al. "En Face" OCT. In: Clinical En Face OCT Atlas. New Delhi: Jaypee Brothers Medical Publisher (P) Ltd.; 2013.
5. Huang D, Lumbroso B, Jia Y, et al. OCT Angiography. In: Optical Coherence Tomography Angiography of the Eye. New Jersey: Slack Inc.; 2018.

Index

Note: Page numbers in **bold** or *italic* refer to tables or figures, respectively.

D

E

F

G

H

I

L

M

N

O

P